Kidney Diseases: Molecular Mechanisms and Clinical Assessment

Kidney Diseases: Molecular Mechanisms and Clinical Assessment

Edited by Jordan Bryan

STATES
ACADEMIC PRESS
www.statesacademicpress.com

States Academic Press,
109 South 5th Street,
Brooklyn, NY 11249, USA

Visit us on the World Wide Web at:
www.statesacademicpress.com

ISBN: 978-1-63989-777-3

Cataloging-in-Publication Data

Kidney diseases : molecular mechanisms and clinical assessment / edited by Jordan Bryan.
p. cm.
Includes bibliographical references and index.
ISBN 978-1-63989-777-3
1. Kidneys--Diseases. 2. Kidneys--Diseases--Case studies.
3. Nephrology. I. Bryan, Jordan.
RC902 .K53 2023
616.61--dc23

Table of Contents

Preface

Every book is a source of knowledge and this one is no exception. The idea that led to the conceptualization of this book was the fact that the world is advancing rapidly; which makes it crucial to document the progress in every field. I am aware that a lot of data is already available, yet, there is a lot more to learn. Hence, I accepted the responsibility of editing this book and contributing my knowledge to the community.

The kidneys are two reddish-brown bean-shaped organs found in vertebrates. They are situated on the right and left sides of the retroperitoneal space. The kidneys are essential for the body's basic physiological activities. Kidney dysfunction disrupts these physiological activities and can result in a variety of diseases. A range of immunological, toxic and ischemic insults can harm kidney cells. This results in inflammation and cell death, which in turn leads to organ damage or complete failure. The damage to renal cells and the subsequent cellular regeneration processes are both influenced by inflammation. However, chronic inflammation can lead to renal fibrosis. The kidneys have the ability to regenerate after injury and can recover completely based on the type of renal lesions. The therapeutic intervention options facilitating the regeneration process are limited to fluid management and extracorporeal kidney support. This book unravels the recent studies on kidney diseases. It attempts to understand the molecular mechanisms and clinical assessment of these diseases. This book will help new researchers by foregrounding their knowledge in this area of study.

While editing this book, I had multiple visions for it. Then I finally narrowed down to make every chapter a sole standing text explaining a particular topic, so that they can be used independently. However, the umbrella subject sinews them into a common theme. This makes the book a unique platform of knowledge.

I would like to give the major credit of this book to the experts from every corner of the world, who took the time to share their expertise with us. Also, I owe the completion of this book to the never-ending support of my family, who supported me throughout the project.

Editor

1

Pigment Nephropathy: Novel Insights into Inflammasome-Mediated Pathogenesis

Kurt T. K. Giuliani [1,2,3], Andrew J. Kassianos [1,2,3,4], Helen Healy [1,2,3] and Pedro H. F. Gois [1,2,3,*]

1 Kidney Health Service, Royal Brisbane and Women's Hospital, Brisbane, QLD 4029, Australia; Kurt.Giuliani@uqconnect.edu.au (K.T.K.G.); Andrew.Kassianos@qimrberghofer.edu.au (A.J.K.); Helen.Healy@health.qld.gov.au (H.H.)
2 Conjoint Kidney Research Laboratory, Chemical Pathology—Pathology Queensland, Brisbane, QLD 4029, Australia
3 Faculty of Medicine, University of Queensland, Brisbane, QLD 4006, Australia
4 Institute of Health and Biomedical Innovation/School of Biomedical Sciences, Queensland University of Technology, Brisbane, QLD 4059, Australia
* Correspondence: Pedro.FrancaGois@health.qld.gov.au

Abstract: Pigment nephropathy is an acute decline in renal function following the deposition of endogenous haem-containing proteins in the kidneys. Haem pigments such as myoglobin and haemoglobin are filtered by glomeruli and absorbed by the proximal tubules. They cause renal vasoconstriction, tubular obstruction, increased oxidative stress and inflammation. Haem is associated with inflammation in sterile and infectious conditions, contributing to the pathogenesis of many disorders such as rhabdomyolysis and haemolytic diseases. In fact, haem appears to be a signalling molecule that is able to activate the inflammasome pathway. Recent studies highlight a pathogenic function for haem in triggering inflammatory responses through the activation of the nucleotide-binding domain-like receptor protein 3 (NLRP3) inflammasome. Among the inflammasome multiprotein complexes, the NLRP3 inflammasome has been the most widely characterized as a trigger of inflammatory caspases and the maturation of interleukin-18 and -1β. In the present review, we discuss the latest evidence on the importance of inflammasome-mediated inflammation in pigment nephropathy. Finally, we highlight the potential role of inflammasome inhibitors in the prophylaxis and treatment of pigment nephropathy.

Keywords: rhabdomyolysis; pigment nephropathy; haem; NLRP3 inflammasome; acute kidney injury

---

1. Introduction

Haem complexes consist of an Fe atom which is coordinated within the centre of a heterocyclic ring known as a protoporphyrin [1]. Haem-containing proteins are a large class of metalloproteins that play a pivotal role in maintaining basic biological functions [2]. Their broad activities range from mitochondrial electron transfer, oxygen transport and storage to signal transduction and control of gene expression [2].

Among the different haem group variants, haem a, b and c are the main biological types [3,4]. Of the haem variants, haem b is the most abundant form and is present biologically within myoglobin and haemoglobin, whilst haem a and c are present in cytochromes. Haem function as a prosthetic group in haemoproteins and are essential for reversible oxygen binding and transport [5,6]. However, under pathological conditions, an excess of circulating free haem may be highly cytotoxic and result in tissue damage, including within the kidney [3,6].

Pigment nephropathy (PN) is an acute decline in kidney function following the breakdown and deposition of endogenous haem pigment-containing proteins (myoglobin, haemoglobin) within renal tissue [7]. Both myoglobin and haemoglobin are freely filtered by glomeruli and when oxidised, release their haem moiety into the urinary space [8,9]. However, within the nephron, excess haem pigments may cause renal vasoconstriction, tubular obstruction, increased oxidative stress and inflammation [10–13].

Inflammation is an essential response of the innate immune system to harmful stimuli [14]. Haem is associated with inflammation in sterile and infectious conditions, contributing to the pathogenesis of many disorders such as rhabdomyolysis and haemolytic diseases [15]. There is an increasing body of evidence that haem trigger the inflammasome signalling cascade and ultimately, the innate immune response [16,17].

In the present review, we discuss the potential role of inflammasome activation as a driver of inflammation in PN. We explore the rationale of translating small molecule inhibitors of inflammasome activation already in clinical use, for diseases outside the kidney, in the prevention and treatment of PN.

2. The Nucleotide-Binding domain-Like Receptor Protein 3 (NLRP3) Inflammasome

The inflammasomes are a family of cytosolic signalling complexes with a central role in the activation of innate immune responses via the maturation and secretion of pro-inflammatory cytokines (interleukin (IL)-1β and IL-18) [18]. In particular, the nucleotide-binding domain-like receptor protein 3 (NLRP3) inflammasome, an extensively characterized inflammasome family member, is widely implicated in a variety of renal injuries, including acute and chronic kidney disease (CKD) [19–21]; oxalate and uric acid crystal nephropathy [22,23]; and diabetic nephropathies [24]. Inflammasomes respond to a diverse range of pathogen-associated molecular patterns (PAMPs) and endogenously derived damage-associated molecular patterns (DAMPs) via a suite of pattern recognition receptors (PRR). Of particular note, endogenous particulate matter, such as haem [16,17], monosodium urate (MSU) [25], oxalate [23,26] and cholesterol crystals [27,28] have all been identified as potent triggers of NLRP3 inflammasome activation and the subsequent release of pro-inflammatory cytokines [24].

Recently, Liston and Masters [29] proposed a mechanism of inflammasome activation in addition to the PAMP-DAMP axis. This mechanism responds to a loss of homeostasis via 'homeostasis-altering molecular processes' (HAMPs). They hypothesized that the PAMP-DAMP-HAMP axis was, collectively, likely to be sufficient for effective immunity and that deficiencies in this axis may cause the pathological inflammatory activation observed in sterile injury [29]. Examples of HAMPs which activate the inflammasome are perturbed membrane potential through K^+ efflux and Ca^{2+} influx [30], extracellular adenosine triphosphate (ATP) [31–33], and mitochondrial damage through reactive oxygen species (ROS) [34], altered mitochondrial membrane potential ($\Delta\Psi_m$) [35] and oxidised mitochondrial DNA (mtDNA) [36]. While their activation triggers may be diverse, the signalling pathways of inflammasome activation can be categorized into either canonical or non-canonical activation.

2.1. Canonical Inflammasome Activation

Following the detection of PAMPs or DAMPs (Signal 1) by PRRs, the NLRP3 inflammasome is canonically activated in an orchestrated cascade of signals [37], see Figure 1. The transmembrane protein family of Toll-like receptors (TLRs) play an important role as PRRs, activating the downstream signalling cascade. This signalling cascade is known as the "priming" phase of inflammasome activation. Once primed, the nuclear factor kappa-light-chain-enhancer of activated B cells (NF-κB) signalling complex translocates to the cell nucleus where it promotes the upregulation of NLRP3 and immature forms of IL-1β and IL-18 [38].

Following the priming phase, a second signal (Signal 2) is required to elicit the activation of the inflammasome, see Figure 1b. These signals can include interrupted phagocytosis [39], extracellular ATP [31–33], K^+ and Ca^{2+} flux [39–41], endoplasmic reticulum stress [42], mitochondrial ROS [34], $\Delta\Psi_m$ [35] and the release of oxidised mtDNA [36]. Particulate matter are also potent secondary signals which can activate the NLRP3 inflammasome via cell-surface contact [39]. The mechanism for detection of these PAMP/DAMP/HAMPs by NLRP3 remains poorly understood.

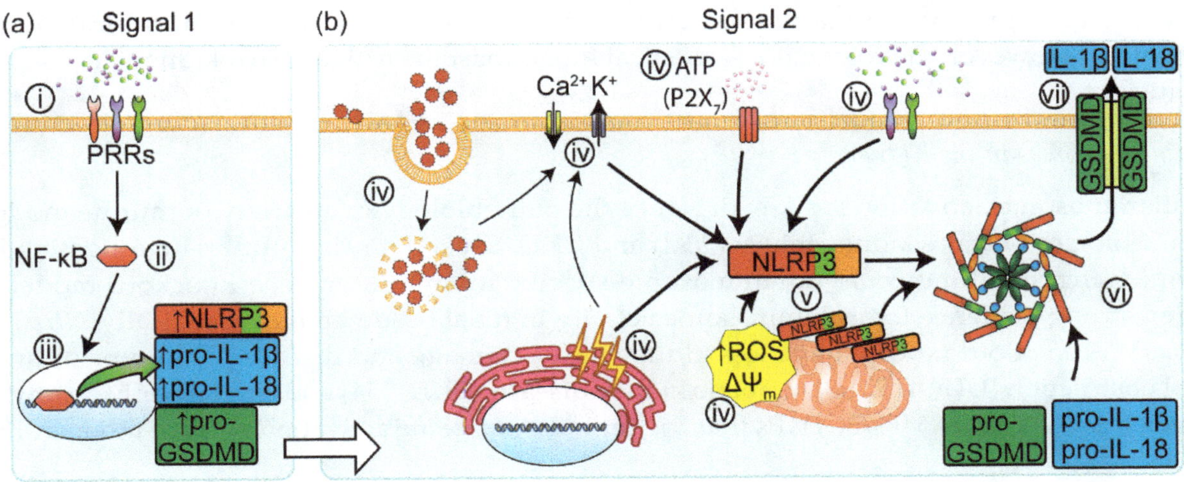

Figure 1. The canonical inflammasome activation signalling cascade is initiated by signal 1 PAMPs and DAMPs. (**a**) Signal 1 elicits the activation of PRRs on the cell surface (i). The activation of PRRs results in a downstream signalling cascade, triggering the translocation of NF-κB into the nucleus (ii), where NF-κB upregulates the expression of NLRP3, pro-GSDMD, pro-IL-1β and pro-IL-18 (iii). (**b**) Signal 2 is provided by an array of PAMPs, DAMPs and HAMPs (iv), including arrested phagocytosis, perturbed membrane potential ($\Delta\Psi_m$), endoplasmic reticulum stress, extracellular ATP, and mitochondrial dysfunction. NLPR3 proteins which have co-localized to the mitochondria (v) are ideally located to rapidly respond to these markers of cellular stress. NLRP3 then oligomerizes with ASC and pro-Caspase-1, forming the NLRP3 inflammasome complex (vi). Caspase-1 undergoes self-cleavage whilst bound to the inflammasome complex (vi), driving the post-translational processing of IL-1β, IL-18 and GSDMD. Once cleaved, GSDMD proteins self-oligomerize to form pores in the cell membrane (vii), allowing for the rapid release of IL-1β and IL-18. In addition, these GSDMD pores may also drive cell-death via pyroptosis. ASC: Apoptosis-associated Speck-like protein containing a Caspase-activation-and-recruitment domain; PRR: pattern recognition receptor; PAMP: pathogen-associated molecular pattern; DAMP: damage-associated molecular pattern; nuclear factor kappa-light-chain-enhancer of activated B cells: NF-κB; NLRP3: nucleotide-binding domain-like receptor protein 3; IL: interleukin; GSDMD: Gasdermin D; ROS: reactive oxygen species; $\Delta\Psi_m$: mitochondrial membrane potential.

Once activated by these molecular signalling patterns, NLRP3 proteins self-oligomerize and nucleate the formation of the NLRP3 inflammasome complex. This inflammasome complex consists of the NLRP3 protein, the ASC (Apoptosis-associated Speck-like protein containing a Caspase-activation-and-recruitment domain) adaptor protein and pro-caspase-1. Boucher, et al. [43] recently showed that pro-caspase-1 proteins dimerize following their recruitment to the inflammasome complex, before self-cleaving into an active state. The transiently active caspase-1 dimer undergoes additional cleavage, forming a proteolytically active holoenzyme with the inflammasome, capable of processing the pro-inflammatory cytokines IL-1β and IL-18 into their active forms [18,43]. Caspase-1 also cleaves Gasdermin-D (GSDMD) into its active form. Active GSDMD translocates to the cell membrane and forms GSDMD pores in the plasma membrane, driving pyroptosis and the consequent rapid release of IL-1β and IL-18 into the surrounding extracellular micro-environment [44–48].

2.2. *Non-Canonical Inflammasome Activation*

Non-canonical activation of the inflammasome differs in that it is dependent on caspase-11 (murine) or caspase-4 (human) activity [49–51]. Gram-negative bacteria-derived PAMPs are established triggers of non-canonical activation, directly sensed by and activating caspase-11/-4 [51]. Active caspase-11/-4 proteolytically cleave pro-GSDMD into its active state, effecting cell death by pyroptosis [49,50]. Kayagaki, et al. [50] showed that murine caspase-11 also triggers an NLRP3-inflammasome response through an as-yet-to-be identified mechanism, resulting in the release of IL-1β and IL-18 [50]. In humans, caspase-4 is required for the maturation and release of IL-18 via a non-canonical inflammasome pathway [51]. However, the role of non-canonical inflammasome activation in kidney disease remains to be elucidated.

2.3. *Inflammasomes in the Kidney*

Inflammasome activation is a key driver of the pathobiology in a variety of murine models and human etiologies of acute kidney injury (AKI) and CKD. Several murine studies investigating NLRP3 function, using small-molecule inflammasome-specific inhibitors or gene knockout models, have provided strong evidence for inflammasome activity in renal tissue injury. Specifically, *Nlrp3*$^{-/-}$, *Asc*$^{-/-}$ and *Casp1*$^{-/-}$ knock-out models have less kidney tissue damage and disease phenotype in unilateral ureteral obstruction (UUO) [52,53], diabetic kidney disease (DKD) [54] and crystal nephropathy [23,26]. However, the PAMPs/DAMPs/HAMPs that trigger inflammasome activation in these models are under active investigation.

Elevated soluble uric acid levels have been reported in the obstructed kidney of UUO mice [53]. Uric acid is an established activator of the inflammasome [55]. Furthermore, ROS derived from the activity of xanthine oxidase (XO), an enzyme which produces uric acid via purine catabolism, has also been reported to elicit an inflammasome response [56]. Allopurinol is a widely prescribed pharmaceutical used in the treatment of gout and directly inhibits XO activity. Notably, UUO mice treated with allopurinol exhibit less NLRP3 and IL-1β expression within the UUO kidney compared to untreated UUO controls [53]. These studies suggest a dual protective role for allopurinol by inhibiting both uric acid production and XO activity, thus preventing inflammasome activation.

Shahzad, et al. [54] reported NLRP3 activation in podocytes, an important cell type in the glomerular filtration barrier, in a murine DKD model [54]. Interestingly, this study demonstrated increased IL-1β and IL-18 expression within plasma and renal cortical extracts of diabetic animals, correlating with the functional kidney biomarker urine albumin/creatinine ratio [54].

IL-1β and IL-18 are produced by infiltrating hematopoietic cells, such as dendritic cells (DC) and macrophages, in mouse kidneys [57]. Supporting this concept, DC depletion in a crystal-induced model of murine renal fibrosis, resulted in reduced fibrosis and improved kidney function [20]. Furthermore, a similar outcome was achieved by treatment with a specific small molecule NLRP3 inflammasome inhibitor (MCC950; detailed below in Section 6.1) that blocked NLRP3 activation in kidney DC, reduced IL-1β and IL-18 production and inhibited the progression of renal fibrosis [20].

In contrast to these murine studies, the examination of inflammasome-mediated renal pathology in humans is less extensive. Whilst human proximal tubular epithelial cells (PTEC) appear to have the necessary inflammasome-related machinery, there is a paucity of evidence for its activation, particularly, whether these cells secrete IL-1β and IL-18 [58]. Intriguingly Kim, et al. [58] recently described an inflammasome-independent role for NLRP3 in human PTEC. In this study, hypoxic injury to PTEC increased NLRP3 expression independent of ASC, caspase-1, and IL-1β. Instead, the NLRP3 protein bound to the mitochondrial antiviral signal (MAVS), resulting in mitochondrial dysfunction (increased mitochondrial ROS) and cell death [58]. There is also emerging evidence that human tubular cells in acute oxalate nephropathy undergo a form of regulated cell death termed necroptosis. Products of necroptosis include DAMPs with the capacity to activate the canonical inflammasome pathway in innate immune cells (DC, macrophages) within the tubulointerstitium [20]. Our group has indeed shown increased numbers of activated human DC within the tubulointerstitium of fibrotic kidney biopsies, accumulating adjacent to injured PTEC [59].

The kidneys play a major role in maintaining homeostasis and regulating blood pressure. Renal inflammation and fibrosis are well-known contributing factors in the pathogenesis of hypertension [60]. In a murine model of salt-induced hypertension, NLRP3 inhibition by treatment with MCC950 reduced hypertension and heart rate, in addition to reduced inflammasome priming, inflammatory cytokines, kidney immune cell infiltration and kidney fibrosis [60]. Nevertheless, the specific mechanisms by which the inflammasome contributes to systemic hypertension are still unclear. Furthermore, the inflammasome-dependent interactions between specialized renal parenchymal and innate immune cells, in particular, the role of NLRP3 signalling in driving the pathobiology of human PN, remains to be elucidated.

3. Haem Catabolism and Role in Immune-Mediated Pathology

Excess haem pigments are highly cytotoxic in the kidney, leading to oxidative stress and inflammation under injurious conditions [61,62]. Our understanding of immune-mediated pathological conditions is that oxidative stress and inflammation are interdependent processes rather than discrete pathways of injury [63].

Free haem catalyses the formation of highly toxic free radicals—hydroxyl radicals (OH·)—from hydrogen peroxide (H_2O_2) via the Fenton reaction. Under homeostatic conditions, excess free cellular haem is catabolized by haem oxygenases (HO)—stress-responsive HO-1 and constitutive HO-2, as summarized in Figure 2. Catabolism of free haem by HO leads to the production of: (1) carbon monoxide (CO); (2) biliverdin (BV), that is converted by biliverdin reductase (BVR) to the antioxidant bilirubin; and (3) the release of labile Fe, which is promptly bound to ferritin (FtH), collectively preventing cellular oxidative stress [64–66]. However, under pathological conditions, the accumulation of intracellular free haem can exceed the rate of haem degradation by the HO-1 isoenzyme. Furthermore, levels of cellular Fe can be greater than the scavenging capacity of FtH. When this occurs, free haem and/or labile Fe accumulate in cells and drive oxidative stress in the micro-environment. The uncontrolled generation of free radicals and the subsequent imbalance between reactive metabolites and endogenous anti-oxidants constitutes the stress response and ultimately lead to cellular damage and inflammation.

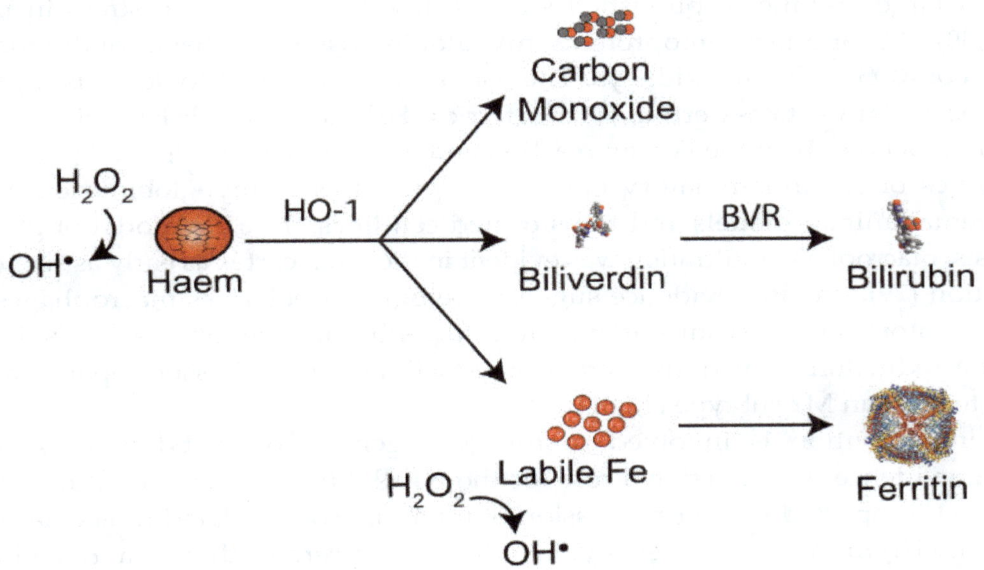

Figure 2. Haem catabolism by HO-1 produces equimolar amounts of carbon monoxide, Biliverdin and labile iron. Biliverdin is converted to bilirubin by biliverdin reductase. Labile Fe can produce ROS, but is rapidly bound to ferritin. Ferritin (PBD ID: 5Z8U) image generated using the RCSB PDB NGL viewer [67]. BVR: Bilirubin reductase; HO-1: Haem oxygenase-1.

Haem directly regulates inflammatory leukocyte migration and retention in vitro and in vivo [68]. In rodent models, intraperitoneal and intrapleural injection of haem results in dose-dependent neutrophil migration into the respective body compartments [68,69]. Haem inhibits neutrophil apoptosis, resulting in the accumulation of neutrophils at sites of haem deposition, and drives expression of proinflammatory cytokines [69–71]. Haem has also been reported to induce surface expression of adhesion molecules—i.e., intercellular adhesion molecule-1 (ICAM-l), vascular adhesion molecule-1 (VCAM-l) and endothelial leukocyte adhesion molecule (E-selectin)—in human endothelial cells, thereby driving the adhesion/retention of leukocytes [72].

Recent evidence suggests haem can trigger activation of innate immune cells via the NLRP3 inflammasome. Dutra et al. showed that haem activation of the NLRP3 inflammasome in bone marrow macrophages was dependent on NADPH oxidases, K^+ efflux and generation of mitochondrial ROS [8]. Notably, NLRP3 activation was independent of haem internalization, lysosomal damage and cell death [8]. Inflammasome activity within immortalized human endothelial cells in response to haem has also been reported in vitro, where haem was sufficient to induce significantly increased IL-1β mRNA transcripts and cytokine release [16]. Intriguingly, HO-1 activity appears to attenuate NLRP3 activity. However, this may be an indirect consequence of haem catabolism by HO-1, rather than direct interactions between HO-1 and NLRP3 [73]. Although recent studies suggest haem is an important trigger of the canonical inflammasome pathway [8,73,74], its functioning via non-canonical NLRP3 inflammasome activation in renal cells has not been explored.

4. Myoglobin-Mediated Pigment Nephropathy

Rhabdomyolysis is a clinical syndrome following physical, thermal, toxic, metabolic, ischaemic, infective and inflammatory insults to muscles [13]. The final step of the skeletal muscle breakdown is the release of toxic intracellular components, such as the hemoprotein myoglobin, into the circulation [10,75].

Myoglobinuric AKI is the most severe complication of rhabdomyolysis [76]. Myoglobin is one of the pathogenic drivers of renal injury following rhabdomyolysis. Myoglobin is cytotoxic, activating both pro-oxidant and inflammatory pathways. Cytotoxicity is augmented in the presence of volume depletion and aciduria, common features of AKI [77,78]. Renal vasoconstriction, tubular obstruction and apoptosis are additional pathological processes in myoglobin toxicity, see Figure 3 [10,12,79].

There is a large volume of published studies describing oxidative stress in myoglobinuric AKI [10,12,13,80]. As for other hemoproteins, myoglobin possesses a haem centre that can catalyse the production of ROS within the kidneys. The haem group within myoglobin is capable of cycling between various oxidative states (ferrous = Fe^{2+}; ferric = Fe^{3+}; and ferryl = Fe^{4+}) that may lead to lipid peroxidation independently of the Fenton reaction and iron release, see Figure 3 [12,13,80].

Most studies of the inflammatory pathogenic processes in myoglobinuric AKI are derived from experimental animal models and transformed cell lines. In a rat model of glycerol-induced rhabdomyolysis, macrophage infiltration was evident in the renal cortex as early as six hours following glycerol injection [79]. In vitro evidence suggests myoglobin polarizes macrophages toward both M1 (pro-inflammatory) and M2 (anti-inflammatory/pro-fibrotic) phenotypes, whilst in vivo research indicates that a reduction in oxidative stress may facilitate kidney tissue repair via a skewing of macrophages toward an M2 subtype [10,81].

Indeed, inflammation is involved in the pathogenesis of rhabdomyolysis-induced AKI, with emerging evidence of a functional role for the NLRP3 inflammasome in this disease process. Komada, et al. [17] reported greater expression of inflammasome-related molecules (NLRP3, ASC, caspase-1 and IL-1β) in the renal parenchyma following glycerol-induced myoglobinuric AKI [17]. Furthermore, activation of the inflammasome pathway correlated with leukocyte infiltration, tubular injury and dysfunction in the diseased kidney. Notably, these endpoints were markedly attenuated in *Nlrp3*$^{-/-}$, *Asc*$^{-/-}$ and *Casp1*$^{-/-}$ knockout mice [17].

At present, many questions regarding the potential triggers of the inflammasome cascade in myoglobinuric AKI remain unanswered. Komada, et al. [17] carried out in vitro experiments using renal tubular epithelial cells incubated with hemin (the oxidised form of haem), ferrous and ferric myoglobin, all potential stimuli of the NLRP3 inflammasome in myoglobinuric AKI. Although these experimental data were not published, the authors reported that these stimuli were insufficient to activate NLRP3 [17]. Although innate immune cells (DC, macrophages) have the required components for canonical inflammasome activation [74,82], the ability of tubular epithelial cells to secrete mature IL-1β via this two-step process remains uncertain [58,74,82]. Therefore, the absence of inflammatory cells in the in vitro experiments of Komada et al. may explain why they failed to demonstrate triggering of canonical inflammasome activation.

Finally, as the pathogenesis of rhabdomyolysis is multifactorial, the role of other concomitant factors, acting either as priming stimuli or directly activating the NLRP3 inflammasome, should not be ignored. For instance, data from several studies suggest that different types of crystals, such as calcium oxalate, monosodium urate and cholesterol, can function as DAMPs to trigger NLRP3 inflammasome activation [22,25,83]. Recently, we highlighted a potential role for urate crystals in generating oxidative stress and activating the NLRP3 inflammasome in an animal model of rhabdomyolysis-associated AKI [10]. Thus, additional research is required to validate this hypothesis as well as to further elucidate the mechanisms underlying inflammation in human myoglobinuric AKI.

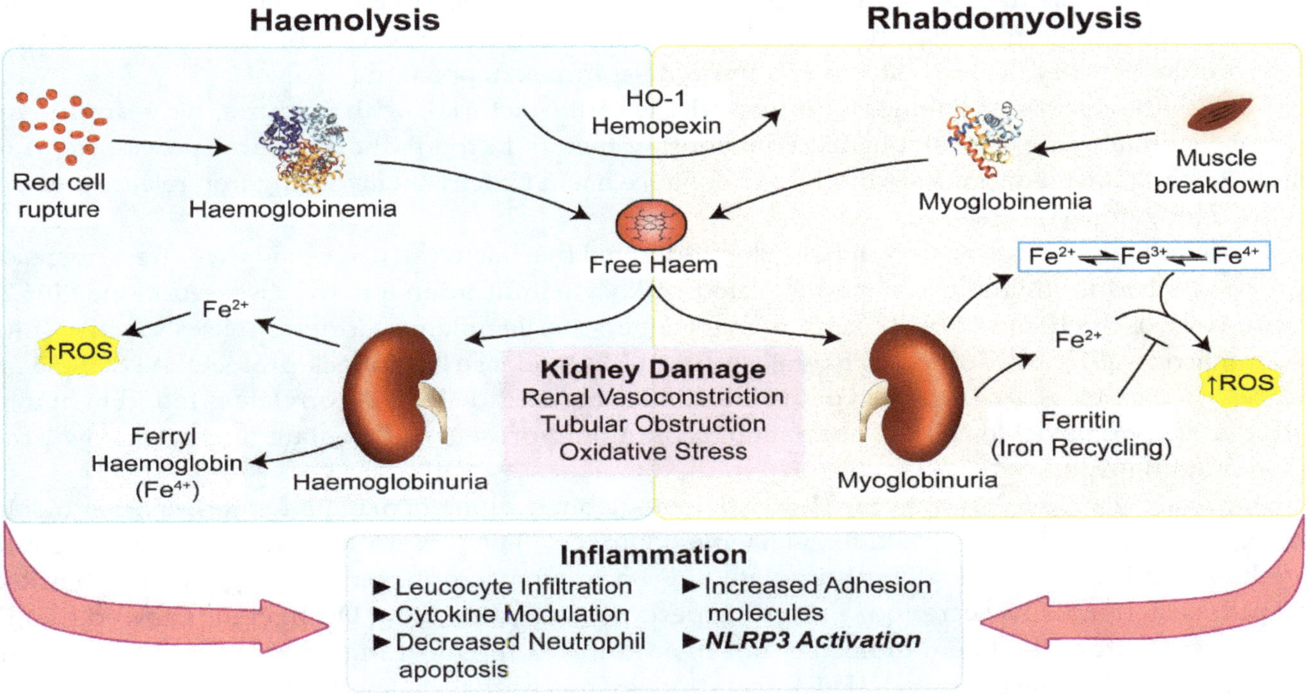

Figure 3. Potential pathways underlying haem-associated kidney injury. Free haem generated by rhabdomyolysis and haemolysis are effectively removed by HO-1 and hemopexin. The binding capacity of these proteins is saturated in pathological conditions and free haem continues to be present. Haemoglobin, myoglobin and plasma free-haem are freely filtered by the glomerulus and can be deposited within the tubules. Oxidative stress, renal vasoconstriction, tubular obstruction by casts, iron-mediated tubular toxicity and inflammation play an important role in acute pigment nephropathy. Myoglobin (PBD ID: 1MBN) and haemoglobin (PBD ID: 1BIJ) structures generated using the RCSB PDB NGL viewer [67]. NLRP3: nucleotide-binding domain-like receptor protein 3; HO-1: Haem Oxygenase-1; ROS: Reactive Oxygen Species.

5. Haemoglobin-Mediated Pigment Nephropathy

Haemolysis is defined as the rupture of red blood cells (RBC) as a result of intrinsic or extrinsic stresses, leading to the release of their intracellular contents, including hemoprotein haemoglobin [84]. Massive intravascular haemolysis is uncommon but occurs in life-threatening conditions such as poisoning, snake and insect envenomation, idiosyncratic drug reactions, haemolytic uraemic syndrome, paroxysmal nocturnal hemoglobinuria, malaria, haemorrhagic fevers, leptospirosis and septic shock [85–91].

In the event of haemolysis, plasma proteins such as haemoglobin-binding haptoglobin and haem-binding hemopexin effectively remove intravascular-produced haemoglobin/haem, thus mitigating haem-mediated deleterious effects [69]. However, under pathological conditions, the binding capacity of these plasma proteins is saturated, resulting in excess free haemoglobin in circulating blood [69]. Haemoglobulin and haem are filtered by the glomerulus, and free haemoglobin in the resultant ultrafiltrate is reabsorbed by the proximal tubules in an endocytic process involving the megalin-cubilin receptor system [65]. However, this absorption transport pathway is also concentration-dependent and large quantities of haemoglobin in the proximal tubules will saturate it, with free haemoglobulin/haem retained in the proximal tubules, leading to nephrotoxicity.

Many diseases featuring massive or recurrent haemolysis are complicated by AKI [9,64,84]. Prior to modern transfusion practices, ABO incompatibility was the most common cause of hemolysis-associated AKI [9]. With the exception of ABO-incompatible blood transfusions, haemolysis is now considered a contributing, rather than sole, trigger in the pathogenesis of haemoglobinuria-related AKI [9]. In fact, some conditions such as poisoning, envenomation and leptospirosis, may present with both haemolysis and rhabdomyolysis [85,92–95]. Furthermore, in malaria-associated AKI, other mechanisms play a greater pathogenic role than haemolysis, including mechanic obstruction by parasitized RBCs, the pro-inflammatory cytokine storm and immune-complex deposition [9,96].

The pathogenesis of haemoglobinuric AKI is multi-factorial, with aciduria, dehydration and renal ischaemia being the established contributing factors in the pathobiological processes [61,62]. These concomitant conditions are thought to enhance haem toxicity by favouring iron release and thus, pro-oxidant cytotoxic conditions [61].

As in myoglobin-derived PN, haemoglobin-derived free haem can drive oxidative stress, increased expression of adhesion molecules and elevated leukocyte infiltration into the diseased kidney [66,72]. Haemolysis also generates DAMP activity that triggers sterile inflammatory responses via the NLRP3 inflammasome [97]. In addition to haem, ruptured RBCs release heat shock proteins, ATP, IL-33 and mtDNA that are recognized triggers of the inflammasome cascade [97]. A correlate is found in humans with the disease of sickle cell, where patients commonly present with a state of chronic low-grade inflammation [69,98].

Intravascular hemolysis may also lead to haemoglobin in different oxidative states, i.e., hemoglobin (Fe^{2+}), methemoglobin (Fe^{3+}), and ferryl haemoglobin (Fe^{4+}) [99]. Nyakundi, et al. [99] demonstrated both haem and ferryl haemoglobin stimulated LPS-primed macrophages to upregulate IL-1β mRNA and induce active IL-1β secretion. Further experiments conducted by Dutra et al. showed that the iron present within the haem molecule, not free iron, was the most important stimulus triggering the NLRP3 inflammasome and IL-1β secretion in macrophages and ultimately contributed to hemolysis-associated lethality [8]. Understanding these molecular pathways triggered by distinct haem motifs may prove useful in identifying novel therapeutic targets for haemoglobin/myoglobin-mediated pigment nephropathies.

6. Inflammasome Inhibition as a Potential Therapeutic Target

The significant pathological role of inflammasome activation in several chronic inflammatory diseases has made it an attractive target for therapeutic intervention. There are two approaches in current strategies inhibiting the inflammasome: (1) Targeting inflammasome activation directly and/or (2) targeting down-stream effects of IL-1β. Here, we review several compounds that could be repurposed, in combination with existing therapies, to ameliorate inflammatory immune responses in PN.

6.1. NLRP3 Inflammasome Inhibitors

Several compounds have been identified and developed for therapeutic inhibition of NLRP3 inflammasome activation. These established inflammasome-inhibiting compounds have been extensively reviewed by Lopez-Castejon and Pelegrin [100] and, more recently, by Baldwin, et al. [101]. Several preclinical studies have already investigated the use of these inflammasome inhibitors in AKI and CKD nephropathies, but their therapeutic efficacy has not been tested in PN.

The second-generation sulfonylurea drug, glyburide (also glibenclamide), is an established compound for the treatment of human type II diabetes mellitus [100,101]. Glyburide blocks K_{ATP} channels, depolarizing the cell membrane, triggering the release of insulin from pancreatic β-cells [100,101]. Glyburide's actions were originally thought to be mediated via its role as a K_{ATP} channel blocker, but emerging evidence suggests that it, in fact, prevents the formation of ASC specks [101]. However, the specific mechanism of the interactions of glyburide and NLRP3 remain poorly understood.

Glyburide has been used in an adenine-rich diet rat model of CKD. In this study, glyburide treatment attenuated NLRP3 expression, improved renal function and ameliorated the CKD histopathology [102]. Unfortunately, glyburide is generally not a recommended treatment in CKD patients due to the increased risk of hypoglycemia [103]. In addition, patients with glucose-6-phosphate dehydrogenase deficiency are susceptible to developing haemolytic anemia following glyburide treatment [104,105].

A novel subclass of sulfonylurea containing compounds, derived from glyburide, was identified by Perregaux, et al. [106]. These compounds inhibited post-translational processing of IL-1β, resulting in little-to-no maturation or extracellular release of the cytokine. One of these compounds, MCC950 (also CP-456,773), was reported by Coll, et al. [107] as a potent, specific inhibitor of the NLRP3 inflammasome. Whilst the mechanism of MCC950-mediated NLRP3 inhibition is still poorly understood, MCC950 has been studied in several disease models, including colitis [108], Parkinson's disease [109], diabetic encephalopathy [110] and non-alcoholic steatohepatitis [111]. Recent studies also evaluated MCC950 in pre-clinical models of AKI and CKD. MCC950 treatment attenuated kidney fibrosis in a murine model of diet-induced oxalate crystal-nephropathy [20]. Furthermore, MCC950 treatment abrogated kidney damage and ameliorated systemic blood pressure in a murine model of hypertension, induced by both surgery (uninephrectomy) and treatment with deoxycorticosterone [60]. MCC950's relatively short half-life and its specificity for the NLRP3 inflammasome [107] make it, and its derivatives, ideal candidates for further investigations in PN.

6.2. Anti-IL-1β and IL-1 Receptor Antagonists

Inhibition of the down-stream IL-1β-signalling pathways has been widely adopted in rheumatology for treatment of auto-inflammatory diseases [112]. Strategies for these therapies involve: (1) Reducing the amount of IL-1β available for activating the endogenous IL-1 receptor (IL-1R) or (2) inhibiting the endogenous receptor directly.

Canakinumab is a potent monoclonal antibody specific for IL-1β [113,114] and an established therapeutic in the treatment of rheumatoid arthritis [112]. Canakinumab has been evaluated in patients with CKD, reducing the risk of major adverse cardiovascular event rates among high-risk atherosclerosis patients [115]. However, no differences in kidney function (as measured by the estimated Glomerulus Filtration Rate) were reported between placebo and Canakinumab-treated CKD patients [115]. A common CKD co-morbidity is gout, which arises as a consequence of increased uric acid. Inflammasome activation is imputed to be the prime mechanism of this auto-inflammatory condition [25]. A clinical trial using Canakinumab showed significantly reduced rates of gout attacks in patients, although no changes in serum uric acid concentrations were observed [116]. Studies such as these provide important foundational evidence for further pre-clinical studies of Canakinumab for the treatment of PN.

Therapeutic strategies targeting the IL-1 receptor (IL-1R) are also used in current clinical practice. Anakinra is a recombinant human IL-1R antagonist, competing with IL-1β for binding with the IL-1R [117]. Anakinra is another established therapeutic in the treatment of auto-inflammatory diseases in rheumatology. Notably, it has been successfully used in patients with Familial Mediterranean Fever (FMF) [118,119], an auto-inflammatory disease associated with mutations in the inflammasome component pyrin that results in triggering inflammasome activation [120,121]. The therapeutic use of anakinra for treating acute gout attacks in CKD patients is currently in clinical trials (ASGARD study), with the results yet to be published [117]. Interestingly, anakinra is being investigated as a third-line therapy in this ASGARD study, following non-response to second-line therapy, where the development of rhabdomyolysis was a reported side-effect [117,122].

Although these IL-1β- and IL-1R-targeting drugs are proving to be effective inflammasome inhibitors, pre-clinical studies investigating their efficacy for the treatment of PN are yet to be performed. These studies need to include in vivo and in vitro models of PN to not only establish therapeutic efficacy but also any unforeseen off-target effects.

7. Concluding Remarks

The release of haem by myoglobin and haemoglobin catabolism is pivotal in the pathogenesis of PN. Whilst haem toxicity is clinically recognized as important, the role of haem in the mechanism of the associated kidney inflammation may be overlooked. Irrespective of its source, haem triggers NLRP3 inflammasome activation, but this mechanistic pathway of disease in PN is still poorly understood. Contemporary studies have shifted to the role of haem driving kidney inflammation via NLRP3 inflammasome activation. The research is focused on the canonical activation of the inflammasome within immune cell populations by haem. The non-canonical activation of the inflammasome in immune cell populations by haem has not been investigated. Furthermore, neither canonical nor non-canonical mechanisms of inflammasome activation within kidney parenchymal cells are fully understood. Well-designed studies are required to address both, focusing on haemolytic driven AKI for which there is currently a lack of information.

The aim of future PN research is to provide evidence to move to pre-clinical studies of potential treatments for both myoglobinuric and haemolytic AKI. Non-renal studies with IL-1R antagonists and direct NLRP3 inflammasome inhibitors are advanced, with small molecules in clinical use for auto-immune rheumatological diseases. Several pre-clinical studies have investigated their therapeutic role in different patterns of kidney disease, but not PN. These studies provide the rationale for translation into clinical trials for the prevention and treatment of PN.

Author Contributions: P.H.F.G, A.J.K, H.H., and K.G. conceptualized the review article. P.H.F.G, K.T.K.G, A.J.K and H.H. contributed in writing, review and editing of the original draft. K.T.K.G. compiled the manuscript and P.H.F.G. supervised the study.

Acknowledgments: The authors wish to thank Madeleine Kersting-Flynn for her advice and assistance with the illustrations presented in this document. The authors also would like to express our profound thanks for the continued support from the staff and patients at the Royal Brisbane and Women's Hospital and Pathology Queensland.

Abbreviations

AKI	Acute Kidney Injury
ASC	Apoptosis-associated speck-like protein containing a CARD domain
ATP	Adenosine Triphosphate
CARD	Caspase activation and recruitment domain
CD	Cluster of differentiation
CKD	Chronic Kidney Disease
DAMPs	Damage-associated molecular patterns
DC	Dendritic cells
DKD	Diabetic kidney disease
ESCRT	Endosomal sorting complexes required for transport
FMF	Familial Mediterranean Fever
GSDMD	Gasdermin-D
HAMPs	Homeostasis-altering molecular processes
HO	Haem Oxygenase
HO-1	Haem Oxygenase-1
ICAM-1	Intercellular Adhesion Molecule-1

IL	Interleukin
IL-1R	IL-1 receptor
LPS	Lipopolysaccharide
MAVS	Mitochondrial antiviral signal
mtDNA	Mitochondrial DNA
NADPH	Dihydronicotinamide-adenine dinucleotide phosphate
NLRP3	Nucleotide-binding domain-like receptor protein 3
PAMPs	Pathogen-associated molecular patterns
PN	Pigment Nephropathy
PRRs	Pattern recognition receptors
PTEC	Proximal Tubule Epithelial Cells
RBC	Red Blood Cells
ROS	Reactive Oxygen Species
TLRs	Toll-like receptors
UUO	Unilateral ureteral obstruction
VCAM-l	Vascular Adhesion Molecule-1
XO	Xanthine Oxidase

References

1. Sikorski, Z.E. *Chemical and Functional Properties of Food Components*; CRC Press: Boc Raton, FL, USA, 2007.
2. Paoli, M.; Marles-Wright, J.; Smith, A. Structure–Function Relationships in Heme-Proteins. *DNA Cell Biol.* **2002**, *21*, 271–280. [CrossRef] [PubMed]
3. Larsen, R.; Gouveia, Z.; Soares, M.P.; Gozzelino, R.; Kapitulnik, J.; Hebrew, T.; Ryter, S.W.; Immenschuh, S. Heme cytotoxicity and the pathogenesis of immune-mediated inflammatory diseases. *Front. Pharmacol.* **2012**. [CrossRef] [PubMed]
4. Smith, L.J.; Kahraman, A.; Thornton, J.M. Heme proteins-Diversity in structural characteristics, function, and folding. *Proteins Struct. Function Bioinform.* **2010**, *78*, 2349–2368. [CrossRef] [PubMed]
5. Mense, S.M.; Zhang, L. Heme: A versatile signaling molecule controlling the activities of diverse regulators ranging from transcription factors to MAP kinases. *Cell Res.* **2006**, *16*, 681–692. [CrossRef] [PubMed]
6. Immenschuh, S.; Vijayan, V.; Janciauskiene, S.; Gueler, F. Heme as a Target for Therapeutic Interventions. *Front Pharmacol.* **2017**, *8*, 146. [CrossRef]
7. Nangaku, M. Hypoxia and Tubulointerstitial Injury: A Final Common Pathway to End-Stage Renal Failure. *Nephron Exp. Nephrol.* **2004**, *98*, e8–e12. [CrossRef] [PubMed]
8. Dutra, F.F.; Alves, L.S.; Rodrigues, D.; Fernandez, P.L.; de Oliveira, R.B.; Golenbock, D.T.; Zamboni, D.S.; Bozza, M.T. Hemolysis-induced lethality involves inflammasome activation by heme. *Proc. Natl. Acad. Sci. USA* **2014**. [CrossRef]
9. Perazella, M.A.; Rosner, M.H. Clinical features and diagnosis of heme pigment-induced acute kidney injury. Available online: https://www.uptodate.com/contents/clinical-features-and-diagnosis-of-heme-pigment-induced-acute-kidney-injury (accessed on 7 February 2019).
10. Gois, P.H.F.; Canale, D.; Volpini, R.A.; Ferreira, D.; Veras, M.M.; Andrade-Oliveira, V.; Câmara, N.O.S.; Shimizu, M.H.M.; Seguro, A.C. Allopurinol attenuates rhabdomyolysis-associated acute kidney injury: Renal and muscular protection. *Free Radic. Biol. Med.* **2016**, *101*, 176–189. [CrossRef] [PubMed]
11. Heyman, S.N.; Rosen, S.; Fuchs, S.; Epstein, F.H.; Brezis, M. Myoglobinuric acute renal failure in the rat: a role for medullary hypoperfusion, hypoxia, and tubular obstruction. *J. Am. Soc. Nephrol.* **1996**, *7*, 1066–1074.
12. Moore, K.P.; Holt, S.G.; Patel, R.P.; Svistunenko, D.A.; Zackert, W.; Goodier, D.; Reeder, B.J.; Clozel, M.; Anand, R.; Cooper, C.E.; et al. A causative role for redox cycling of myoglobin and its inhibition by alkalinization in the pathogenesis and treatment of rhabdomyolysis-induced renal failure. *J. Biol. Chem.* **1998**, *273*, 31731–31737. [CrossRef] [PubMed]
13. Zager, R.A.; Burkhart, K. Myoglobin toxicity in proximal human kidney cells: Roles of Fe, Ca2+, H2O2, and terminal mitochondrial electron transport. *Kidney Int.* **1997**, *51*, 728–738. [CrossRef] [PubMed]

14. Guo, H.; Callaway, J.B.; Ting, J.P.Y. Inflammasomes: Mechanism of action, role in disease, and therapeutics. *Nat. Med.* **2015**, *21*, 677–687. [CrossRef] [PubMed]
15. Dutra, F.F.; Bozza, M.T. Heme on innate immunity and inflammation. *Front. Pharmacol.* **2014**, *5*, 115. [CrossRef]
16. Erdei, J.; Tóth, A.; Balogh, E.; Nyakundi, B.B.; Bányai, E.; Ryffel, B.; Paragh, G.; Cordero, M.D.; Jeney, V. Induction of NLRP3 Inflammasome Activation by Heme in Human Endothelial Cells. *Oxid. Med. Cell. Longev.* **2018**. [CrossRef] [PubMed]
17. Komada, T.; Usui, F.; Kawashima, A.; Kimura, H.; Karasawa, T.; Inoue, Y.; Kobayashi, M.; Mizushina, Y.; Kasahara, T.; Taniguchi, S.I.; et al. Role of NLRP3 inflammasomes for rhabdomyolysis-induced acute kidney injury. *Sci. Rep.* **2015**. [CrossRef]
18. Schroder, K.; Tschopp, J. The Inflammasomes. *Cell* **2010**, *140*, 821–832. [CrossRef]
19. Brähler, S.; Zinselmeyer, B.H.; Raju, S.; Nitschke, M.; Suleiman, H.; Saunders, B.T.; Johnson, M.W.; Böhner, A.M.C.; Viehmann, S.F.; Theisen, D.J.; et al. Opposing Roles of Dendritic Cell Subsets in Experimental GN. *J. Am. Soc. Nephrol.* **2017**. [CrossRef]
20. Ludwig-Portugall, I.; Bartok, E.; Dhana, E.; Evers, B.D.G.; Primiano, M.J.; Hall, J.P.; Franklin, B.S.; Knolle, P.A.; Hornung, V.; Hartmann, G.; et al. An NLRP3-specific inflammasome inhibitor attenuates crystal-induced kidney fibrosis in mice. *Kidney Int.* **2016**, *90*, 525–539. [CrossRef]
21. Anders, H.J.; Muruve, D.A. The Inflammasomes in Kidney Disease. *J. Am. Soc. Nephrol.* **2011**, *22*, 1007–1018. [CrossRef]
22. Wilson, G.J.; Gois, P.H.F.; Zhang, A.; Wang, X.; Law, B.M.P.; Kassianos, A.J.; Healy, H.G. The Role of Oxidative Stress and Inflammation in Acute Oxalate Nephropathy Associated with Ethylene Glycol Intoxication. *Kidney Int. Rep.* **2018**, *3*, 1217–1221. [CrossRef]
23. Knauf, F.; Asplin, J.R.; Granja, I.; Schmidt, I.M.; Moeckel, G.W.; David, R.J.; Flavell, R.A.; Aronson, P.S. NALP3-mediated inflammation is a principal cause of progressive renal failure in oxalate nephropathy. *Kidney Int.* **2013**, *84*, 895–901. [CrossRef] [PubMed]
24. Yaribeygi, H.; Katsiki, N.; Butler, A.E.; Sahebkar, A. Effects of antidiabetic drugs on NLRP3 inflammasome activity, with a focus on diabetic kidneys. *Drug Discov. Today* **2018**. [CrossRef]
25. Martinon, F.; Pétrilli, V.; Mayor, A.; Tardivel, A.; Tschopp, J. Gout-associated uric acid crystals activate the NALP3 inflammasome. *Nature* **2006**, *440*, 237. [CrossRef] [PubMed]
26. Mulay, S.R.; Kulkarni, O.P.; Rupanagudi, K.V.; Migliorini, A.; Darisipudi, M.N.; Vilaysane, A.; Muruve, D.; Shi, Y.; Munro, F.; Liapis, H.; et al. Calcium oxalate crystals induce renal inflammation by NLRP3-mediated IL-1β secretion. *J. Clin. Investig.* **2013**, *123*, 236–246. [CrossRef]
27. Rajamäki, K.; Lappalainen, J.; Öörni, K.; Välimäki, E.; Matikainen, S.; Kovanen, P.T.; Eklund, K.K. Cholesterol Crystals Activate the NLRP3 Inflammasome in Human Macrophages: A Novel Link between Cholesterol Metabolism and Inflammation. *PLoS ONE* **2010**, *5*, e11765. [CrossRef]
28. Duewell, P.; Kono, H.; Rayner, K.J.; Sirois, C.M.; Vladimer, G.; Bauernfeind, F.G.; Abela, G.S.; Franchi, L.; Nuñez, G.; Schnurr, M.; et al. NLRP3 inflammasomes are required for atherogenesis and activated by cholesterol crystals. *Nature* **2010**, *464*, 1357. [CrossRef] [PubMed]
29. Liston, A.; Masters, S.L. Homeostasis-altering molecular processes as mechanisms of inflammasome activation. *Nat. Rev. Immunol.* **2017**, *17*, 208. [CrossRef] [PubMed]
30. He, Y.; Zeng, M.Y.; Yang, D.; Motro, B.; Núñez, G. NEK7 is an essential mediator of NLRP3 activation downstream of potassium efflux. *Nature* **2016**, *530*, 354–357. [CrossRef]
31. Amores-Iniesta, J.; Barberà-Cremades, M.; Martínez, C.M.; Pons, J.A.; Revilla-Nuin, B.; Martínez-Alarcón, L.; Di Virgilio, F.; Parrilla, P.; Baroja-Mazo, A.; Pelegrín, P. Extracellular ATP Activates the NLRP3 Inflammasome and Is an Early Danger Signal of Skin Allograft Rejection. *Cell Rep.* **2017**, *21*, 3414–3426. [CrossRef] [PubMed]
32. Chen, K.; Zhang, J.; Zhang, W.; Zhang, J.; Yang, J.; Li, K.; He, Y. ATP-P2X4 signaling mediates NLRP3 inflammasome activation: A novel pathway of diabetic nephropathy. *Int. J. Biochem. Cell Biol.* **2013**, *45*, 932–943. [CrossRef]
33. Sadatomi, D.; Nakashioya, K.; Mamiya, S.; Honda, S.; Tanimura, S.; Yamamura, Y.; Kameyama, Y.; Takeda, K. Mitochondrial function is required for extracellular ATP-induced NLRP3 inflammasome activation. *J. Biochem.* **2017**, *161*, 503–512. [CrossRef]
34. Elliott, E.I.; Miller, A.N.; Banoth, B.; Iyer, S.S.; Stotland, A.; Weiss, J.P.; Gottlieb, R.A.; Sutterwala, F.S.; Cassel, S.L. Cutting Edge: Mitochondrial Assembly of the NLRP3 Inflammasome Complex Is Initiated at Priming. *J. Immunol.* **2018**, *200*, 3047. [CrossRef] [PubMed]

35. Zhou, R.; Tardivel, A.; Thorens, B.; Choi, I.; Tschopp, J. Thioredoxin-interacting protein links oxidative stress to inflammasome activation. *Nat. Immunol.* **2010**, *11*, 136–140. [CrossRef] [PubMed]

36. Zhong, Z.; Liang, S.; Sanchez-Lopez, E.; He, F.; Shalapour, S.; Lin, X.j.; Wong, J.; Ding, S.; Seki, E.; Schnabl, B.; et al. New mitochondrial DNA synthesis enables NLRP3 inflammasome activation. *Nature* **2018**. [CrossRef] [PubMed]

37. Lin, K.-M.; Hu, W.; Troutman, T.D.; Jennings, M.; Brewer, T.; Li, X.; Nanda, S.; Cohen, P.; Thomas, J.A.; Pasare, C. IRAK-1 bypasses priming and directly links TLRs to rapid NLRP3 inflammasome activation. *Proc. Natl. Acad. Sci. USA* **2014**, *111*, 775–780. [CrossRef]

38. Liu, T.; Zhang, L.; Joo, D.; Sun, S.-C. NF-κB signaling in inflammation. *Signal Transduct. Target. Ther.* **2017**, *2*, 17023. [CrossRef]

39. Hari, A.; Zhang, Y.; Tu, Z.; Detampel, P.; Stenner, M.; Ganguly, A.; Shi, Y. Activation of NLRP3 inflammasome by crystalline structures via cell surface contact. *Sci. Rep.* **2014**, *4*, 7281. [CrossRef] [PubMed]

40. He, Y.; Hara, H.; Núñez, G. Mechanism and Regulation of NLRP3 Inflammasome Activation. *Trends Biochem. Sci.* **2016**, *41*, 1012–1021. [CrossRef]

41. Hornung, V.; Bauernfeind, F.; Halle, A.; Samstad, E.O.; Kono, H.; Rock, K.L.; Fitzgerald, K.A.; Latz, E. Silica crystals and aluminum salts activate the NALP3 inflammasome through phagosomal destabilization. *Nat. Immunol.* **2008**, *9*, 847. [CrossRef] [PubMed]

42. Bronner, D.N.; Abuaita, B.H.; Chen, X.; Fitzgerald, K.A.; Nuñez, G.; He, Y.; Yin, X.-M.; O'Riordan, M.X.D. Endoplasmic Reticulum Stress Activates the Inflammasome via NLRP3- and Caspase-2-Driven Mitochondrial Damage. *Immunity* **2015**, *43*, 451–462. [CrossRef]

43. Boucher, D.; Monteleone, M.; Coll, R.C.; Chen, K.W.; Ross, C.M.; Teo, J.L.; Gomez, G.A.; Holley, C.L.; Bierschenk, D.; Stacey, K.J.; et al. Caspase-1 self-cleavage is an intrinsic mechanism to terminate inflammasome activity. *J. Exp. Med.* **2018**. [CrossRef]

44. Monteleone, M.; Stanley, A.C.; Chen, K.W.; Brown, D.L.; Bezbradica, J.S.; von Pein, J.B.; Holley, C.L.; Boucher, D.; Shakespear, M.R.; Kapetanovic, R.; et al. Interleukin-1β Maturation Triggers Its Relocation to the Plasma Membrane for Gasdermin-D-Dependent and -Independent Secretion. *Cell Rep.* **2018**, *24*, 1425–1433. [CrossRef] [PubMed]

45. Sborgi, L.; Rühl, S.; Mulvihill, E.; Pipercevic, J.; Heilig, R.; Stahlberg, H.; Farady, C.J.; Müller, D.J.; Broz, P.; Hiller, S. GSDMD membrane pore formation constitutes the mechanism of pyroptotic cell death. *EMBO J.* **2016**, *35*, 1766–1778. [CrossRef] [PubMed]

46. Liu, X.; Zhang, Z.; Ruan, J.; Pan, Y.; Magupalli, V.G.; Wu, H.; Lieberman, J. Inflammasome-activated gasdermin D causes pyroptosis by forming membrane pores. *Nature* **2016**, *535*, 153–158. [CrossRef] [PubMed]

47. Rühl, S.; Shkarina, K.; Demarco, B.; Heilig, R.; Santos, J.C.; Broz, P. ESCRT-dependent membrane repair negatively regulates pyroptosis downstream of GSDMD activation. *Science* **2018**, *362*, 956–960. [CrossRef]

48. Sun, G.; Guzman, E.; Balasanyan, V.; Conner, C.M.; Wong, K.; Zhou, H.R.; Kosik, K.S.; Montell, D.J. A molecular signature for anastasis, recovery from the brink of apoptotic cell death. *J. Cell Biol.* **2017**, *216*, 3355–3368. [CrossRef]

49. Pellegrini, C.; Antonioli, L.; Lopez-Castejon, G.; Blandizzi, C.; Fornai, M. Canonical and non-canonical activation of NLRP3 inflammasome at the crossroad between immune tolerance and intestinal inflammation. *Front. Immunol.* **2017**, *8*, 36. [CrossRef]

50. Kayagaki, N.; Stowe, I.B.; Lee, B.L.; O'Rourke, K.; Anderson, K.; Warming, S.; Cuellar, T.; Haley, B.; Roose-Girma, M.; Phung, Q.T.; et al. Caspase-11 cleaves gasdermin D for non-canonical inflammasome signalling. *Nature* **2015**, *526*, 666–671. [CrossRef]

51. Knodler, L.A.; Crowley, S.M.; Sham, H.P.; Yang, H.; Wrande, M.; Ma, C.; Ernst, R.K.; Steele-Mortimer, O.; Celli, J.; Vallance, B.A. Noncanonical Inflammasome Activation of Caspase-4/Caspase-11 Mediates Epithelial Defenses against Enteric Bacterial Pathogens. *Cell Host Microbe* **2014**, *16*, 249–256. [CrossRef]

52. Vilaysane, A.; Chun, J.; Seamone, M.E.; Wang, W.; Chin, R.; Hirota, S.; Li, Y.; Clark, S.A.; Tschopp, J.; Trpkov, K.; et al. The NLRP3 Inflammasome Promotes Renal Inflammation and Contributes to CKD. *J. Am. Soc. Nephrol.* **2010**, *21*, 1732–1744. [CrossRef]

53. Braga, T.T.; Forni, M.F.; Correa-Costa, M.; Ramos, R.N.; Barbuto, J.A.; Branco, P.; Castoldi, A.; Hiyane, M.I.; Davanso, M.R.; Latz, E.; et al. Soluble Uric Acid Activates the NLRP3 Inflammasome. *Sci. Rep.* **2017**, *7*, 39884. [CrossRef]

54. Shahzad, K.; Bock, F.; Dong, W.; Wang, H.; Kopf, S.; Kohli, S.; Al-Dabet, M.D.M.; Ranjan, S.; Wolter, J.;

Wacker, C.; et al. Nlrp3-inflammasome activation in non-myeloid-derived cells aggravates diabetic nephropathy. *Kidney Int.* **2015**, *87*, 74–84. [CrossRef] [PubMed]

55. Gersch, M.S.; Johnson, R.J. Uric acid and the immune response. *Nephrol. Dial. Transplant.* **2006**, *21*, 3046–3047. [CrossRef] [PubMed]
56. Ives, A.; Nomura, J.; Martinon, F.; Roger, T.; LeRoy, D.; Miner, J.N.; Simon, G.; Busso, N.; So, A. Xanthine oxidoreductase regulates macrophage IL1β secretion upon NLRP3 inflammasome activation. *Nat. Commun.* **2015**, *6*, 6555. [CrossRef] [PubMed]
57. Garlanda, C.; Dinarello, C.A.; Mantovani, A. The Interleukin-1 Family: Back to the Future. *Immunity* **2013**, *39*, 1003–1018. [CrossRef]
58. Kim, S.M.; Kim, Y.G.; Kim, D.J.; Park, S.H.; Jeong, K.H.; Lee, Y.H.; Lim, S.J.; Lee, S.H.; Moon, J.Y. Inflammasome-Independent Role of NLRP3 Mediates Mitochondrial Regulation in Renal Injury. *Front. Immunol.* **2018**, *9*, 2563. [CrossRef] [PubMed]
59. Kassianos, A.J.; Wang, X.; Sampangi, S.; Muczynski, K.; Healy, H.; Wilkinson, R. Increased tubulointerstitial recruitment of human CD141hi CLEC9A+ and CD1c+ myeloid dendritic cell subsets in renal fibrosis and chronic kidney disease. *AJP Renal Physiol.* **2013**, *305*, F1391–F1401. [CrossRef] [PubMed]
60. Krishnan, S.M.; Ling, Y.H.; Huuskes, B.M.; Ferens, D.M.; Saini, N.; Chan, C.T.; Diep, H.; Kett, M.M.; Samuel, C.S.; Kemp-Harper, B.K.; et al. Pharmacological inhibition of the NLRP3 inflammasome reduces blood pressure, renal damage, and dysfunction in salt-sensitive hypertension. *Cardiovasc. Res.* **2019**, *115*, 776–787. [CrossRef]
61. Paller, M.S. Hemoglobin- and myoglobin-induced acute renal failure in rats: Role of iron in nephrotoxicity. *Am. J. Physiol.* **1988**, *255*, F539–F544. [CrossRef]
62. Zager, R.A.; Gamelin, L.M. Pathogenetic mechanisms in experimental hemoglobinuric acute renal failure. *Am. J. Physiol.* **1989**, *256*, F446–F455. [CrossRef]
63. Biswas, S.K. Does the Interdependence between Oxidative Stress and Inflammation Explain the Antioxidant Paradox? *Oxid. Med. Cell. Longev.* **2016**. [CrossRef]
64. Qian, Q.; Nath, K.A.; Wu, Y.; Daoud, T.M.; Sethi, S. Hemolysis and acute kidney failure. *Am. J. Kidney Dis.* **2010**. [CrossRef] [PubMed]
65. Tracz, M.J.; Alam, J.; Nath, K.A. Physiology and Pathophysiology of Heme: Implications for Kidney Disease. *J. Am. Soc. Nephrol.* **2007**. [CrossRef]
66. Wagener, F.A.D.T.G.; Eggert, A.; Boerman, O.C.; Oyen, W.J.G.; Verhofstad, A.; Abraham, N.G.; Adema, G.; Van Kooyk, Y.; De Witte, T.; Figdor, C.G. Heme is a potent inducer of inflammation in mice and is counteracted by heme oxygenase. *Blood* **2001**. [CrossRef]
67. Rose, A.S.; Bradley, A.R.; Valasatava, Y.; Duarte, J.M.; Prlić, A.; Rose, P.W. NGL viewer: Web-based molecular graphics for large complexes. *Bioinformatics* **2018**, *34*, 3755–3758. [CrossRef] [PubMed]
68. Porto, B.N.; Alves, L.S.; Fernández, P.L.; Dutra, T.P.; Figueiredo, R.T.; Graça-Souza, A.V.; Bozza, M.T. Heme induces neutrophil migration and reactive oxygen species generation through signaling pathways characteristic of chemotactic receptors. *J. Biol. Chem.* **2007**. [CrossRef]
69. Graça-Souza, A.V.; Arruda, M.A.B.; De Freitas, M.S.; Barja-Fidalgo, C.; Oliveira, P.L. Neutrophil activation by heme: Implications for inflammatory processes. *Blood* **2002**. [CrossRef]
70. Arruda, M.A.; Rossi, A.G.; de Freitas, M.S.; Barja-Fidalgo, C.; Graça-Souza, A.V. Heme inhibits human neutrophil apoptosis: Involvement of phosphoinositide 3-kinase, MAPK, and NF-κB. *J. Immunol.* **2004**, *173*, 2023–2030. [CrossRef]
71. Figueiredo, R.T.; Fernandez, P.L.; Mourao-Sa, D.S.; Porto, B.N.; Dutra, F.F.; Alves, L.S.; Oliveira, M.F.; Oliveira, P.L.; Graça-Souza, A.V.; Bozza, M.T. Characterization of heme as activator of toll-like receptor 4. *J. Biolog. Chem.* **2007**. [CrossRef]
72. Wagener, F.A.; Feldman, E.; de Witte, T.; Abraham, N.G. Heme induces the expression of adhesion molecules ICAM-1, VCAM-1, and E selectin in vascular endothelial cells. *Proc. Soc. Exp. Biol. Med. Soc. Exp. Biol. Med.* **1997**, *216*, 456–463. [CrossRef]
73. Lv, J.; Su, W.; Yu, Q.; Zhang, M.; Di, C.; Lin, X.; Wu, M.; Xia, Z. Heme oxygenase-1 protects airway epithelium against apoptosis by targeting the proinflammatory NLRP3–RXR axis in asthma. *J. Biol. Chem.* **2018**, *293*, 18454–18465. [CrossRef]
74. Lorenz, G.; Darisipudi, M.N.; Anders, H.J. Canonical and non-canonical effects of the NLRP3 inflammasome in kidney inflammation and fibrosis. *Nephrol. Dial. Transplant.* **2014**, *29*, 41–48. [CrossRef]
75. Bosch, X.; Poch, E.; Grau, J.M. Rhabdomyolysis and Acute Kidney Injury. *N. Engl. J. Med.* **2009**, *361*, 62–72.

[CrossRef]
76. Korrapati, M.C.; Shaner, B.E.; Schnellmann, R.G. Recovery from Glycerol-Induced Acute Kidney Injury Is Accelerated by Suramin. *J. Pharmacol. Exp. Ther.* **2012**. [CrossRef]
77. Desforges, J.F.; Better, O.S.; Stein, J.H. Early Management of Shock and Prophylaxis of Acute Renal Failure in Traumatic Rhabdomyolysis. *N. Engl. J. Med.* **1990**, *322*, 825–829. [CrossRef]
78. Zager, R.A. Rhabdomyolysis and myohemoglobinuric acute renal failure. *Kidney Int* **1996**, *49*, 314–326. [CrossRef] [PubMed]
79. Homsi, E.; Janino, P.; De Faria, J.B.L. Role of caspases on cell death, inflammation, and cell cycle in glycerol-induced acute renal failure. *Kidney Int.* **2006**, *69*, 1385–1392. [CrossRef]
80. Zager, R.A.; Foerder, C.A. Effects of inorganic iron and myoglobin on in vitro proximal tubular lipid peroxidation and cytotoxicity. *J. Clin. Investig.* **1992**, *89*, 989–995. [CrossRef] [PubMed]
81. Belliere, J.; Casemayou, A.; Ducasse, L.; Zakaroff-Girard, A.; Martins, F.; Iacovoni, J.S.; Guilbeau-Frugier, C.; Buffin-Meyer, B.; Pipy, B.; Chauveau, D.; et al. Specific macrophage subtypes influence the progression of rhabdomyolysis-induced kidney injury. *J. Am. Soc. Nephrol.* **2015**, *26*, 1363–1377. [CrossRef]
82. Lichtnekert, J.; Kulkarni, O.P.; Mulay, S.R.; Rupanagudi, K.V.; Ryu, M.; Allam, R.; Vielhauer, V.; Muruve, D.; Lindenmeyer, M.T.; Cohen, C.D.; et al. Anti-GBM Glomerulonephritis Involves IL-1 but Is Independent of NLRP3/ASC Inflammasome-Mediated Activation of Caspase-1. *PLoS ONE* **2011**, *6*, e26778. [CrossRef] [PubMed]
83. Karasawa, T.; Takahashi, M. The crystal-induced activation of NLRP3 inflammasomes in atherosclerosis. *Inflamm. Regen.* **2017**, *37*, 18. [CrossRef] [PubMed]
84. Nath, K.A.; Murali, N.S. *Myoglobinuric and Hemoglobinuric Acute Kidney Injury*, 5th ed.; Saunders Elsevier: Philadelphia, PA, USA, 2009; pp. 298–304.
85. Anuradha, S.; Arora, S.; Mehrotra, S.; Arora, A.; Kar, P. Acute renal failure following para-phenylenediamine (PPD) poisoning: A case report and review. *Renal Fail.* **2004**, *26*, 329–332. [CrossRef]
86. Fernandez, P.L.; Dutra, F.F.; Alves, L.; Figueiredo, R.T.; Mourão-Sa, D.; Fortes, G.B.; Bergstrand, S.; Lönn, D.; Cevallos, R.R.; Pereira, R.M.S.; et al. Heme Amplifies the Innate Immune Response to Microbial Molecules through Spleen Tyrosine Kinase (Syk)-dependent Reactive Oxygen Species Generation. *J. Biol. Chem.* **2010**, *285*, 32844–32851. [CrossRef]
87. Gois, P.H.F.; Martines, M.S.; Ferreira, D.; Volpini, R.; Canale, D.; Malaque, C.; Crajoinas, R.; Girardi, A.C.C.; Massola Shimizu, M.H.; Seguro, A.C. Allopurinol attenuates acute kidney injury following Bothrops jararaca envenomation. *PLoS Negl. Trop. Dis.* **2017**, *11*, e0006024. [CrossRef]
88. Mate-Kole, M.O.; Yeboah, E.D.; Affram, R.K.; Adu, D. Blackwater fever and acute renal failure in expatriates in Africa. *Renal Fail.* **1996**, *18*, 525–531. [CrossRef]
89. Schrier, S.L. Diagnosis of Hemolytic Anemia in the Adult. Available online: https://www.uptodate.com/contents/diagnosis-of-hemolytic-anemia-in-the-adult (accessed on 12 March 2019).
90. Viraraghavan, R.; Chakravarty, A.G.; Soreth, J. Cefotetan-induced haemolytic anaemia: A review of 85 cases. *Adverse Drug React. Toxicol. Rev.* **2002**, *21*, 101–107. [CrossRef]
91. Chapman, A.B.; Rahbari-Oskoui, F.F.; Bennett, W.M. Acquired cystic disease of the kidney in adults. Available online: https://www.uptodate.com/contents/acquired-cystic-disease-of-the-kidney-in-adults (accessed on 11 March 2019).
92. Abreu, P.A.E.; Seguro, A.C.; Canale, D.; Silva, A.M.G.d.; Matos, L.d.R.B.; Gotti, T.B.; Monaris, D.; Jesus, D.A.d.; Vasconcellos, S.A.; de Brito, T.; et al. Lp25 membrane protein from pathogenic Leptospira spp. is associated with rhabdomyolysis and oliguric acute kidney injury in a guinea pig model of leptospirosis. *PLoS Negl. Trop. Dis.* **2017**, *11*, e0005615. [CrossRef] [PubMed]
93. Albuquerque, P.L.; Jacinto, C.N.; Silva Junior, G.B.; Lima, J.B.; Veras, M.d.S.B.; Daher, E.F.; Daher, E.F. Acute kidney injury caused by Crotalus and Bothrops snake venom: A review of epidemiology, clinical manifestations and treatment. *Rev. Inst. Med. Trop. Sao Paulo* **2013**, *55*, 295–301. [CrossRef]
94. De Bragança, A.C.; Moreau, R.L.M.; De Brito, T.; Shimizu, M.H.M.; Canale, D.; De Jesus, D.A.; Silva, A.M.G.; Gois, P.H.; Seguro, A.C.; Magaldi, A.J. Ecstasy induces reactive oxygen species, kidney water absorption and rhabdomyolysis in normal rats. Effect of N-acetylcysteine and Allopurinol in oxidative stress and muscle fiber damage. *PLoS ONE* **2017**, *12*, e0179199. [CrossRef]
95. Trowbridge, A.A.; Green, J.B.; Bonnett, J.D.; Shohet, S.B.; Ponnappa, B.D.; McCombs, W.B. Hemolytic anemia associated with leptospirosis. Morphologic and lipid studies. *Am. J. Clin. Pathol.* **1981**, *76*, 493–498. [CrossRef]

96. Da Silva Junior, G.B.; Pinto, J.R.; Barros, E.J.G.; Farias, G.M.N.; Daher, E.D.F. Kidney involvement in malaria: An update. *Rev. Inst. Med. Trop. Sao Paulo* **2017**. [CrossRef]
97. Mendonça, R.; Silveira, A.A.A.; Conran, N. Red cell DAMPs and inflammation. *Inflamm. Res.* **2016**. [CrossRef]
98. Wagener, F.A.; Abraham, N.G.; Van Kooyk, Y.; De Witte, T.; Figdor, C.G. Heme-induced cell adhesion in the pathogenesis of sickle-cell disease and inflammation. *Trends Pharmacol. Sci.* **2001**. [CrossRef]
99. Nyakundi, B.B.; Tóth, A.; Balogh, E.; Nagy, B.; Erdei, J.; Ryffel, B.; Paragh, G.; Cordero, M.D.; Jeney, V. Oxidized hemoglobin forms contribute to NLRP3 inflammasome-driven IL-1β production upon intravascular hemolysis. *Biochim. Biophys. Acta Mol. Basis Dis.* **2019**. [CrossRef]
100. López-Castejón, G.; Pelegrín, P. Current status of inflammasome blockers as anti-inflammatory drugs. *Expert Opin. Investig. Drugs* **2012**, *21*, 995–1007. [CrossRef] [PubMed]
101. Baldwin, A.G.; Brough, D.; Freeman, S. Inhibiting the Inflammasome: A Chemical Perspective. *J. Med. Chem.* **2016**, *59*, 1691–1710. [CrossRef] [PubMed]
102. Diwan, V.; Gobe, G.; Brown, L. Glibenclamide improves kidney and heart structure and function in the adenine-diet model of chronic kidney disease. *Pharmacol. Res.* **2014**, *79*, 104–110. [CrossRef] [PubMed]
103. Berns, J.S.; Glickman, J.D. Management of Hyperglycemia in Patients with Type 2 Diabetes and Pre-Dialysis Chronic Kidney Disease or End-Stage Renal Disease. Available online: https://www.uptodate.com/contents/management-of-hyperglycemia-in-patients-with-type-2-diabetes-and-pre-dialysis-chronic-kidney-disease-or-end-stage-renal-disease (accessed on 15 March 2019).
104. Meloni, G.; Meloni, T. Glyburide-induced acute haemolysis in a G6PD-deficient patient with NIDDM. *Br. J. Haematol.* **1996**, *92*, 159–160. [CrossRef] [PubMed]
105. Vinzio, S.; Andrès, E.; Perrin, A.-E.; Schlienger, J.-L.; Goichot, B. Glibenclamide-induced acute haemolytic anaemia revealing a G6PD-deficiency. *Diabetes Res. Clin. Pract.* **2004**, *64*, 181–183. [CrossRef]
106. Perregaux, D.G.; McNiff, P.; Laliberte, R.; Hawryluk, N.; Peurano, H.; Stam, E.; Eggler, J.; Griffiths, R.; Dombroski, M.A.; Gabel, C.A. Identification and characterization of a novel class of interleukin-1 post-translational processing inhibitors. *J. Pharmacol. Exp. Ther.* **2001**, *299*, 187–197. [PubMed]
107. Coll, R.C.; Robertson, A.A.B.; Chae, J.J.; Higgins, S.C.; Muñoz-Planillo, R.; Inserra, M.C.; Vetter, I.; Dungan, L.S.; Monks, B.G.; Stutz, A.; et al. A small-molecule inhibitor of the NLRP3 inflammasome for the treatment of inflammatory diseases. *Nat. Med.* **2015**, *21*, 248–255. [CrossRef] [PubMed]
108. Perera, A.P.; Fernando, R.; Shinde, T.; Gundamaraju, R.; Southam, B.; Sohal, S.S.; Robertson, A.A.B.; Schroder, K.; Kunde, D.; Eri, R. MCC950, a specific small molecule inhibitor of NLRP3 inflammasome attenuates colonic inflammation in spontaneous colitis mice. *Sci. Rep.* **2018**, *8*, 8618. [CrossRef] [PubMed]
109. Gordon, R.; Albornoz, E.A.; Christie, D.C.; Langley, M.R.; Kumar, V.; Mantovani, S.; Robertson, A.A.B.; Butler, M.S.; Rowe, D.B.; O'Neill, L.A.; et al. Inflammasome inhibition prevents α-synuclein pathology and dopaminergic neurodegeneration in mice. *Sci. Transl. Med.* **2018**, *10*, eaah4066. [CrossRef]
110. Zhai, Y.; Meng, X.; Ye, T.; Xie, W.; Sun, G.; Sun, X. Inhibiting the NLRP3 Inflammasome Activation with MCC950 Ameliorates Diabetic Encephalopathy in db/db Mice. *Molecules* **2018**, *23*, 1–14. [CrossRef]
111. Mridha, A.R.; Wree, A.; Robertson, A.A.B.; Yeh, M.M.; Johnson, C.D.; Van Rooyen, D.M.; Haczeyni, F.; Teoh, N.C.H.; Savard, C.; Ioannou, G.N.; et al. NLRP3 inflammasome blockade reduces liver inflammation and fibrosis in experimental NASH in mice. *J. Hepatol.* **2017**, *66*, 1037–1046. [CrossRef]
112. Vitale, A.; Insalaco, A.; Sfriso, P.; Lopalco, G.; Emmi, G.; Cattalini, M.; Manna, R.; Cimaz, R.; Priori, R.; Talarico, R.; et al. A Snapshot on the On-Label and Off-Label Use of the Interleukin-1 Inhibitors in Italy among Rheumatologists and Pediatric Rheumatologists: A Nationwide Multi-Center Retrospective Observational Study. *Front. Pharmacol.* **2016**, *7*, 380. [CrossRef]
113. Alten, R.; Gram, H.; Joosten, L.A.; Berg, W.B.v.d.; Sieper, J.; Wassenberg, S.; Burmester, G.; van Riel, P.; Diaz-Lorente, M.; Bruin, G.J.M.; et al. The human anti-IL-1β monoclonal antibody ACZ885 is effective in joint inflammation models in mice and in a proof-of-concept study in patients with rheumatoid arthritis. *Arthritis Res. Ther.* **2008**, *10*, R67. [CrossRef]
114. Rondeau, J.-M.; Ramage, P.; Zurini, M.; Gram, H. The molecular mode of action and species specificity of canakinumab, a human monoclonal antibody neutralizing IL-1β. *mAbs* **2015**, *7*, 1151–1160. [CrossRef]
115. Ridker, P.M.; MacFadyen, J.G.; Glynn, R.J.; Koenig, W.; Libby, P.; Everett, B.M.; Lefkowitz, M.; Thuren, T.; Cornel, J.H. Inhibition of Interleukin-1beta by Canakinumab and Cardiovascular Outcomes in Patients With Chronic Kidney Disease. *J. Am. Coll. Cardiol.* **2018**, *71*, 2405–2414. [CrossRef] [PubMed]
116. Solomon, D.H.; Glynn, R.J.; MacFadyen, J.G.; Libby, P.; Thuren, T.; Everett, B.M.; Ridker, P.M. Relationship

of Interleukin-1β Blockade With Incident Gout and Serum Uric Acid Levels: Exploratory Analysis of a Randomized Controlled TrialInterleukin-1β Blockade, Incident Gout, and Serum Uric Acid Levels. *Ann. Intern. Med.* **2018**, *169*, 535–542. [CrossRef] [PubMed]

117. Balasubramaniam, G.; Parker, T.; Turner, D.; Parker, M.; Scales, J.; Harnett, P.; Harrison, M.; Ahmed, K.; Bhagat, S.; Marianayagam, T.; et al. Feasibility randomised multicentre, double-blind, double-dummy controlled trial of anakinra, an interleukin-1 receptor antagonist versus intramuscular methylprednisolone for acute gout attacks in patients with chronic kidney disease (ASGARD): Protocol study. *BMJ Open* **2017**, *7*, e017121. [PubMed]
118. Ben-Zvi, I.; Kukuy, O.; Giat, E.; Pras, E.; Feld, O.; Kivity, S.; Perski, O.; Bornstein, G.; Grossman, C.; Harari, G.; et al. Anakinra for Colchicine-Resistant Familial Mediterranean Fever: A Randomized, Double-Blind, Placebo-Controlled Trial. *Arthritis Rheumatol.* **2017**, *69*, 854–862. [CrossRef] [PubMed]
119. Ugurlu, S.; Ergezen, B.; Ozdogan, H. Anakinra treatment in patients with Familial Mediterranean Fever: A single-center experience. *Pediatr. Rheumatol.* **2015**, *13*, P123. [CrossRef]
120. Moghaddas, F.; Llamas, R.; De Nardo, D.; Martinez-Banaclocha, H.; Martinez-Garcia, J.J.; Mesa-del-Castillo, P.; Baker, P.J.; Gargallo, V.; Mensa-Vilaro, A.; Canna, S.; et al. A novel Pyrin-Associated Autoinflammation with Neutrophilic Dermatosis mutation further defines 14-3-3 binding of pyrin and distinction to Familial Mediterranean Fever. *Ann. Rheum. Dis.* **2017**, *76*, 2085–2094. [CrossRef] [PubMed]
121. Masters, S.L.; Lagou, V.; Jéru, I.; Baker, P.J.; Van Eyck, L.; Parry, D.A.; Lawless, D.; De Nardo, D.; Garcia-Perez, J.E.; Dagley, L.F.; et al. Familial autoinflammation with neutrophilic dermatosis reveals a regulatory mechanism of pyrin activation. *Sci. Transl. Med.* **2016**, *8*, 332–345. [CrossRef] [PubMed]
122. Curiel, R.V.; Guzman, N.J. Challenges Associated with the Management of Gouty Arthritis in Patients with Chronic Kidney Disease: A Systematic Review. *Semin. Arthritis Rheum.* **2012**, *42*, 166–178. [CrossRef] [PubMed]

2

Molecular Mechanisms of the Acute Kidney Injury to Chronic Kidney Disease Transition

Francesco Guzzi [1,2,3,*], Luigi Cirillo [3], Rosa Maria Roperto [3], Paola Romagnani [1,2,3] and Elena Lazzeri [1,2]

1 Excellence Centre for Research, Transfer and High Education for the development of DE NOVO Therapies (DENOTHE), University of Florence, 50139 Florence, Italy; paola.romagnani@unifi.it (P.R.); elena.lazzeri@unifi.it (E.L.)

2 Department of Experimental and Clinical Biomedical Sciences "Mario Serio", University of Florence, 50134 Florence, Italy

3 Nephrology and Dialysis Unit, Meyer Children's University Hospital, 50139 Florence, Italy; cirlui89@gmail.com (L.C.); rosa.roperto@meyer.it (R.M.R.)

* Correspondence: francesco.guzzi@gmail.com

Abstract: Increasing evidence has demonstrated the bidirectional link between acute kidney injury (AKI) and chronic kidney disease (CKD) such that, in the clinical setting, the new concept of a unified syndrome has been proposed. The pathophysiological reasons, along with the cellular and molecular mechanisms, behind the ability of a single, acute, apparently self-limiting event to drive chronic kidney disease progression are yet to be explained. This acute injury could promote progression to chronic disease through different pathways involving the endothelium, the inflammatory response and the development of fibrosis. The interplay among endothelial cells, macrophages and other immune cells, pericytes and fibroblasts often converge in the tubular epithelial cells that play a central role. Recent evidence has strengthened this concept by demonstrating that injured tubules respond to acute tubular necrosis through two main mechanisms: The polyploidization of tubular cells and the proliferation of a small population of self-renewing renal progenitors. This alternative pathophysiological interpretation could better characterize functional recovery after AKI.

Keywords: acute kidney injury; chronic kidney disease; renal progenitors; polyploidization

---

1. AKI Is Not a Self-Limiting Event

Despite the common belief of a generally benign nature, the profound, long-term implications of acute kidney injury (AKI) are appearing more and more evident. In particular, the emergent finding of a progression to various degrees of chronic kidney disease (CKD) after apparently self-limiting AKI episodes, independent from the etiology, has attracted great attention.

In the last decade, the assumption of an existing association between AKI and CKD has gradually spread in the nephrology and intensive care fields with evidence of a tight link between even mild serum creatinine elevation and long-term CKD [1–3]. The classic teaching case regarding acute renal failure, in particular acute tubular necrosis (ATN), has been that those patients generally achieve full or nearly full recovery [4,5]. The consensus on a new definition of AKI has helped to improve the understanding of its long-term clinical consequences and to demonstrate a clear link between AKI episodes, their severity, and their outcome [6]. With the help of standardized criteria for the definition of AKI and CKD, diverse observational studies collecting data from large administrative databases have increasingly showed a possible association between these two clinical entities [7–9]. Indeed, the more recent assumption is now to consider AKI and CKD as two interconnected syndromes where CKD is a risk factor for AKI and, in the meantime, AKI is a risk factor for the development and progression of CKD [3]. A recent systematic review and meta-analysis by See et al. [7] aimed to quantify the association between AKI and CKD by evaluating the results from 82 studies comprising more than 2 million patients experiencing AKI. The authors confirmed an increase in the risk of new or progressive CKD after AKI (HR 2.67, 95% CI 1.99–3.58) with a gradient of risk across AKI stages, an increased risk of end stage renal disease (ESRD) (HR 4.81, 95% CI 3.04–7.62), and an increased risk of death (HR 1.80, 95% CI 1.61–2.02) [7]. Moreover, previous studies have demonstrated that AKI severity [10], duration [11] and frequency [12] are associated with an increased risk of CKD progression. The AKI–CKD link has also been highlighted in pediatric studies [13–15].

Despite continuous progresses in the field and the recent ability to better identify the molecular signature of different renal cell types following acute injury, the mechanisms that drive the transition to chronic disease remain debated [16,17]. The traditional beliefs are now challenged by clinical observations and new advances in experimental transgenic models. Researchers have made significant effort trying to elucidate the pathophysiological link from AKI to CKD on cellular and molecular levels by using experimental models. CKD can occur through several pathologic mechanisms involving one or more of the kidney compartments: Vasculature, the tubule-interstitium or the glomerulus. Microvascular loss occurs along with increased fibrosis, worsening relative hypoxia within the kidney and in particular within the outer medulla. This is associated with changes in pericytes to adopt a pro-fibrotic myofibroblast phenotype. Moreover, consequent to altered oxygen availability, tubular injury and necrosis cause tubular dysfunction, oliguria and reduced glomerular filtration via tubulo-glomerular feedback. Thus, after an ischemic injury, the loss of nephronic mass, with remnant nephron hyperfiltration, renin-angiotensin system (RAS) activation, systemic hypertension and subsequent glomerulosclerosis have been described to pave the way from AKI to CKD [18–20]. Regardless of the initial insult, evidence of tubular cell loss and replacement by collagen scars and infiltrating macrophages are associated with further renal functional loss and progression towards end stage renal failure. Experimental models have shown that selective epithelial injury could drive capillary rarefaction, interstitial fibrosis, glomerulosclerosis and progression to CKD, substantiating a direct role for damaged tubular epithelial cells (TECs) [21]. Therefore, tubular epithelial cells have attracted increasing attention [22,23].

A new interpretation of this pathophysiology is that the epithelial tubular cell may allow for a better understanding of this somehow unexpected turn in the AKI natural history. Altogether, there is a need for the further investigation of the AKI-to-CKD transition as a public health priority.

2. Pathophysiology of the AKI-to-CKD Transition

From a pathophysiological point of view, microvascular integrity, changes in leukocyte and pericyte behavior, and tubular cell survival and function are all features of both AKI and CKD, and several cellular and molecular pathways have been considered to define the transition process. The main pathological mechanisms which concur to explain the AKI-to-CKD transition include: (i) Endothelial dysfunction, vasoconstriction and vascular congestion [24,25]; (ii) interstitial inflammation and the associated infiltration of monocytes/macrophages, neutrophils, T- and B-cells [26–30]; (iii) fibrosis via myofibroblasts recruitment and matrix deposition [31–33]; and (iv) tubular epithelial injury and dysregulated repair [23,34,35] (Figure 1). After a brief description of the main molecular pathways of the endothelial, inflammatory and fibrotic response to injury, we focus on the proximal tubular epithelial cell, the main player of the AKI-to-CKD transition [35].

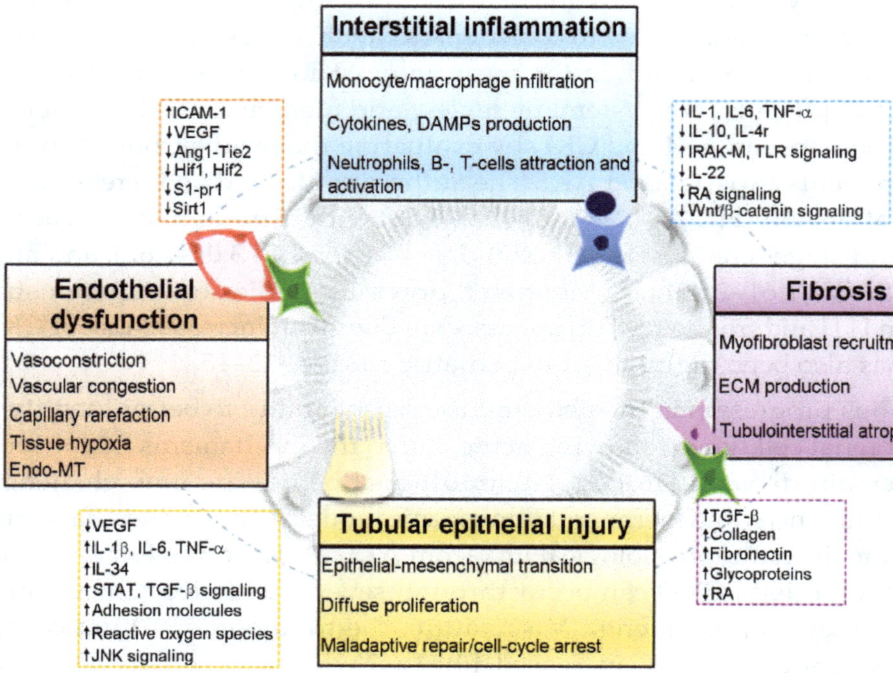

Figure 1. The interplay between endothelial dysfunction, interstitial inflammation, fibrosis and tubular epithelial injury concur to explain the acute kidney injury-to-chronic kidney disease (AKI-to-CKD) transition.

2.1. *Endothelial Dysfunction*

Capillary rarefaction has been extensively described as a consistent feature of the acutely injured nephron and has been linked to progression as a potential initiator of chronic nephropathy. A reduction in regional renal oxygen delivery leads to inflammation, ischemia, and necrosis, thus reflecting an imbalance between arterial pressure and vascular resistance, with a particularly vulnerable area in the outer stripe of the outer medulla. The existence of a putative bone marrow-derived endothelial progenitor cell (EPC) population has been hypothesized and linked to progression to chronic disease [36]. However, a recent study that combined bone marrow and kidney transplantation in a transgenic murine model demonstrated that no extra-renal cells substantially contribute to endothelial repair after selective injury [37].

Once capillary rarefaction is established, tissue hypoxia, mitochondrial dysfunction, inflammation and subsequent fibrosis occur [24]. The cellular and molecular pathways that underlie capillary rarefaction—in particular, the interplay between hypoxia, anti-angiogenic, and angiogenic factors—have yet to be explained [38]. Among angiogenic factors, vascular endothelial growth factor (VEGF), an endogenous cytokine produced by epithelial cells and directed to endothelial cells, is crucial for the preservation of vascular networks. Its reduced production could promote microvascular dysfunction and morphologic changes in the nephron [39,40]. The effects of its exogenous administration, with restoration of the microvascular density, improved renal blood flow, and reduced fibrogenic activity have been described in swine kidneys [41]. Similar effects, with improved endothelial cell survival and prevention of capillary leakage, resulted from the activation of the endothelium-specific receptor Tie2 through angiopoietin-1 (Ang-1)—a protein produced by vasculature support cells and specialized pericytes [42]. Moreover, the transgenic murine inactivation of endothelial hypoxia-inducible factors (Hif1-α and Hif2-α), as well as the deletion of endothelial sphingosine 1-phosphate receptor 1 (S1-pr1), resulted in increased acute and chronic inflammation and fibrosis after injury without affecting capillary permeability [43,44]. Therefore, there is considerable interest in the potential for Hif-stabilizing agents as therapeutic tools in renal injury [45]. In two models of folic acid-induced AKI and ureteral obstruction, Sirtuin 1 (Sirt 1) inactivation in endothelial cells caused impaired recovery, increased fibrosis, and disease progression [46,47].

Endothelial-to-mesenchymal transition (EndoMT) has been proposed as a contributor to capillary rarefaction, interstitial fibrosis, and, therefore, chronic damage [48]. Indeed, the reduction of EndoMT, obtained by reducing endothelium-specific transforming growth factor β (TGF-β) in a transgenic mouse model, was followed by the preservation of renal blood flow and microvasculature, less tissue hypoxia and tubulointerstitial fibrosis, thereby supporting the hypothesis of a link between EndoMT and chronic changes [49]. Moreover, the renal pericyte is now recognized as a key contributor to vascular stability in response to kidney injury [50].

Pericytes sit in close proximity to the endothelial cells within many organs, where they maintain vascular stability and release factors, including PDGF (platelet-derived growth factor) [51], angiopoietin [52], TGF-β [53], VEGF [54] and sphingosine-1-phosphate [55]. There is now an increasing understanding of the role played by these cells in acute and chronic kidney injury, where they leave their perivascular site in response to injury and differentiate to become myofibroblasts. Thus, either injuries or defects in pericyte function induce their detachment, contributing to both vascular rarefaction and increased fibrosis. In the end, recent advances have elucidated a contribution of endothelial cells and their products to capillary rarefaction, inflammation and tubulogenic pathways in a complex cellular interplay [43,44].

2.2. *Interstitial Inflammation*

Both resident and infiltrating immune cells participate in inflammation, injury and repair in the acute phase of kidney injury; through a tight cross-talk with endothelial cells, epithelial cells, and pericytes, they also contribute to disease progression [56]. The recent identification of a particular subset of renal resident macrophages, located at the abluminal side of the peritubular capillaries and capable of monitoring endothelial transport, has provided a perfect paradigm of the interplay between endothelium and immune system [57]. Resident macrophages seem to form a distinct anatomical and functional unit with the peritubular capillary endothelial cells that have the ability to detect and scavenge small immune complexes, possibly explaining the further recruitment of monocytes and neutrophils, as well as tissue injury in immune complex diseases [57]. This macrophage-endothelial functional unit, with a specific cross-talk at both the cellular and molecular levels, is also likely to be involved in the response to AKI [38].

The link between endothelial cells and inflammation is also suggested by CD169+ monocytes/macrophages that counteract the inflammatory response induced by intercellular adhesion molecule-1 (ICAM-1) expression after ischemic AKI [58]. Because they regulate inflammation, neutrophils infiltration, and because of their paracrine effects on tubular epithelial cells, macrophages can play an important role as determinants of AKI outcomes. Two populations of macrophages have been proposed by in vitro studies on behalf of their chemokine receptor repertoire: Pro-inflammatory or M1-subtype (interleukin (IL)-1, IL-6, and tumor necrosis factor-α (TNF-α)) and anti-inflammatory or M2-subtype (arginase, mannose receptor, IL-10, and IL-4 receptor-α), the first classically activated and the latter alternatively activated [59]. Despite being recently revised in regards to these two populations' in vivo behavior [60,61], this classification has been useful to identify different responses after acute injury in the kidney and a putative role for these cells in disease progression [28]. Macrophages have contrasting roles in renal injury and repair, first increasing the number of M1-polarized cells and then switching to an M2 phenotype supporting epithelial cell repair. Indeed, the depletion of M2 macrophages in mice with established AKI has resulted in prolongation of renal injury [62].

In a post-ischemic transgenic murine model, IL-1 receptor-associated kinase-M (IRAK-M), specifically expressed by monocyte/macrophages, has been demonstrated to influence the progression of AKI to CKD. IRAK-M expression induces the healing phase by inhibiting the toll-like receptor (TLR) and IL-1 receptor signaling, resolving TNF-α-dependent inflammation, and dampening the M1 pro-inflammatory response, all of which have been found to allow for improved functional recovery and structural regeneration [26]. Macrophages also participate in endogenous repair by secreting cytokines, such as IL-22, and providing ligands for retinoic acid (RA) and Wnt/β-catenin. In an ischemia-reperfusion injury (IRI) transgenic murine model, the administration or overexpression of IL-22 has been found to preserve renal function by increasing signal transducer and transcription factor 3 (STAT3) and protein kinase B (Akt) phosphorylation in proximal tubular epithelial cells, upregulating anti-apoptotic genes (e.g., *Bcl-2*), and downregulating pro-apoptotic genes (e.g., *Bad*) [63]. Retinoic acid (RA) signaling, activated in macrophages and tubular epithelial cells within hours of injury, has been found to reduce macrophage-dependent injury and fibrosis after AKI [64]. In zebrafish and murine models, the activation of RA signaling between epithelial cells and macrophages after AKI has been found to limit the injury extent by promoting the activation of M2 macrophages and tubular epithelial cell repair [64]. Wnt/β-catenin is another important pathway in recovery from AKI. Its activation by macrophages has been found to stimulate repair [65], and its early intervention is required to minimize renal damage after AKI in the initial phase [66]. However, its persistent activation and Wnt1 overexpression have been shown to play a role in progression to CKD through uncontrolled fibroblasts activation and inflammation [66,67]. Therefore, while important in facilitating repair after AKI, the presence of macrophages is also correlated with fibrosis and adverse outcomes. Moreover, the reciprocal expression of colony-stimulating factor-1 (CSF-1) and its receptor between macrophages and tubular epithelial cells could enhance cell proliferation and stimulate the anti-inflammatory M2 subtype [68]. Interestingly, to highlight the complexity of the interplay between these cells upon injury, IL-34 produced by injured TECs may have a pro-inflammatory ability despite sharing the same macrophage receptor of CSF-1 [69].

After the initial phase of injury, early inflammation is followed by the infiltration of circulating immune cells (T- and B-cells) attracted by cytokines and damage-associated molecular patterns (DAMPs) released by injured cells [27]. While interacting with activated monocytes/macrophages, injured TECs, and endothelial cells, DAMPs participate in the development of a pro-fibrotic milieu which activates pericytes to proliferate and evolve into myofibroblasts, thereby inducing matrix deposition, renal fibrosis, and CKD [70]. In contrast, a subset of regulatory T-cells (Treg) may act like self-tolerance inducers and suppress inflammation by enhancing immune homeostasis [71]. Together with their positive effects, Treg depletion has been shown to aggravate ischemic AKI [72]. Interestingly, the protective role of CD4+ and CD8+ T-cells in a murine model of toxic nephropathy (aristolochic acid nephropathy) has recently been described after treatment with selective monoclonal antibodies [73]. Concerning B-cells, immunoglobulins production, antigen presentation, and subsequent complement activation have been described as possible contributors to the progression from acute to chronic renal injury [74].

2.3. Fibrosis

Several obstructive, ischemia-reperfusion and nephrotoxic animal models have investigated the link between AKI and CKD by focusing on the development of interstitial fibrosis [31–33]. Myofibroblasts, whether derived from activated resident fibroblasts or from pericytes, are responsible for extracellular matrix (ECM) production, with the deposition of collagens, fibronectins and other glycoproteins, which, together with TGF-β, contribute to fibrosis [32,75]. The expression of α-smooth muscle actin (α-SMA), usually confined to the vascular compartment, and platelet-derived growth factor receptor-β (PDGFR-β), identifies these cells in the interstitium of injured kidneys [75]. A number of studies have consistently linked peritubular capillaries rarefaction, pericytes detachment, interstitial hypoxia and tubular epithelial injury as triggers of renal fibrosis [21,50]. In particular, whereas an ischemic injury could be responsible for capillary rarefaction and pericyte detachment, pericyte loss could be a trigger for endothelial damage and capillary rarefaction followed by tubular epithelial injury and fibrosis [50]. Though the severity of interstitial fibrosis in renal biopsies has been recognized as the major prognostic factor for CKD/ESRD, fibrosis has been considered a self-sustaining process [76], and a causal relationship between ECM deposition, fibrosis and chronic kidney injury has not yet been identified.

Recent studies have suggested that fibrosis could also be beneficial for the healing processes [34]. During repair from experimental AKI, tubules that fail to recover become atrophic, and fibrosis surrounds them in well-demarcated areas that separate the injured parenchyma from restored or not injured tubules [34]. In this view, fibrosis is itself essentially a self-limiting repair process that restricts injury, and it is not autonomously progressive. Indeed, many other experimental data do not support a major role of self-perpetuating tubulointerstitial fibrosis in the transition from AKI to CKD and highlight that progressive renal fibrosis requires additional injuries—unless primary interstitial disease is itself the triggering factor for fibrosis [23,77]. Recently, in a transgenic mouse model expressing diphtheria toxin receptor on renal fibroblasts, Nakamura et al. showed that fibroblasts depletion could worsen the expression of tubular injury markers, with a marked increase after unilateral ureteral obstruction [33]. While the transition of resident fibroblasts to myofibroblasts has been described to trigger fibrosis [78], myofibroblasts can also acquire retinoic acid-production ability—lost by the injured tubular epithelial cells—supporting epithelial integrity and repair [33] and dampening pro-inflammatory macrophages [64]. In the aged kidney, the ability of resident fibroblasts to support repair is less pronounced [79].

Altogether, a deeper understanding of the cellular and molecular pathways involving fibrosis in different types of acute kidney injury will be of great importance for the development of therapeutic strategies to halt the progression of AKI to CKD [80,81].

2.4. *Tubular Epithelial Injury*

The most sensitive cells to acute ischemic and nephrotoxic injury are the proximal S3 segment tubular epithelial cells of the outer stripe of the outer medulla due to their intense workload, high metabolic demand, and limited capacity for anaerobic energy production [82]. In fact, this region accounts for a unique microvascular environment which is extremely vulnerable to hypoperfusion, renal hypoxia, and mitochondrial damage [82,83]. Recently, a shift from a victim to the driving force of the AKI-to-CKD transition has been proposed for the tubular epithelial cell [35]. Indeed, injured TECs have been shown to act as drivers of both inflammation and fibrosis. They produce a large variety of cytokines (e.g., IL-6, IL-1β, and TNF-α), thereby gaining a pro-inflammatory phenotype and directly influencing macrophage behavior [84,85], and they are an important source of chemokines—via several pathways including STAT signaling and TGF-β signaling—adhesion molecules and reactive oxygen species [35]. Traditionally, injured TECs have been thought to undergo a process of dedifferentiation, a partial epithelial–mesenchymal transition (EMT) [86,87], i.e., the de novo expression of mesenchymal marker such as vimentin in TECs [88] induced by the injury-mediated reactivation of snail family zinc finger 1 (Snail1) [89,90]. This transient dedifferentiation is also characterized by the re-expression of developmental genes such as *Pax2* and cell cycle markers such as proliferating cell nuclear antigen (PCNA)—thus suggesting extensive proliferation—followed by a loss of mesenchymal markers, which has been interpreted as re-differentiation into fully viable epithelial cells [91,92]. This extensive proliferative ability could be responsible for rapid repair upon acute injury.

This proliferative capacity is thought to explain why young and mildly injured patients regain normal (or near-normal) renal function within days from acute injury, regardless of etiology. According to this view, the kidney's reparative potential is counterbalanced by maladaptive repair, as if they are on a balance pan. Shifting from proliferation to maladaptive repair would explain disease progression. In one toxic and one obstructive nephropathy models, Yang et al. demonstrated a causal association between cell cycle arrest and fibrosis [93]. Due to abnormal repair processes, TECs can become atrophic and gain a pro-fibrotic phenotype after AKI. G2/M-arrested TECs may activate the JNK signaling to induce the production of pro-fibrotic cytokines (e.g., TGF-β and connective tissue growth factor (CTGF)) [22]. Altogether, whereas favorable cell cycle events could be responsible for repair, cell cycle arrest could determine the progression of injury. Dysregulated and inefficient (i.e., maladaptive) tubular repair has been related to the persistence of an inflammatory milieu, ECM deposition and subsequent tubular cells convergence towards a pro-fibrotic and senescent phenotype [94]. Indeed, dedifferentiated TECs acquire pro-fibrotic characteristics that elicit CKD progression [23].

An alternative pathophysiological interpretation of cell cycle events after acute injury has recently been proposed [95,96]. Indeed, several studies have recently pointed toward the existence of a scattered population of undifferentiated, self-renewing, renal progenitors with the ability to regenerate fully differentiated TECs rather than acquire a dedifferentiation state [97–102]. After their identification in the human kidney, further studies were able to provide detailed characterization in both humans and mice [100] and to identify these cells as a source of tubular regeneration after AKI [103]. This strategy for kidney regeneration appears to be highly conserved across species [104] and involved in kidney development, maintenance, and regeneration [105]. New experimental evidence provided by lineage tracing studies has strengthened the concept that tubular epithelial cell regeneration is mostly due to a scattered progenitors' population rather than to the majority of remnant cells [95]. Renal progenitors are more numerous in the proximal tubule S3 segment, the segment which is more sensitive to ischemic and nephrotoxic injury and from where tubular cells detach in large numbers, thus explaining the high proliferation of tubular epithelial cells observed in this area (Figure 2) [95]. The intense immunoreactivity of nuclear proliferation markers (such as proliferating cell nuclear antigen-PCNA and Ki-67) has also been observed after acute injury in the proximal tubule S2 segment and other uninjured areas of the nephron [88,106]. Regardless, although such cell cycle markers confirm the cell's entry in the cell cycle, they do not entail its completion with the formation of two new differentiated daughter cells. Thanks to simultaneous cell cycle phase lineage tracing analysis and DNA content measurement with FUCCI (fluorescent ubiquitination-based cell cycle indicator) technology, it has been shown that the majority of remnant TECs do enter the cell cycle, but they undergo endoreplication-mediated hypertrophy (Figure 2). Endoreplication is an evolutionary conserved cell cycle program by which cells replicate their genome without division, resulting in polyploid cells (i.e., polyploidization). Polyploidization increases the gene copy number in response to the need to quickly support increased functional requests for a higher metabolic output while persistently maintaining differentiated and specialized cell functions. This permits hypertrophy and function recovery [95,96].

In mammals, endoreplication-induced polyploidy has been observed in multiple tissue and organs (including the skin, placenta, liver, and blood) during normal development and under stressful conditions [107]. In the kidney, tubular cell polyploidization has frequently been observed in the proximal convoluted tubule S2 segment that is not directly injured during ATN (Figure 2). Accordingly, a new interpretation could follow: i) AKI causes TEC loss; ii) a small subset of progenitor cells showing resistance to death and proliferative ability are responsible for parenchymal regeneration; and iii) remnant TECs enter the cell cycle but undergo endoreplication-mediated polyploidy rather than mitosis, thus rapidly compensating for function loss [95].

According to this new hypothesis, the physiological response to AKI could imply a limited regeneration mediated by scattered renal progenitors and a polyploidization response by remnant TECs [96]. Polyploid TECs do not truly reconstitute parenchymal loss; thus, they might be a marker of irreversible loss and elicit progression towards chronic disease. In this view, a response to AKI is a costly process which cannot endlessly repeat without any consequence; rather, the tubular epithelium is more susceptible to further damage after every hit, better mirroring the clinical spectrum of the AKI-to-CKD transition.

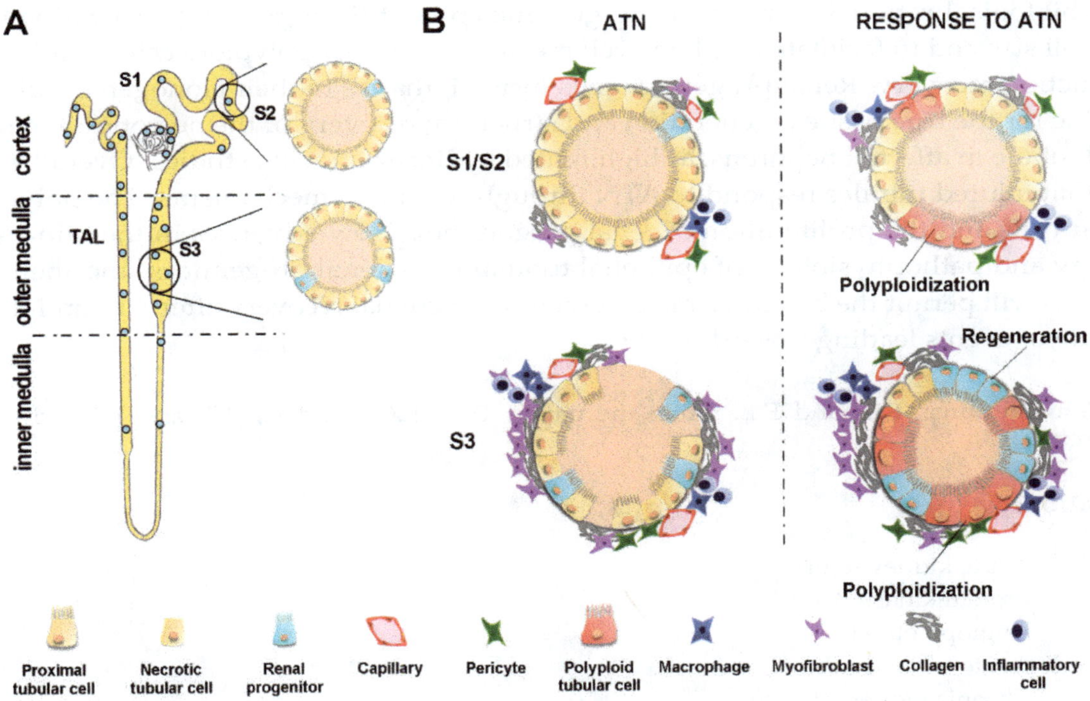

Figure 2. A new pathophysiological interpretation of tubular response to AKI leading towards CKD: The proliferation of renal progenitors and polyploidization of tubular cells. (**A**) Schematic localization of renal progenitors scattered along the S1–S2 segment, the S3 segment, and thick ascending limb (TAL) in the nephron. (Figure modified from Lazzeri et al., Trends Mol Med, 2019); (**B**) Top: In the uninjured proximal tubule S1–S2 segment, tubular epithelial cells enhance their working capacity by entering the cell cycle to increase their DNA content without division, resulting in polyploid tubular cells (i.e., polyploidization). Bottom: In the necrotic proximal tubule S3 segment, renal progenitors proliferate and complete cell division to drive regeneration, while the remnant tubular epithelial cells undergo polyploidization rather than mitosis. ATN: Acute tubular necrosis.

3. Conclusions

A tight link between AKI and CKD is now becoming evident, both in the clinical and experimental settings. AKI severity, duration and frequency are associated with the development of CKD, but even mild episodes are associated with an increased risk of disease progression. Recent experimental findings have provided new insight into the cellular and molecular mechanisms of the AKI-to-CKD transition; these experiments have been trying to unveil the relative contribution of endothelial dysfunction, immune cell response, pericytes and fibroblasts activation. Regardless of the AKI etiology, endothelial dysfunction and subsequent hypoxia (as well as death of tubular cells from a toxic injury) trigger a cascade of self-sustaining events involving myofibroblast activation derived from resident fibroblasts or pericytes, extracellular matrix deposition, and interstitial inflammation. The overall view has shown that all the molecular and cellular mechanisms converge to the tubular epithelial cell dysfunction. Indeed, the lack of recovery of the tubular structure's integrity sustains the above-mentioned events, thus promoting the progression of interstitial injury. The direct increase in the risk of CKD development and progression, which mirrors the severity of the acute episode, suggests a causative role of the final effector of acute function loss, i.e., epithelial cell injury. In several highly specialized organs, widespread parenchymal proliferation is likely to be a counterproductive strategy. Indeed, the mitosis and cytokinesis of highly specialized parenchymal cells determines a temporary loss of function that might become critical for the organ's survival. It is now becoming evident that, to minimize the mitotic ability of specialized parenchymal cells without losing their functional performance, evolution has selected an alternative type of response: Hypertrophy via polyploidization.

The biological rationale for increasing genome content through polyploidization could be to increase cell size and to facilitate amplified cell metabolism so that polyploid cells could sustain acute organ function recovery. Renal progenitor cells instead, thanks to their clonogenic ability, could be responsible for the true tissue regeneration and structural recovery of the necrotic S3 segment of the proximal tubule in affected nephrons, as highlighted by lineage tracing studies. Overall, these results suggest that injured tubules respond to ATN through two main mechanisms: The polyploidization of tubular cells and the proliferation of renal progenitors. New advances in the understanding of the biology and pathophysiology of epithelial tubular cells, renal progenitors, and their adaptation mechanisms will permit the better characterization of functional recovery after AKI and the tracing of the cascade of events leading towards CKD.

Author Contributions: F.G. and E.L. wrote the paper; F.G., L.C., R.M.R., P.R. and E.L. critically revised the manuscript.

Abbreviations

AKI	Acute kidney injury
Akt	Protein kinase B
Ang-1	Angiopoietin-1
ATN	Acute tubular necrosis
CKD	Chronic kidney disease
CSF-1	Colony-stimulating factor-1
CTGF	Connective tissue growth factor
DAMPs	Damage-associated molecular patterns
ECM	Extracellular matrix
EMT	Epithelial-mesenchymal transition
EndoMT	Endothelial to mesenchymal transition
EPC	Endothelial progenitor cells
ESRD	End stage renal disease
FUCCI	Fluorescent ubiquitination-based cell cycle indicator
Hif	Hypoxia-inducible factor
ICAM-1	Intercellular adhesion molecule-1
IL	Interleukin
IRAK-M	IL-1 receptor-associated kinase-M
IRI	Ischemia-reperfusion injury
PCNA	Proliferating cell nuclear antigen
PDGF	Platelet-derived growth factor
PDGFR-β	Platelet-derived growth factor receptor-β
RA	Retinoic acid
RAS	Renin-angiotensin system
S1-pr1	Sphingosine 1-phosphate receptor 1
Sirt 1	Sirtuin 1
Snail1	Snail family zinc finger 1
STAT3	Signal transducer and transcription factor 3
TEC	Tubular epithelial cell
TGF-β	Transforming growth factor β
TLR	Toll-like receptor
TNF-α	Tumor necrosis factor-α
VEGF	Vascular endothelial growth factor
α-SMA	α-smooth muscle actin

References

1. Ponte, B.; Felipe, C.; Muriel, A.; Tenorio, M.T.; Liaño, F. Long-term functional evolution after an acute kidney injury: A 10-year study. *Nephrol. Dial. Transplant. Off. Publ. Eur. Dial. Transpl. Assoc.—Eur. Ren. Assoc.* **2008**, *23*, 3859–3866. [CrossRef] [PubMed]

2. Coca, S.G.; Singanamala, S.; Parikh, C.R. Chronic kidney disease after acute kidney injury: A systematic review and meta-analysis. *Kidney Int.* **2012**, *81*, 442–448. [CrossRef] [PubMed]
3. Chawla, L.S.; Eggers, P.W.; Star, R.A.; Kimmel, P.L. Acute kidney injury and chronic kidney disease as interconnected syndromes. *N. Engl. J. Med.* **2014**, *371*, 58–66. [CrossRef] [PubMed]
4. Lowe, K.G. The late prognosis in acute tubular necrosis. *Lancet* **1952**, *259*, 1086–1088. [CrossRef]
5. Liaño, F.; Felipe, C.; Tenorio, M.-T.; Rivera, M.; Abraira, V.; Sáez-de-Urturi, J.-M.; Ocaña, J.; Fuentes, C.; Severiano, S. Long-term outcome of acute tubular necrosis: A contribution to its natural history. *Kidney Int.* **2007**, *71*, 679–686. [CrossRef] [PubMed]
6. Ricci, Z.; Cruz, D.N.; Ronco, C. Classification and staging of acute kidney injury: Beyond the RIFLE and AKIN criteria. *Nat. Rev. Nephrol.* **2011**, *7*, 201–208. [CrossRef] [PubMed]
7. See, E.J.; Jayasinghe, K.; Glassford, N.; Bailey, M.; Johnson, D.W.; Polkinghorne, K.R.; Toussaint, N.D.; Bellomo, R. Long-term risk of adverse outcomes after acute kidney injury: A systematic review and meta-analysis of cohort studies using consensus definitions of exposure. *Kidney Int.* **2019**, *95*, 160–172. [CrossRef]
8. Ishani, A.; Xue, J.L.; Himmelfarb, J.; Eggers, P.W.; Kimmel, P.L.; Molitoris, B.A.; Collins, A.J. Acute kidney injury increases risk of ESRD among elderly. *J. Am. Soc. Nephrol.* **2009**, *20*, 223–228. [CrossRef]
9. Amdur, R.L.; Chawla, L.S.; Amodeo, S.; Kimmel, P.L.; Palant, C.E. Outcomes following diagnosis of acute renal failure in U.S. veterans: Focus on acute tubular necrosis. *Kidney Int.* **2009**, *76*, 1089–1097. [CrossRef]
10. Ishani, A.; Nelson, D.; Clothier, B.; Schult, T.; Nugent, S.; Greer, N.; Slinin, Y.; Ensrud, K.E. The Magnitude of Acute Serum Creatinine Increase After Cardiac Surgery and the Risk of Chronic Kidney Disease, Progression of Kidney Disease, and Death. *Arch. Intern. Med.* **2011**, *171*, 226–233. [CrossRef]
11. Mehta, S.; Chauhan, K.; Patel, A.; Patel, S.; Pinotti, R.; Nadkarni, G.N.; Parikh, C.R.; Coca, S.G. The prognostic importance of duration of AKI: A systematic review and meta-analysis. *BMC Nephrol.* **2018**, *19*, 91. [CrossRef] [PubMed]
12. Thakar, C.V.; Christianson, A.; Himmelfarb, J.; Leonard, A.C. Acute kidney injury episodes and chronic kidney disease risk in diabetes mellitus. *Clin. J. Am. Soc. Nephrol.* **2011**, *6*, 2567–2572. [CrossRef] [PubMed]
13. Devarajan, P.; Jefferies, J.L. Progression of chronic kidney disease after acute kidney injury. *Prog. Pediatr. Cardiol.* **2016**, *41*, 33–40. [CrossRef] [PubMed]
14. Uber, A.M.; Sutherland, S.M. Acute kidney injury in hospitalized children: Consequences and outcomes. *Pediatr. Nephrol. Berl. Ger.* **2018**, 1–8. [CrossRef] [PubMed]
15. Sigurjonsdottir, V.K.; Chaturvedi, S.; Mammen, C.; Sutherland, S.M. Pediatric acute kidney injury and the subsequent risk for chronic kidney disease: Is there cause for alarm? *Pediatr. Nephrol. Berl. Ger.* **2018**, *33*, 2047–2055. [CrossRef]
16. Basile, D.P.; Bonventre, J.V.; Mehta, R.; Nangaku, M.; Unwin, R.; Rosner, M.H.; Kellum, J.A.; Ronco, C.; ADQI XIII Work Group. Progression after AKI: Understanding Maladaptive Repair Processes to Predict and Identify Therapeutic Treatments. *J. Am. Soc. Nephrol.* **2016**, *27*, 687–697. [CrossRef]
17. Bellomo, R.; Kellum, J.A.; Ronco, C. Acute kidney injury. *Lancet* **2012**, *380*, 756–766. [CrossRef]
18. Venkatachalam, M.A.; Griffin, K.A.; Lan, R.; Geng, H.; Saikumar, P.; Bidani, A.K. Acute kidney injury: A springboard for progression in chronic kidney disease. *Am. J. Physiol. Renal Physiol.* **2010**, *298*, F1078–F1094. [CrossRef]
19. Rodriguez-Romo, R.; Benitez, K.; Barrera-Chimal, J.; Perez-Villalva, R.; Gomez, A.; Aguilar-Leon, D.; Rangel-Santiago, J.F.; Huerta, S.; Gamba, G.; Uribe, N.; et al. AT1 receptor antagonism before ischemia prevents the transition of acute kidney injury to chronic kidney disease. *Kidney Int.* **2016**, *89*, 363–373. [CrossRef]
20. Chou, Y.-H.; Chu, T.-S.; Lin, S.-L. Role of renin-angiotensin system in acute kidney injury-chronic kidney disease transition. *Nephrol. Carlton Vic* **2018**, *23*, 121–125. [CrossRef]
21. Grgic, I.; Campanholle, G.; Bijol, V.; Wang, C.; Sabbisetti, V.S.; Ichimura, T.; Humphreys, B.D.; Bonventre, J.V. Targeted proximal tubule injury triggers interstitial fibrosis and glomerulosclerosis. *Kidney Int.* **2012**, *82*, 172–183. [CrossRef] [PubMed]
22. Ferenbach, D.A.; Bonventre, J.V. Mechanisms of maladaptive repair after AKI leading to accelerated kidney ageing and CKD. *Nat. Rev. Nephrol.* **2015**, *11*, 264–276. [CrossRef] [PubMed]
23. Venkatachalam, M.A.; Weinberg, J.M.; Kriz, W.; Bidani, A.K. Failed Tubule Recovery, AKI-CKD Transition, and Kidney Disease Progression. *J. Am. Soc. Nephrol.* **2015**, *26*, 1765–1776. [CrossRef] [PubMed]
24. Basile, D.P. The endothelial cell in ischemic acute kidney injury: Implications for acute and chronic function.

Kidney Int. **2007** *72*, 151–156. [CrossRef] [PubMed]

25. Basile, D.P.; Collett, J.A.; Yoder, M.C. Endothelial colony-forming cells and pro-angiogenic cells: Clarifying definitions and their potential role in mitigating acute kidney injury. *Acta. Physiol. Oxf. Engl.* **2018**, *222*, e12914. [CrossRef] [PubMed]
26. Lech, M.; Gröbmayr, R.; Ryu, M.; Lorenz, G.; Hartter, I.; Mulay, S.R.; Susanti, H.E.; Kobayashi, K.S.; Flavell, R.A.; Anders, H.-J. Macrophage phenotype controls long-term AKI outcomes—Kidney regeneration versus atrophy. *J. Am. Soc. Nephrol.* **2014**, *25*, 292–304. [CrossRef] [PubMed]
27. Anders, H.-J.; Schaefer, L. Beyond Tissue Injury—Damage-Associated Molecular Patterns, Toll-Like Receptors, and Inflammasomes Also Drive Regeneration and Fibrosis. *J. Am. Soc. Nephrol.* **2014**, *25*, 1387–1400. [CrossRef]
28. Belliere, J.; Casemayou, A.; Ducasse, L.; Zakaroff-Girard, A.; Martins, F.; Iacovoni, J.S.; Guilbeau-Frugier, C.; Buffin-Meyer, B.; Pipy, B.; Chauveau, D.; et al. Specific Macrophage Subtypes Influence the Progression of Rhabdomyolysis-Induced Kidney Injury. *J. Am. Soc. Nephrol.* **2015**, *26*, 1363–1377. [CrossRef] [PubMed]
29. Jang, H.R.; Rabb, H. Immune cells in experimental acute kidney injury. *Nat. Rev. Nephrol.* **2015**, *11*, 88–101. [CrossRef]
30. Sato, Y.; Yanagita, M. Immune cells and inflammation in AKI to CKD progression. *Am. J. Physiol. Renal Physiol.* **2018**, *315*, 1501–1512. [CrossRef]
31. Gomez, I.G.; Duffield, J.S. The FOXD1 lineage of kidney perivascular cells and myofibroblasts: Functions and responses to injury. *Kidney Int. Suppl.* **2014**, *4*, 26–33. [CrossRef] [PubMed]
32. Mack, M.; Yanagita, M. Origin of myofibroblasts and cellular events triggering fibrosis. *Kidney Int.* **2015**, *87*, 297–307. [CrossRef] [PubMed]
33. Nakamura, J.; Sato, Y.; Kitai, Y.; Wajima, S.; Yamamoto, S.; Oguchi, A.; Yamada, R.; Kaneko, K.; Kondo, M.; Uchino, E.; et al. Myofibroblasts acquire retinoic acid–producing ability during fibroblast-to-myofibroblast transition following kidney injury. *Kidney Int.* **2019**, *95*, 526–539. [CrossRef] [PubMed]
34. Kaissling, B.; Lehir, M.; Kriz, W. Renal epithelial injury and fibrosis. *Biochim. Biophys. Acta* **2013**, *1832*, 931–939. [CrossRef] [PubMed]
35. Liu, B.-C.; Tang, T.-T.; Lv, L.-L.; Lan, H.-Y. Renal tubule injury: A driving force toward chronic kidney disease. *Kidney Int.* **2018**, *93*, 568–579. [CrossRef]
36. Patschan, D.; Kribben, A.; Müller, G.A. Postischemic microvasculopathy and endothelial progenitor cell-based therapy in ischemic AKI: Update and perspectives. *Am. J. Physiol.-Ren. Physiol.* **2016**, *311*, 382–394. [CrossRef]
37. Sradnick, J.; Rong, S.; Luedemann, A.; Parmentier, S.P.; Bartaun, C.; Todorov, V.T.; Gueler, F.; Hugo, C.P.; Hohenstein, B. Extrarenal Progenitor Cells Do Not Contribute to Renal Endothelial Repair. *J. Am. Soc. Nephrol.* **2016**, *27*, 1714–1726. [CrossRef]
38. Kumar, S. Cellular and molecular pathways of renal repair after acute kidney injury. *Kidney Int.* **2018**, *93*, 27–40. [CrossRef]
39. Tanaka, S.; Tanaka, T.; Nangaku, M. Hypoxia as a key player in the AKI-to-CKD transition. *Am. J. Physiol. Renal Physiol.* **2014**, *307*, 1187–1195. [CrossRef]
40. Chade, A.R. Vascular Endothelial Growth Factor Therapy for the Kidney: Are We There Yet? *J. Am. Soc. Nephrol.* **2016**, *27*, 1–3. [CrossRef]
41. Chade, A.R.; Tullos, N.A.; Harvey, T.W.; Mahdi, F.; Bidwell, G.L. Renal Therapeutic Angiogenesis Using a Bioengineered Polymer-Stabilized Vascular Endothelial Growth Factor Construct. *J. Am. Soc. Nephrol.* **2016**, *27*, 1741–1752. [CrossRef] [PubMed]
42. Hörbelt, M.; Lee, S.-Y.; Mang, H.E.; Knipe, N.L.; Sado, Y.; Kribben, A.; Sutton, T.A. Acute and chronic microvascular alterations in a mouse model of ischemic acute kidney injury. *Am. J. Physiol.-Ren. Physiol.* **2007**, *293*, 688–695. [CrossRef] [PubMed]
43. Kapitsinou, P.P.; Sano, H.; Michael, M.; Kobayashi, H.; Davidoff, O.; Bian, A.; Yao, B.; Zhang, M.-Z.; Harris, R.C.; Duffy, K.J.; et al. Endothelial HIF-2 mediates protection and recovery from ischemic kidney injury. *J. Clin. Invest.* **2014**, *124*, 2396–2409. [CrossRef] [PubMed]
44. Perry, H.M.; Huang, L.; Ye, H.; Liu, C.; Sung, S.J.; Lynch, K.R.; Rosin, D.L.; Bajwa, A.; Okusa, M.D. Endothelial Sphingosine 1-Phosphate Receptor-1 Mediates Protection and Recovery from Acute Kidney Injury. *J. Am. Soc. Nephrol.* **2016**, *27*, 3383–3393. [CrossRef] [PubMed]
45. Tanaka, T.; Wiesener, M.; Bernhardt, W.; Eckardt, K.-U.; Warnecke, C. The human *HIF* (hypoxia-inducible factor)-3α gene is a HIF-1 target gene and may modulate hypoxic gene induction. *Biochem. J.* **2009**, *424*, 143–151. [CrossRef] [PubMed]

46. Vasko, R.; Xavier, S.; Chen, J.; Lin, C.H.S.; Ratliff, B.; Rabadi, M.; Maizel, J.; Tanokuchi, R.; Zhang, F.; Cao, J.; et al. Endothelial Sirtuin 1 Deficiency Perpetrates Nephrosclerosis through Downregulation of Matrix Metalloproteinase-14: Relevance to Fibrosis of Vascular Senescence. *J. Am. Soc. Nephrol.* **2014**, *25*, 276–291. [CrossRef] [PubMed]
47. Kida, Y.; Zullo, J.A.; Goligorsky, M.S. Endothelial sirtuin 1 inactivation enhances capillary rarefaction and fibrosis following kidney injury through Notch activation. *Biochem. Biophys. Res. Commun.* **2016**, *478*, 1074–1079. [CrossRef] [PubMed]
48. Basile, D.P.; Friedrich, J.L.; Spahic, J.; Knipe, N.; Mang, H.; Leonard, E.C.; Changizi-Ashtiyani, S.; Bacallao, R.L.; Molitoris, B.A.; Sutton, T.A. Impaired endothelial proliferation and mesenchymal transition contribute to vascular rarefaction following acute kidney injury. *Am. J. Physiol.-Ren. Physiol.* **2011**, *300*, 721–733. [CrossRef]
49. Xavier, S.; Vasko, R.; Matsumoto, K.; Zullo, J.A.; Chen, R.; Maizel, J.; Chander, P.N.; Goligorsky, M.S. Curtailing Endothelial TGF-β Signaling Is Sufficient to Reduce Endothelial-Mesenchymal Transition and Fibrosis in CKD. *J. Am. Soc. Nephrol.* **2015**, *26*, 817–829. [CrossRef]
50. Kramann, R.; Wongboonsin, J.; Chang-Panesso, M.; Machado, F.G.; Humphreys, B.D. Gli1$^+$ Pericyte Loss Induces Capillary Rarefaction and Proximal Tubular Injury. *J. Am. Soc. Nephrol.* **2017**, *28*, 776–784. [CrossRef]
51. Betsholtz, C. Insight into the physiological functions of PDGF through genetic studies in mice. *Cytokine Growth Factor Rev.* **2004**, *15*, 215–228. [CrossRef] [PubMed]
52. Sundberg, C.; Kowanetz, M.; Brown, L.F.; Detmar, M.; Dvorak, H.F. Stable expression of angiopoietin-1 and other markers by cultured pericytes: Phenotypic similarities to a subpopulation of cells in maturing vessels during later stages of angiogenesis in vivo. *Lab. Investig. J. Tech. Methods Pathol.* **2002**, *82*, 387–401. [CrossRef]
53. Carvalho, R.L.C. Defective paracrine signalling by TGF in yolk sac vasculature of endoglin mutant mice: A paradigm for hereditary haemorrhagic telangiectasia. *Development* **2004**, *131*, 6237–6247. [CrossRef] [PubMed]
54. Benjamin, L.E.; Hemo, I.; Keshet, E. A plasticity window for blood vessel remodelling is defined by pericyte coverage of the preformed endothelial network and is regulated by PDGF-B and VEGF. *Dev. Camb. Engl.* **1998**, *125*, 1591–1598.
55. Chae, S.-S.; Paik, J.-H.; Allende, M.L.; Proia, R.L.; Hla, T. Regulation of limb development by the sphingosine 1-phosphate receptor S1p1/EDG-1 occurs via the hypoxia/VEGF axis. *Dev. Biol.* **2004**, *268*, 441–447. [CrossRef] [PubMed]
56. Anders, H.-J. Immune system modulation of kidney regeneration—mechanisms and implications. *Nat. Rev. Nephrol.* **2014**, *10*, 347–358. [CrossRef]
57. Stamatiades, E.G.; Tremblay, M.-E.; Bohm, M.; Crozet, L.; Bisht, K.; Kao, D.; Coelho, C.; Fan, X.; Yewdell, W.T.; Davidson, A.; et al. Immune Monitoring of Trans-endothelial Transport by Kidney-Resident Macrophages. *Cell* **2016**, *166*, 991–1003. [CrossRef]
58. Karasawa, K.; Asano, K.; Moriyama, S.; Ushiki, M.; Monya, M.; Iida, M.; Kuboki, E.; Yagita, H.; Uchida, K.; Nitta, K.; et al. Vascular-Resident CD169-Positive Monocytes and Macrophages Control Neutrophil Accumulation in the Kidney with Ischemia-Reperfusion Injury. *J. Am. Soc. Nephrol.* **2015**, *26*, 896–906. [CrossRef]
59. Mantovani, A.; Sica, A.; Sozzani, S.; Allavena, P.; Vecchi, A.; Locati, M. The chemokine system in diverse forms of macrophage activation and polarization. *Trends Immunol.* **2004**, *25*, 677–686. [CrossRef]
60. Martinez, F.O.; Gordon, S. The M1 and M2 paradigm of macrophage activation: Time for reassessment. *F1000Prime Rep.* **2014**, *6*, 13. [CrossRef]
61. Clements, M.; Gershenovich, M.; Chaber, C.; Campos-Rivera, J.; Du, P.; Zhang, M.; Ledbetter, S.; Zuk, A. Differential Ly6C Expression after Renal Ischemia-Reperfusion Identifies Unique Macrophage Populations. *J. Am. Soc. Nephrol.* **2016**, *27*, 159–170. [CrossRef] [PubMed]
62. Jang, H.-S.; Kim, J.; Park, Y.-K.; Park, K.M. Infiltrated Macrophages Contribute to Recovery after Ischemic Injury But Not to Ischemic Preconditioning in Kidneys. *Transplantation* **2008**, *85*, 447–455. [CrossRef] [PubMed]
63. Xu, M.-J.; Feng, D.; Wang, H.; Guan, Y.; Yan, X.; Gao, B. IL-22 Ameliorates Renal Ischemia-Reperfusion Injury by Targeting Proximal Tubule Epithelium. *J. Am. Soc. Nephrol.* **2014** *25*, 967–977. [CrossRef] [PubMed]
64. Chiba, T.; Skrypnyk, N.I.; Skvarca, L.B.; Penchev, R.; Zhang, K.X.; Rochon, E.R.; Fall, J.L.; Paueksakon, P.; Yang, H.; Alford, C.E.; et al. Retinoic Acid Signaling Coordinates Macrophage-Dependent Injury and Repair after AKI. *J. Am. Soc. Nephrol.* **2016**, *27*, 495–508. [CrossRef] [PubMed]

65. Lin, S.-L.; Li, B.; Rao, S.; Yeo, E.-J.; Hudson, T.E.; Nowlin, B.T.; Pei, H.; Chen, L.; Zheng, J.J.; Carroll, T.J.; et al. Macrophage Wnt7b is critical for kidney repair and regeneration. *Proc. Natl. Acad. Sci. USA* **2010**, *107*, 4194–4199. [CrossRef] [PubMed]
66. Zhou, D.; Tan, R.J.; Fu, H.; Liu, Y. Wnt/β-catenin signaling in kidney injury and repair: A double-edged sword. *Lab. Invest.* **2016**, *96*, 156–167. [CrossRef]
67. Tan, R.J.; Zhou, D.; Zhou, L.; Liu, Y. Wnt/β-catenin signaling and kidney fibrosis. *Kidney Int. Suppl.* **2014**, *4*, 84–90. [CrossRef] [PubMed]
68. Zhang, M.-Z.; Yao, B.; Yang, S.; Jiang, L.; Wang, S.; Fan, X.; Yin, H.; Wong, K.; Miyazawa, T.; Chen, J.; et al. CSF-1 signaling mediates recovery from acute kidney injury. *J. Clin. Invest.* **2012**, *122*, 4519–4532. [CrossRef]
69. Baek, J.-H.; Zeng, R.; Weinmann-Menke, J.; Valerius, M.T.; Wada, Y.; Ajay, A.K.; Colonna, M.; Kelley, V.R. IL-34 mediates acute kidney injury and worsens subsequent chronic kidney disease. *J. Clin. Invest.* **2015**, *125*, 3198–3214. [CrossRef]
70. Lee, S.A.; Noel, S.; Sadasivam, M.; Hamad, A.R.A.; Rabb, H. Role of Immune Cells in Acute Kidney Injury and Repair. *Nephron* **2017**, *137*, 282–286. [CrossRef]
71. Kim, M.-G.; Koo, T.Y.; Yan, J.-J.; Lee, E.; Han, K.H.; Jeong, J.C.; Ro, H.; Kim, B.S.; Jo, S.-K.; Oh, K.H.; et al. IL-2/Anti-IL-2 Complex Attenuates Renal Ischemia-Reperfusion Injury through Expansion of Regulatory T Cells. *J. Am. Soc. Nephrol.* **2013**, *24*, 1529–1536. [CrossRef] [PubMed]
72. Gandolfo, M.T.; Jang, H.R.; Bagnasco, S.M.; Ko, G.-J.; Agreda, P.; Satpute, S.R.; Crow, M.T.; King, L.S.; Rabb, H. Foxp3$^+$ regulatory T cells participate in repair of ischemic acute kidney injury. *Kidney Int.* **2009**, *76*, 717–729. [CrossRef] [PubMed]
73. Baudoux, T.; Husson, C.; De Prez, E.; Jadot, I.; Antoine, M.-H.; Nortier, J.L.; Hougardy, J.-M. CD4+ and CD8+ T Cells Exert Regulatory Properties During Experimental Acute Aristolochic Acid Nephropathy. *Sci. Rep.* **2018**, *8*, 5334. [CrossRef] [PubMed]
74. Renner, B.; Strassheim, D.; Amura, C.R.; Kulik, L.; Ljubanovic, D.; Glogowska, M.J.; Takahashi, K.; Carroll, M.C.; Holers, V.M.; Thurman, J.M. B Cell Subsets Contribute to Renal Injury and Renal Protection after Ischemia/Reperfusion. *J. Immunol.* **2010**, *185*, 4393–4400. [CrossRef] [PubMed]
75. Klingberg, F.; Hinz, B.; White, E.S. The myofibroblast matrix: Implications for tissue repair and fibrosis: The myofibroblast matrix. *J. Pathol.* **2013**, *229*, 298–309. [CrossRef] [PubMed]
76. Mackensen-Haen, S.; Bader, R.; Grund, K.E.; Bohle, A. Correlations between renal cortical interstitial fibrosis, atrophy of the proximal tubules and impairment of the glomerular filtration rate. *Clin. Nephrol.* **1981**, *15*, 167–171. [PubMed]
77. Picken, M.; Long, J.; Williamson, G.A.; Polichnowski, A.J. Progression of Chronic Kidney Disease After Acute Kidney Injury: Role of Self-Perpetuating Versus Hemodynamic-Induced Fibrosis. *Hypertens. Dallas Tex 1979* **2016**, *68*, 921–928. [CrossRef] [PubMed]
78. Takaori, K.; Nakamura, J.; Yamamoto, S.; Nakata, H.; Sato, Y.; Takase, M.; Nameta, M.; Yamamoto, T.; Economides, A.N.; Kohno, K.; et al. Severity and Frequency of Proximal Tubule Injury Determines Renal Prognosis. *J. Am. Soc. Nephrol.* **2016**, *27*, 2393–2406. [CrossRef]
79. Sato, Y.; Mii, A.; Hamazaki, Y.; Fujita, H.; Nakata, H.; Masuda, K.; Nishiyama, S.; Shibuya, S.; Haga, H.; Ogawa, O.; et al. Heterogeneous fibroblasts underlie age-dependent tertiary lymphoid tissues in the kidney. *JCI Insight* **2016**, *1*, e87680. [CrossRef]
80. Allinovi, M.; de Chiara, L.; Angelotti, M.L.; Becherucci, F.; Romagnani, P. Anti-fibrotic treatments: A review of clinical evidence. *Matrix Biol.* **2018**, *68–69*, 333–354. [CrossRef]
81. De Chiara, L.; Romagnani, P. Tubule repair: With a little help from my "unexpected" friends. *Kidney Int.* **2019**, *95*, 487–489. [CrossRef] [PubMed]
82. Sharfuddin, A.A.; Molitoris, B.A. Pathophysiology of ischemic acute kidney injury. *Nat. Rev. Nephrol.* **2011**, *7*, 189–200. [CrossRef] [PubMed]
83. Funk, J.A.; Schnellmann, R.G. Persistent disruption of mitochondrial homeostasis after acute kidney injury. *Am. J. Physiol. Renal Physiol.* **2012**, *302*, 853–864. [CrossRef] [PubMed]
84. Wang, Y.; Chang, J.; Yao, B.; Niu, A.; Kelly, E.; Breeggemann, M.C.; Abboud Werner, S.L.; Harris, R.C.; Zhang, M.-Z. Proximal tubule-derived colony stimulating factor-1 mediates polarization of renal macrophages and dendritic cells, and recovery in acute kidney injury. *Kidney Int.* **2015**, *88*, 1274–1282. [CrossRef] [PubMed]
85. Huen, S.C.; Huynh, L.; Marlier, A.; Lee, Y.; Moeckel, G.W.; Cantley, L.G. GM-CSF Promotes Macrophage Alternative Activation after Renal Ischemia/Reperfusion Injury. *J. Am. Soc. Nephrol.* **2015**, *26*, 1334–1345. [CrossRef]

86. Kramann, R.; Kusaba, T.; Humphreys, B.D. Who regenerates the kidney tubule? *Nephrol. Dial. Transplant. Off. Publ. Eur. Dial. Transpl. Assoc. -Eur. Ren. Assoc.* **2015**, *30*, 903–910. [CrossRef] [PubMed]
87. Chang-Panesso, M.; Humphreys, B.D. Cellular plasticity in kidney injury and repair. *Nat. Rev. Nephrol.* **2017**, *13*, 39–46. [CrossRef]
88. Witzgall, R.; Brown, D.; Schwarz, C.; Bonventre, J.V. Localization of proliferating cell nuclear antigen, vimentin, c-Fos, and clusterin in the postischemic kidney. Evidence for a heterogenous genetic response among nephron segments, and a large pool of mitotically active and dedifferentiated cells. *J. Clin. Invest.* **1994**, *93*, 2175–2188. [CrossRef]
89. Grande, M.T.; Sánchez-Laorden, B.; López-Blau, C.; De Frutos, C.A.; Boutet, A.; Arévalo, M.; Rowe, R.G.; Weiss, S.J.; López-Novoa, J.M.; Nieto, M.A. Snail1-induced partial epithelial-to-mesenchymal transition drives renal fibrosis in mice and can be targeted to reverse established disease. *Nat. Med.* **2015**, *21*, 989–997. [CrossRef]
90. Lovisa, S.; LeBleu, V.S.; Tampe, B.; Sugimoto, H.; Vadnagara, K.; Carstens, J.L.; Wu, C.-C.; Hagos, Y.; Burckhardt, B.C.; Pentcheva-Hoang, T.; et al. Epithelial-to-mesenchymal transition induces cell cycle arrest and parenchymal damage in renal fibrosis. *Nat. Med.* **2015**, *21*, 998–1009. [CrossRef]
91. Vogetseder, A.; Karadeniz, A.; Kaissling, B.; Le Hir, M. Tubular cell proliferation in the healthy rat kidney. *Histochem. Cell Biol.* **2005**, *124*, 97–104. [CrossRef] [PubMed]
92. Vogetseder, A.; Picard, N.; Gaspert, A.; Walch, M.; Kaissling, B.; le Hir, M. Proliferation capacity of the renal proximal tubule involves the bulk of differentiated epithelial cells. *Am. J. Physiol.-Cell Physiol.* **2008**, *294*, 22–28. [CrossRef] [PubMed]
93. Yang, L.; Besschetnova, T.Y.; Brooks, C.R.; Shah, J.V.; Bonventre, J.V. Epithelial cell cycle arrest in G2/M mediates kidney fibrosis after injury. *Nat. Med.* **2010**, *16*, 535–543. [CrossRef] [PubMed]
94. Canaud, G.; Bonventre, J.V. Cell cycle arrest and the evolution of chronic kidney disease from acute kidney injury. *Nephrol. Dial. Transplant.* **2015**, *30*, 575–583. [CrossRef] [PubMed]
95. Lazzeri, E.; Angelotti, M.L.; Peired, A.; Conte, C.; Marschner, J.A.; Maggi, L.; Mazzinghi, B.; Lombardi, D.; Melica, M.E.; Nardi, S.; et al. Endocycle-related tubular cell hypertrophy and progenitor proliferation recover renal function after acute kidney injury. *Nat. Commun.* **2018**, *9*, 1344. [CrossRef] [PubMed]
96. Lazzeri, E.; Angelotti, M.L.; Conte, C.; Anders, H.-J.; Romagnani, P. Surviving Acute Organ Failure: Cell Polyploidization and Progenitor Proliferation. *Trends Mol. Med.* **2019**, *25*, 366–381. [CrossRef] [PubMed]
97. Lombardi, D.; Becherucci, F.; Romagnani, P. How much can the tubule regenerate and who does it? An open question. *Nephrol. Dial. Transplant.* **2016**, *31*, 1243–1250. [CrossRef] [PubMed]
98. Lindgren, D.; Boström, A.-K.; Nilsson, K.; Hansson, J.; Sjölund, J.; Möller, C.; Jirström, K.; Nilsson, E.; Landberg, G.; Axelson, H.; et al. Isolation and characterization of progenitor-like cells from human renal proximal tubules. *Am. J. Pathol.* **2011**, *178*, 828–837. [CrossRef] [PubMed]
99. Angelotti, M.L.; Ronconi, E.; Ballerini, L.; Peired, A.; Mazzinghi, B.; Sagrinati, C.; Parente, E.; Gacci, M.; Carini, M.; Rotondi, M.; et al. Characterization of renal progenitors committed toward tubular lineage and their regenerative potential in renal tubular injury. *Stem Cells Dayt. Ohio* **2012**, *30*, 1714–1725. [CrossRef]
100. Smeets, B.; Boor, P.; Dijkman, H.; Sharma, S.V.; Jirak, P.; Mooren, F.; Berger, K.; Bornemann, J.; Gelman, I.H.; Floege, J.; et al. Proximal tubular cells contain a phenotypically distinct, scattered cell population involved in tubular regeneration: Phenotypically distinct proximal tubular cells. *J. Pathol.* **2013**, *229*, 645–659. [CrossRef]
101. Kumar, S.; Liu, J.; Pang, P.; Krautzberger, A.M.; Reginensi, A.; Akiyama, H.; Schedl, A.; Humphreys, B.D.; McMahon, A.P. Sox9 Activation Highlights a Cellular Pathway of Renal Repair in the Acutely Injured Mammalian Kidney. *Cell Rep.* **2015**, *12*, 1325–1338. [CrossRef] [PubMed]
102. Kang, H.M.; Huang, S.; Reidy, K.; Han, S.H.; Chinga, F.; Susztak, K. Sox9-Positive Progenitor Cells Play a Key Role in Renal Tubule Epithelial Regeneration in Mice. *Cell Rep.* **2016**, *14*, 861–871. [CrossRef] [PubMed]
103. Berger, K.; Bangen, J.-M.; Hammerich, L.; Liedtke, C.; Floege, J.; Smeets, B.; Moeller, M.J. Origin of regenerating tubular cells after acute kidney injury. *Proc. Natl. Acad. Sci. USA* **2014**, *111*, 1533–1538. [CrossRef] [PubMed]
104. Romagnani, P.; Lasagni, L.; Remuzzi, G. Renal progenitors: An evolutionary conserved strategy for kidney regeneration. *Nat. Rev. Nephrol.* **2013**, *9*, 137–146. [CrossRef] [PubMed]
105. Rinkevich, Y.; Montoro, D.T.; Contreras-Trujillo, H.; Harari-Steinberg, O.; Newman, A.M.; Tsai, J.M.; Lim, X.; Van-Amerongen, R.; Bowman, A.; Januszyk, M.; et al. In Vivo Clonal Analysis Reveals Lineage-Restricted Progenitor Characteristics in Mammalian Kidney Development, Maintenance, and Regeneration. *Cell Rep.* **2014**, *7*, 1270–1283. [CrossRef] [PubMed]
106. Humphreys, B.D.; Valerius, M.T.; Kobayashi, A.; Mugford, J.W.; Soeung, S.; Duffield, J.S.; McMahon, A.P.;

Bonventre, J.V. Intrinsic Epithelial Cells Repair the Kidney after Injury. *Cell Stem Cell* **2008**, *2*, 284–291. [CrossRef] [PubMed]

107. Shu, Z.; Row, S.; Deng, W.-M. Endoreplication: The Good, the Bad, and the Ugly. *Trends Cell Biol.* **2018**, *28*, 465–474. [CrossRef]

3

Arachidonic Acid Metabolism and Kidney Inflammation

Tianqi Wang [1,2,†], Xianjun Fu [2,3,†], Qingfa Chen [4], Jayanta Kumar Patra [5], Dongdong Wang [6,7], Zhenguo Wang [2,*] and Zhibo Gai [3,*]

1 Traditional Chinese Medicine History and Literature, Institute for Literature and Culture of Chinese Medicine, Shandong University of Traditional Chinese Medicine, Jinan 250355, China
2 Institute for Literature and Culture of Chinese Medicine, Shandong University of Traditional Chinese Medicine, Jinan 250355, China
3 Key Laboratory of Traditional Chinese Medicine for Classical Theory, Ministry of Education, Shandong University of Traditional Chinese Medicine, Jinan 250355, China
4 The Institute for Tissue Engineering and Regenerative Medicine, The Liaocheng University, Liaocheng 252000, China
5 Research Institute of Biotechnology & Medical Converged Science, Dongguk University-Seoul, Goyangsi 10326, Korea
6 Institute of Clinical Chemistry, University Hospital Zurich, University of Zurich, Wagistrasse 14, 8952 Schlieren, Switzerland
7 Guizhou University of Traditional Chinese Medicine, Fei Shan Jie 32, Guiyang 550003, China
* Correspondence: zhenguow@126.com (Z.W.); zhibo.gai@usz.ch (Z.G.)

† These authors contributed equally to this work.

Abstract: As a major component of cell membrane lipids, Arachidonic acid (AA), being a major component of the cell membrane lipid content, is mainly metabolized by three kinds of enzymes: cyclooxygenase (COX), lipoxygenase (LOX), and cytochrome P450 (CYP450) enzymes. Based on these three metabolic pathways, AA could be converted into various metabolites that trigger different inflammatory responses. In the kidney, prostaglandins (PG), thromboxane (Tx), leukotrienes (LTs) and hydroxyeicosatetraenoic acids (HETEs) are the major metabolites generated from AA. An increased level of prostaglandins (PGs), TxA_2 and leukotriene B4 (LTB_4) results in inflammatory damage to the kidney. Moreover, the LTB_4-leukotriene B4 receptor 1 (BLT1) axis participates in the acute kidney injury via mediating the recruitment of renal neutrophils. In addition, AA can regulate renal ion transport through 19-hydroxystilbenetetraenoic acid (19-HETE) and 20-HETE, both of which are produced by cytochrome P450 monooxygenase. Epoxyeicosatrienoic acids (EETs) generated by the CYP450 enzyme also plays a paramount role in the kidney damage during the inflammation process. For example, 14 and 15-EET mitigated ischemia/reperfusion-caused renal tubular epithelial cell damage. Many drug candidates that target the AA metabolism pathways are being developed to treat kidney inflammation. These observations support an extraordinary interest in a wide range of studies on drug interventions aiming to control AA metabolism and kidney inflammation.

Keywords: arachidonic acid; cyclooxygenase; lipoxygenase; cytochrome P450; kidney inflammation; therapeutic target

---

1. Introduction

Arachidonic acid (AA), also named eicosa-5,8,11,14-tetraenoic acid, is a ω-6 polyunsaturated fatty acid (PFA) and is mainly present in the form of phospholipids in the cell membrane. When cells are under stress, AA is released from the phospholipids by phospholipase A_2 (PLA_2) and phospholipase

C (PLC) as free arachidonic acids [1–3], which become the precursor of proinflammatory bioactive mediators through three metabolic pathways. Through the cyclooxygenase (COX) pathway, AA can be metabolized into prostaglandins (PGs) and thromboxanes (TXs). AA can also be converted into leukotrienes (LTs) and lipoxins (LXs) by the lipoxygenase (LOX) pathway [4–6]. Moreover, AA also generates epoxyeicosatrienoic acids (EETs) or hydroxyeicosatetraenoic acids (HETEs) through the cytochrome P450 (CYP450) pathway. Together, these AA metabolites are referred as eicosanoids, which are effective autocrine and paracrine bioactive mediators, and are widely involved in a variety of physiological and pathological processes [7–10].

Kidney inflammation, characterized by hematuria, proteinuria, edema, hypertension, etc., is caused by immune-mediated inflammatory mediators (such as complement, cytokines, reactive oxygen species, etc.), resulting in a group of kidney diseases with a varying degree of renal dysfunction. Without prompt treatment, it will lead to thromboembolism, acute renal failure (and even chronic nephritis), chronic renal failure and finally uremia [11].

The relationship between AA and inflammation attracts our interest in the effect of AA metabolism on kidney inflammation. Therefore, we systematically summarized the effect of AA-derived bioactive mediators on kidney inflammation by discussing the regulatory mechanism of AA metabolism in the kidney, followed by the mechanism of AA-induced renal inflammation and a potential treatment targeting the AA metabolism.

2. Regulation of the AA Metabolism in the Kidney

2.1. The Release of AA

Normally, AA exists in the cell membrane in the form of phospholipids. When the cell membrane is subjected to stimuli, especially the inflammatory reaction, the phospholipids are released from the cell membrane. Through the hydrolysis of phospholipids by PLA_2 and PLC [1,3,12], AA is released and then transformed into a bioactive metabolite with the help of different enzymes, thus promoting inflammatory cascades. At present, it is well known that at least three metabolic pathways (the COX pathway, LOX pathway and CYP450 pathway) are involved in the metabolism of AA, which are closely related to the occurrence, development, and regression of renal inflammation (Figure 1) [1].

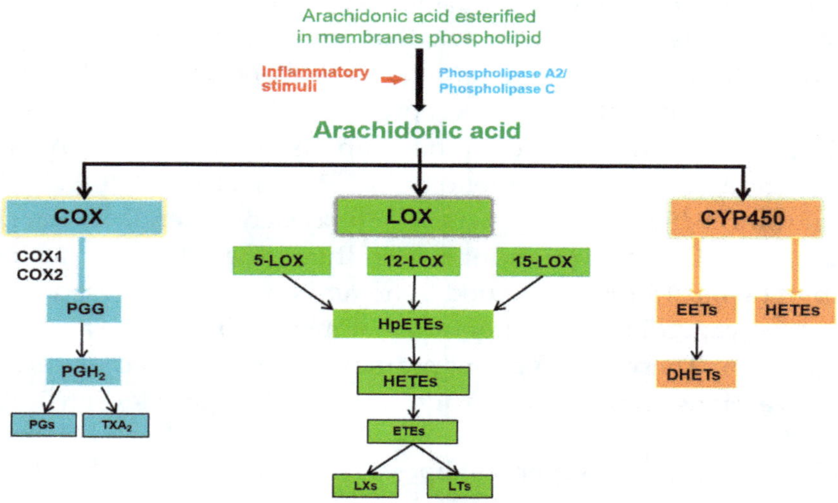

Figure 1. Scheme of eicosanoids biosynthesis pathways from arachidonic acid.

2.2. COX Pathway

COX-1/2, also called prostaglandin H synthase (PGHS), is one of the key enzymes involved in the AA metabolism [13]. The constitutive enzyme COX-1 is responsible for the expression of prostaglandin E_2 (PGE_2) at the background level or the expression of PG under hypotonic swelling stimulation [14]. COX-2 is almost not expressed at normal physiological conditions; however, it is highly expressed when the kidney is under the influence of stimuli, such as chronic sodium deficiency and ultrafiltration [15]. It is important to note that COX-2 is the dominating source of prostacyclin [16]. Once AA is released, it can be metabolized by two isozymes of PGHS, PGHS-1 and PGHS-2 [17]. PGHSs have two different but complementary enzyme activities, one is cyclooxygenase (dioxygenase) activity, which catalyzes the production of PGG_2 from arachidonic acid, and the other is peroxidase activity, which promotes the reduction of PGG_2 to PGH_2 [18]. In general, the COX protein contains a cyclooxygenase site and a peroxidase site. AA is converted to the endogenous hydrogen peroxide PGG_2 by the cyclooxygenase site, and the peroxidase site is responsible for reducing PGG_2 to PGH_2 [19]. COXs initially metabolize AA to unstable PGG_2 by their COX function and then convert it to PGH_2 by their peroxidase function. PGH_2, like cell-and tissue-selective prostanoid synthases and isomerases, is not stable, and can easily generate many bioactive prostaglandins, such as prostaglandins D2, E2, F2α, and I_2, and TXA_2, depending on the differential expression of these synthetases in different tissues [20–23]. PGH_2 can also be decomposed into malonaldehyde (MDA) and 12L-hydroxy-5,8,10-heptadecatrienoic acid (HHT) by thromboxane synthase [24]. The process of converting PGH_2 to PGD requires two PGD synthetases, namely hematopoietic PGD synthase (H-PGDS) and lipocalin-type PGD synthase (L-PGDS). Then the PGD_2 is metabolized to 15-deoxy-Δ 12,14-prostaglandin J 2 (15d-PGJ 2) [25]. PGI_2 is extremely unstable, with a half-life of only two to three minutes, and is easily converted to 6-keto-prostaglandin F1α spontaneously [26,27]. In particular, PGH_2 is produced in most cells by the action of microsomal PGE_2 synthase (mPGES). PGE_2 is synthesized in almost all human cells and exerts extremely complex physiological effects in the inflammatory response through the signaling pathway which is composed of four G protein-coupled receptors: E-type prostanoid receptors (EP)1, EP2, EP3 and EP4 [28–30]. As for TXA_2, AA can generate TXA_2 via the action of thromboxane synthase [31], which has a half-life of only about 30 s and is then spontaneously converted to thromboxane B_2 (TXB_2) [32,33]. Three things that need to be especially pointed out are that platelets mainly form TXA_2, endothelial cells mainly form PGI_2, and PGE_2 is the main prostatic body produced by renal collecting tubule cells [34]. In recent years, another variant of the COX family, COX-3 (or CX-1b), which is an allosteric splice variant of COX-1, has been discovered, and its gene sequence differs from COX-2 in such a way that the COX-3 retains the intron 1 sequences [35]. COX-3 also catalyzes the production of PGH_2, its activity can be inhibited by crude aminophenol, and it is mainly expressed in the microvessels of the brain and heart [36–38]. Hence, its role in AA metabolism and kidney inflammation needs to be further explored.

2.3. LOX Pathway

Under the catalysis of lipoxygenase, AA is metabolized into hydroperoxyeicosatetraenoic acid (HpETE). Current research suggests that at least four enzymes, namely 5-LOX, 8-LOX, 12-LOX, and 15-LOX are involved in the metabolism of AA in the LOX pathway. However, the 5-, 12-, and 15-positions are the main oxidation sites of AA, leading to oxidation reactions that are based on the catalysis of 5-LOX, 12-LOX, and 15-LOX enzymes. In this review, we focus on the 5-LOX, 12-LOX and 15-LOX pathways (Figure 2).

Human 5-LOX holds a major function in kidney inflammation, ranging from kidney tubules to glomeruli. In this pathway, AA forms 5-hydroperoxyeicosatetraenoic acid (5-HpETE) by dioxygenase [39], and then 95% is generated into 5-hydroxyeicosatetraenoic acid (5-hydroxy-6,8,11,15-eicosatetraenoic acid, 5-HETE) at C7 and 5% is generated into 8-HETE at C10, which are the first two steps during the conversion process of AA to proinflammatory LTs [40]. Besides, Oxo-ETE is generated via the LOX product, HETEs by the microsomal dehydrogenase in the human polymorphonuclear leukocytes (PMNLs) [39,41]. Then, oxo-ETEs are formed through the oxidation of HETEs [42,43], which is the strongest eosinophil chemoattractant among bioactive mediators. From here, AA metabolites are further converted to LTA_4 and LXs via 5-LOX activator protein (5-FLAP) and dehydrase [44]. Basically, the catalytic function of the 5-LOX enzyme is mainly manifested in the following two aspects: one is the insertion of molecular oxygen by dioxygenase activity and the other is the formation of epoxide by LTA_4 synthase activity. Regarding 5-HpETE, it is generated from AA through homolytic cleavage and removal of hydrogen on the pro-S hydrogen at carbon-7 [39]. 5-LOX can generate LTA_4 by removing the C10 hydrogen atom from 5-HpETE [45]. LTA_4 is unstable and can be hydrolyzed or combined with glutathione or transcellularly transferred to generate bioactive eicosanoids. In neutrophils and other inflammatory cells of kidney tissue, LTA_4 is catalyzed by epoxide hydrolase to form LTB_4 [46]. LTA_4 and glutathione (GSH) catalyze the production of LTC_4 using glutathione S-transferase (GST) and then remove glutamic acid to form LTD_4 via γ-glutamyl transferase, which is further metabolized by dipeptidase to form LTE_4. Then, LTF_4 is synthesized from LTE_4 by γ-glutamyl transferase [47].

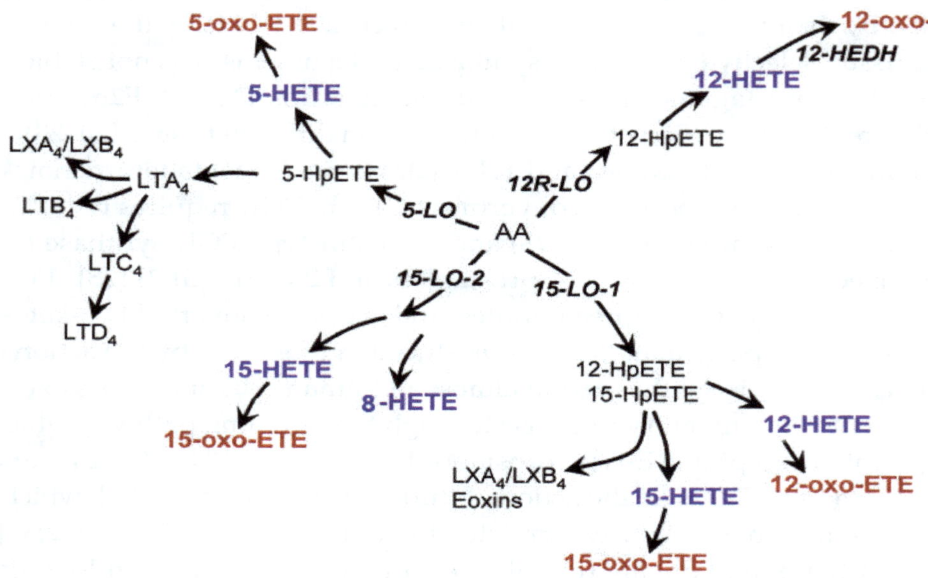

Figure 2. Lipoxygenase, and dehydrogenase pathways for the formation of HETEs, oxo-ETEs, and related eicosanoids.

The roles of the 12-LOX and 15-LOX pathways are mainly in the production of HETEs and LXs. The 12-LOX pathway is similar to the 5-LOX pathway. AA first generates 12-HpETE and 12-hydroxyeicosatetraenoic acid (12-HETE) via 12-LOX [48,49]. But there is a difference between them, as in addition to the conversion of AA to 12-HETE, 12-LOX can also convert 5(S)-HETE to 5(S),12(S)-dihydroxyeicosatetraenoic acid (-diHETE) as well as metabolize 15(S)-HETE to 14(R),15(S)-diHETE in the leukocytes. These products ultimately convert into extra-platelet LTA_4 [50,51]. Another biosynthetic pathway for LXs involves 5-LOX in neutrophils and 12-LOX in the platelets. 5-LOX generates LTA_4 in the neutrophil, which is then transferred to the platelet, where 12-LOX subsequently generates either LXA_4 or LXB_4 [45,52,53]. Same as the 12-LOX pathway, the principal effect of the 15-LOX pathway is to ultimately generate HETEs, ETEs and LXs. There are two isoforms in mammalian cells: 15-LOX-1 and 15-LOX-2. 15-LOX-1 (12/15-LOX), which is encoded by the arachidonate 15-lipoxygenase (ALOX15) gene, could metabolize AA into LXA_4, LXB_4 and 15-oxo-ETEs [43,45], while 15-LOX-2 will metabolize AA into 15-oxo-ETE and 8SHETE. HpETEs. In particular, when using 5, 15-diHpETE as a substrate, the primary product catalyzed by 12-LOX and 15-LOX-1 is LXB_4, and the efficiency of 15-LOX-1 is 20 times higher than that of 12-LOX [45]. In humans, 15-LOX-1 and leukocyte 12-LOX have high homology and can form 12(S)-HETE and 15(S)-HETE simultaneously, so these two pathways can be collectively called 12/15-LOX (12/15-LOX). When 15-LOX-2 metabolizes AA to produce only 15-HETE, 15-LOX-1 also metabolizes linoleic acid to synthesize hydroxyoctadecadienoic acid [54]. Then, 15-HETE is rapidly converted into LXA_4 or LXB_4 by hydrolase [55].

2.4. *Cytochrome P450 (CYP450) Pathway*

The CYP450 pathway is the major metabolic pathway of AA in the kidney [56]. CYP450 can be detected in the endoplasmic reticulum, mitochondria and nuclear membrane of the kidney [57,58]. In general, AA produces corresponding metabolites mainly through three kinds of reduced triphosphopyridine nucleotide (NADPH, or reduced coenzyme II)-dependent oxidation in the CYP450 pathway. The first is the formation of 5,6-; 8,9-; 11,12-; and 14,15-epoxyeicosatrienoic acids (EETs) through surface oxidation [59–63]. The kidney is an organ with high expoxygenase activity, which, like the liver, also produces enantioselective EETs. In the case of lipoxygenase and cyclooxygenase, AA is first converted to hydrogen peroxide (HpETEs) [43], and then through CYP450 isozymes, oxo-ETEs can also be formed directly from HpETEs (just like the common process of forming HETEs via enzymatic oxidation) [42]. 14,15-EET is the main epoxy compound formed by kidney, and most of the isomers in this region are in (R,S) configuration. CYP2 is the main CYP450 epoxygenase family, and more importantly, CYP2C8 is the most paramount and plays a central epoxygenase role in the metabolism of AA to biologically active EETs in human kidney [64,65]. In addition, the CYP2J family also contributes to the formation of EETs in human and mouse kidneys [64,65]. Early research of CYP2C epoxygenases suggested that CYP2C29 and CYP2C39 produced 14,15-EET, and the CYP2C38 produced 11,12-EET [66]. In particularly, human CYP2J2 isoforms are extremely efficient at epoxidation of AA at the 14,15-position [67]. CYP2J5 is an epoxygenase enzyme that is confined in tubular cells and metabolizes AA to 8,9-EET; 11,12-EET; and 14,15-EET in the mouse kidney [68]. Therefore, different vascular smooth muscle cells and epithelial transport processes controlled by EETs have led to the differential localization and regulation of renal vascular and tubular CYP450 cyclooxygenase, and these conclusions are consistent throughout [69]. Then, EETs are mainly hydrolyzed by soluble epoxide hydrolase (sEH) to form 5,6-; 8,9-; 11,12-; and 14,15-dihydroxyepoxyeicosatrienoic acids (DHETs), which possess weak biological activity [70]. Recent research has confirmed that sEH is one of the key enzymes in the metabolism of EETs, and the regulation of sEH activity and can change the level of EETs in vivo [70].

The other two CYP450 pathways ultimately produce HETEs. One is the formation of 5-, 8-, 9-, 11-, 12-, or 15-HETEs by propylene oxidation. HpETEs produced by lipoxygenase and cyclooxygenase can be reduced to monohydroxy fatty acids (HETEs) by peroxidase [43], which means the hydroxyl group is adjacent to a conjugated diene system. CYP2J5 can also facilitate the process, which has been confirmed in tubular cells, and metabolizes AA to 11-HETE and 15-HETE in mouse kidney [68]. The other is the formation of 19- and 20-Hydroxyeicosatetraenoic (19- and 20-HETE) by ω-1 hydroxylation. The CYP ω-hydroxylase that has been discovered so far is mainly in the CYP4 family. In kidney, proximal straight tubules are capable of converting AA to 20-HETE and 19(S)-HETE by ω-hydroxylase [71]. What's more, 20-HETE is the main product of AA catalyzed by CYP ω-hydroxylase, and in the human kidney, 20-HETE formation is mediated by both CYP4F2 and CYP4A11 [56,72]. Then, 20-HETE can be further oxidized to 20-carboxy arachidonic acid (20-COOH-AA) by alcohol dehydrogenase [73]. It is now well established from a few studies that, CYP4A1, CYP4A2, and CYP4A3 have remarkable AA ω-hydroxylase activity [74]. Moreover, CYP4A1 as an arachidonate ω-hydroxylase has a higher catalytic efficiency, with a turnover rate 20 times higher than that of CYP4A2 or CYP4A3 [74]. Besides, CYP4A1 can also convert AA to 11,12-EET in the mouse kidney [74].

3. Mechanism of AA-induced Renal Inflammation

3.1. *PGs and Renal Inflammation*

PGs produced by the COX pathway, function differently in case of renal vascular disease. The impact of PGs on renal inflammation is mainly focused in the field of lupus nephritis (LN). In mice and humans, urinary prostaglandin D synthase (uPGDS) is considered as a biomarker of LN, which makes the role of PGD_2 important in the development of LN [75]. PGD_2 are considered as an inflammatory marker, while lipocalin-like-prostaglandin-D synthase (L-PGDS) is considered as a urinary biomarker for human active lupus nephritis [76]. One study of 184 longitudinal observations in 80 patients showed that lipocalin-like-prostaglandin-D synthase could predict the onset/remission of LN [77]. In patients with systemic lupus erythematosus (SLE), increased expression of PGD_2 receptors (PTGDRs) in blood basophils causes an increase of PGD_2 metabolites in the plasma [78]. PGD_2 regulates the inflammatory response through two receptors, PTGDR-1 and PTGDR-2, which are also called D prostanoid receptor-1 (DP-1) and D prostanoid receptor-2 (DP-2). DP-2 also functions as the chemo-attractant receptor-homologous molecule, which is expressed on the T helper type 2 (TH2) cells (CRTH2) [79,80]. Under in vivo condition, the targeted cells of PGD_2 are mainly basophils, and the two PTGDRs are expressed at the highest level in the peripheral blood leukocytes. Interestingly, PTGDR-1 is ubiquitously expressed in the leukocytes, whereas PTGDR-2 only mediates the activation and chemotaxis of basophils, eosinophils, and $CD4^+$ TH2 cells [81]. PGD_2 and PTGDR induce the activation and infiltration of basophils in the kidneys of patients with SLE via mediating C-X-C motif ligand 12 (CXCL12) [78]. CXCL12 plays a biological role mainly through the chemokine receptor CXCR4, and regulates the physiological distribution of neutrophils in the kidney [82,83]. Inflammatory tissues and secondary lymphoid organs (SLOs) are associated with high levels of CXCL12, and CXCL12 mediates immune cell recruitment, which are the factors associated with the pathogenesis of SLE [78]. More importantly, basophil autocrine PGD_2 is the main factor of PGD2-induced CXCR4 epoxidation. In humans and mice, the CXCL12-CXCR4 axis promotes the accumulation of basophils in SLOs during lupus through its mediating effect on the PGD_2-PTGDR axis [78]. At the same time, we also can't deny the bad consequence caused by PGE_2 and TXB_2 in the LN. High levels of PGE_2 and TXB_2 promoted the activation of T cells and the production of IL-4 and IL-10 cytokines, which in turn leads to glomerulosclerosis in LN [84].

In addition, a potential link between PGs and tubulointerstitial lesions and glomerulonephritis was well studied. In the kidney with unilateral ureteral obstruction (UUO), PGD_2 has penetrated all the sides of tubulointerstitial lesions by DP-2 expressed on CD4-positive T cells to activate Th2 lymphocytes. High levels of L-PGDS increased the degree of tubular fibrosis, while L-PGDS-knockout mice and prostaglandin D2 receptor CRTH2-knockout mice revealed a reduction in renal fibrosis, which may be related to the reduced infiltration of Th2 lymphocytes as well as reduced generation of the Th2 cytokines IL-4 and IL-13 [85]. In contrast, the PGD_2 metabolite, 15d-PGJ2, can activate PPARγ and modulate the adhesion process via inhibiting the TNFα-triggered IKK-NFκB pathway, which eventually suppresses inflammation in mouse renal tubular epithelial cells [86]. Moreover, PGs are also regulators of renal ischemia and vasoconstriction. Conversely, PGl_2 and PGE_1 have the effect of relaxing blood vessels and preventing hypoxia-mediated renal tissue damage. More importantly, in the case of renal artery stenosis, PGl_2 and PGE_1 selectively prevent tissue contraction and inhibit the decline of GFR [87,88].

It is well known that PGE_2 is the major product of the COX-2 pathway in the kidneys, which mediates kidney damage [89]. PGE2 play a crucial role in renal hemodynamics, renin release, and renal tubular sodium/water resorption [90,91]. In pathological environments such as diabetic nephropathy, PGE2 synthesis is increased, which may affect cell proliferation, differentiation or apoptosis [92,93]. Current studies indicate that four different EP receptors for PGE_2 are closely associated with rapidly progressive glomerulonephritis (RPGN) [94]. In humans, EP1 receptor mRNA is predominantly expressed in the glomerulus [95]. In diabetic mouse models, activation of EP1 promotes the progression of diabetic nephropathy [96]. On the other hand, deletion of EP1 inhibited the down-regulation of nephrin, and improved glomerular basement membrane thickening and foot process regression [96]. In contrast, a few studies have shown that EP1 deficiency caused severe renal impairment in mice with glomerulonephritis, and the cause of this difference has not yet been discovered [97]. Interestingly, PGE_2 has both vasodilation and vasoconstriction effects on renal afferent arterioles. Treatment with high concentrations of PGE_2 (between 1 and 10 nmol/L) caused arterial vasodilation, and at lower concentrations (0.100 nmol/L), PGE_2 leads to vasoconstriction and aggravates hydronephrosis, which may be due to the binding of the EP3 receptor to the pertussis toxin (PTX)-sensitive G protein $G\alpha_i$. [98]. Glomerular hypertrophy caused by unilateral nephrectomy in mice may be associated with increased expression of EP2 [99]. In netrin-1-deficient mice, proximal tubular injury can be attributed to the COX-2-PGE_2-mediated inflammatory response [100]. Further studies have confirmed that activation of the COX-2-PGE_2-EP2 axis may be a specific response of podocytes to fluid flow shear stress. This appears to provide a mechanistic basis for changes in podocyte structure and glomerular filtration barrier, leading to proteinuria in high filtration-mediated renal injury [99]. EP3 also plays a paramount role in the progression of renal diseases. $Ep3^{-/-}$ -STZ mice have less volume of urine and higher urine osmotic pressure compared with wild-type STZ (WT-STZ) mice, indicating enhanced water reabsorption. In parallel, the expressions of aquaporin-1, aquaporin-2, and urea transporter A1 in $Ep3^{-/-}$ -STZ mice were increased, so the presence of EP3 was an important promoting factor in the progression of renal disease [101]. EP4 is abundant in almost all types of kidney cells [95], and plays different roles at the glomeruli [102] and tubules [103]. The $G\alpha_s$-conjugated EP4 receptor directly activates adenylate cyclase, increases cAMP, and also activates phosphoinositide kinase 3 [94,104]. In addition, EP4 also stimulates AMP-activated protein kinase and COX2 in mouse podocytes in a p38-dependent manner [105]. When the rats were treated with a low-salt diet, EP4 transcripts in the glomeruli increased significantly, which in turn mediated PGE_2-induced renin secretion and maintained renal blood flow [106]. More importantly, the overexpression of EP4 contributed to podocyte injury and compromised the glomerular filtration barrier in podocyte-specific EP4 receptor transgenic ($EP4^{pod+}$) mice after 5/6 nephrectomy [107]. On the other hand, in a rat model of cisplatin-induced renal failure, the COX1-PGE2-EP4 axis plays more important roles than dose COX-2 in regulating renal epithelial regeneration [108]. The endogenous PGE_2-EP4 system is involved in tubule-interstitial fibrosis in a mouse UUO model. EP4 knockout significantly augmented obstruction-induced histological alterations. The effects of EP4 agonist are controversial. Use of EP4-sepicific agonist down-regulated the expression of renal macrophage chemokines and pro-fibrinogen growth factors, and inhibited the progression of renal inflammation [103]. In the rat model of acute renal failure, EP4 agonist reduces serum creatinine level and improve survival rate [109]. Moreover, in chronic kidney failure both EP2 and EP4 receptors are shown to be equally important in preserving the progression of chronic kidney disease [109]. In addition, PGE2 can alter renal cell growth, matrix transformation, fibrosis, and apoptosis by activating the EP4 receptor [89]. However, in a STZ-induced diabetic mouse model, the level of cytokines (TNFα and IL-6) and chemokines (MCP-1 and IP-10) in urine of EP4 agonist-treated mice were remarkably higher than those of vehicle-treated diabetes mice, which aggravated glomerular sclerosis and renal tubular interstitial fibrosis [110]. The exact mechanisms of EP4 agonists for the treatment of different kidney diseases need to be further studied.

3.2. HETEs and Renal Inflammation

It has been argued that the regulatory effects of HETEs on platelet function by autocrine or paracrine play a crucial role in the renal inflammation. In view of renal inflammation, which is often associated with renal vascular disease, HETEs have a dual role of anti-thrombotic and pro-thrombotic effects. 5-HETE, 12-HETE and 15-HETE inhibited platelet PLA_2 activity [111]. Platelets are more sensitive to ADP-induced aggregation, and mouse platelets disrupted by gene targeting 12-lipoxygenase ($P\text{-}12LO^{-/-}$) of the 12-LOX gene exhibit selective hypersensitivity to ADP [112]. Current study found that in patients with type 2 diabetes, exogenous 12-HpETE activates platelet p38 mitogen-activated protein kinase (p38 MAPK), which in turn promotes the platelet activation in the oxidative stress-related pathophysiological states [113]. Under oxidative stress, a decrease in the glutathione peroxidase activity promotes the formation of 12-HpETE and further causes an increase in the phosphorylation level of p38 MAPK, which further activates platelets [113], exacerbating the kidney damage [114]. Therefore, HETE-induced renal inflammation can be achieved through the regulation of platelets.

In recent years, increasing literatures reveal the activation of peroxisome proliferator-activated receptors (PPARs) by HETEs. PPARs, with three isotypes (PPARα, PPARδ, and PPARγ), are all transcriptional factors for lipogenesis and mainly expressed in the adipocytes and immune cells that regulate the expression of a quantity of genes associated with renal inflammation [115–117]. In macrophages, high concentrations of HETEs activate PPARγ [118,119], the latter gives rise to the increasing expression of CD36, which induces the apoptosis of tubule-interstitial cells, and ultimately leads to the inflammation and fibrosis of renal tubules [120]. In addition, HETEs can also activate PPARα [121], which has an important effect on renal inflammation by participating in the regulation of lipid metabolism [122,123]. Moreover, the metabolite of 20-HETE, 20-COOH-AA, is an endogenous dual activator of PPARα and PPARγ, and its efficiency to activate PPARγ is twice than that of 20-HETE, revealing the potential modulatory effects of 20-COOH-AA on renal inflammation via activation of PPARs.

The roles of HETEs are also of interest in regulating the renal ion transport during renal inflammation. 20-HETE has a wide range of biological effects, including cell proliferation and angiogenesis, and is a relevant factor that regulates the renal function [124]. 20-HETE is widely synthesized in the renal tubules, including proximal tubules, thick ascending rings, small arteries of the renal cortex and the outer medulla. 20-HETE can fully bind to major vasoconstrictors, such as angiotensin II [125], adrenaline, and endothelin [126]. As early as 1991, Escalante had pointed out that both 20-HETE and 20-COOH-AA, acting similarly to furosemide, reduce the Na^+ and K^+ concentrations of medullary thick ascending limb of Henle (mTALH) cells, suggesting the potential impact of HETEs on renal blood flow, GFR and urinary sodium excretion rates [127]. CYP4A11 is a key enzyme in the synthesis of 20-HETE. Both CYP4A and CYP4F belong to the CYP4 gene family, which catalyzes the conversion of arachidonic acid to 20-HETE [128]. The expression of CYP4A protein and the production of 20-HETE were significantly higher in the renal cortex and outer medulla of Dahl S salt-sensitive rats that fed either a low-salt or high-salt diet, indicating that the increased levels of renal 20-HETE in Dahl S rats promoted sodium retention and the development of salt sensitive hypertension [129]. Normalization of the 20-HETE levels with fibrates or transfer of wild-type CYP4A genes in congenic Dahl S strains is of great significance for inhibiting the progression of proteinuria and renal injury [129–131]. In the kidney, especially in the renal cortex, CYP4A also increases pressure natriuresis in the Dahl salt-sensitive rat [132]. The amount of 20-HETE metabolites in the CYP450 pathway produced by the extra renal medullary microsomes of salt-sensitive (SS/Jr) rats was significantly lower than that of salt-resistant (SR/Jr) rats [133].

In contrast, pharmacological inhibition of 20-HETE production in the outer medulla of the kidney in Lewis rats renders salt-sensitive [134], which means 20-HETE is a powerful vasoconstrictor in the kidney [135,136]. In renal microvessels, 20-HETE can strongly inhibit the activity of Na^+/K^+-ATPase and is a highly effective vasoconstrictor [137]. Increased production of 20-HETE in the renal microcirculation will decrease glomerular capillary pressure and GFR [124,138]. More importantly, 20-HETE can also reduce the pressure of post-glomerular circulation and ultimately promote the development of hypertension [138]. Interestingly though, 20-HETE-mediated increases in renal vascular resistance also reduce stress during glomerular circulation, thereby preventing the occurrence of glomerular damage caused by hypertension [139]. Therefore, when the synthesis of 20-HETE in the kidney is disturbed, the self-regulation of renal blood flow and the renal tubule-glomerular feedback system will be affected, resulting in reduced ion transport, increasing the difficulty of blood pressure control, and eventually aggravating glomerulonephritis and renal tubular interstitial nephritis [124]. The effect of 20-HETE on vascular function causes an ischemia-reperfusion injury (IRI) change that prolongs vasoconstriction after reperfusion and increased I/R injury [140]. It is well known that IRI is the most common cause of AKI, and 20-HETE production is elevated after renal ischemia (I/R) [141–143]. Use of 20-HETE analogues at a lower dosage can reduce the elevated plasma creatinine levels after I/R injury. In addition, 20-HETE analogues preconditioning reduced the area of tubular epithelial necrosis after I/R injury [143]. Moreover, 20-HETE can also be used to attenuate IRI by increasing medullary oxygen cooperation because it increases medullary blood flow and inhibits the renal tubular sodium transport [143,144]. On the other hand, in the kidney, 20-HETE overexpression significantly aggravated cell damage caused by I/R damage, which was mediated by the activation of caspase-3 and partly by enhanced CYP4A-producing free radicals [140]. Thus, the relationship between 20-HETE and AKI may be further clarified. 20-HETE may also promote the progression of renal inflammation by mediating apoptosis [145,146]. Studies have proved that CYP4A and NADPH oxidase expression was up-regulated in glomeruli of diabetic OVE26 mice [145]. And hyperglycemia increases 20-HETE production and enhances 20-HETE-dependent ROS formation and apoptosis in the mouse podocytes and rat tubuli epithelial cells, while 20-HETE blockade reduces ROS and improves apoptosis and albuminuria [145,146]. Recent research indicated that 20-HETE can increase the TRPC6 activity in podocytes, secondary to podocytes and activate ROS production [147]. Activation of TRPC6 results in the disappearance of the foot processes, but eliminates the detachment of podocyte [148]. Similar to 20-HETE, the correlation between 19-HETE and renal inflammation is mainly achieved through its effects on renal hemodynamics and blood pressure, which will not be repeated here [149].

3.3. LTs/LXs and Renal Inflammation

As the major metabolite of the LOX pathway, LTs and LXs both play considerable roles in kidney inflammation. LTs are a class of powerful chemotactic molecules that regulate leukocyte migration and activation [150]. Current studies have confirmed increases of LTs and LXs in the kidneys after ischemia, which further mediates a series of inflammatory reactions leading to the kidney damage [151]. More importantly, studies have shown that renal tissue can produce LTs without relying on circulating inflammatory cells [152]. The action of LTB_4 on neutrophil aggregation and infiltration and kidney tissue damage in the rat iARF model was first reported. In the rat kidney ischemia-reperfusion (I/R) model, LTB_4 played a leading role in the polymorphonuclear neutrophils (PMNs) [153]. LTB_4-dependent cells migrate to ischemic renal parenchyma and activate neutrophils, which can rapidly up-regulate leukocyte adhesion molecules, and then promote the initial infiltration of PMNs. Activated neutrophils induce endothelial cell injury, and vasodilation is blocked, further aggravating ischemic tubulointerstitial damage and causing a vicious circle of renal tissue damage [153]. A recent study by Landgraf on LTB_4-mediated renal tissue inflammation has found that LTB_4 and LTD_4 inhibited the endocytosis of albumin in LLC-PK1 cells (pig kidney cells), attenuating the activation of protein kinase C (PKC) and protein kinase B (PKB) and thereby reducing the absorption of albumin. Meanwhile, in mice models, LTs inhibited the secretion of the anti-inflammatory cytokine IL-10, hindered the PI-3K/PKB pathway, and caused albumin overload that finally gave rise to tubule-interstitial damage [154,155]. After a few minutes of reperfusion, PMNs were recruited and LTA_4 was immediately transformed into LTB_4 in the kidney. Once PMNs entered the interstitial space, the above mechanism will be performed at high speed, thus accelerating the extensive migration of PMNs and forming a vicious cycle of tissue damage [153]. The role of LTs in glomerular injury has also been demonstrated in the nephrotoxic serum-induced glomerular injury model, due to increased recruitment/activation of polymorphonuclear cells and increased LTB_4 production in the kidney, which eventually amplifies the reduction of glomerular filtration rate [156]. Moreover, LTB_4 and $LTC_4/D_4/E_4$ levels are both increased in patients with nephrotic syndrome (NS), and this may be the reason why the serum creatinine, diastolic blood pressure, and protein/creatinine ratio of patients are significantly reduced [157].

As another major metabolite of the LOX pathway, LXs are important endogenous anti-inflammatory lipid transmitters that have been discovered earlier and can act on a variety of cells, including neutrophils, mononuclear macrophages, mesangial cells etc., to exert complex anti-inflammatory effects [158–160]. In glomerulonephritis, LXA_4 inhibits LTs and reduces further infiltration of leukocytes [161,162]. In acute poststreptococcal glomerulonephritis (APSGN), one of the crucial pathological effects is the infiltration of neutrophils and monocytes in the glomeruli during the acute phase [163]. In vitro experiments with human mesangial cells showed that very low concentrations of LXA_4 (1–10 nmol/L) inhibited the expression of cell fibrosis-related genes induced by platelet-derived growth factor and connective tissue growth factor [164]. Leukocytes infiltrate and LTB_4 synthesis increases in rat kidneys at the early stage after nephrotoxic serum injection. At the same time, IL-4 and IL-13 produced by Th2 cells stimulate glomerular expression of LOX and synthesis of 15S-HETE and LXA_4. The later inhibits LTB_4 signaling, reduces leukocyte chemotaxis and transforms neutrophil infiltration into mononuclear macrophage infiltration, resulting in removal of apoptotic neutrophils and repairmen of tissue damage [165,166]. Another nephritis involving LXs is Henoch-Schonlein purpura nephritis (HSPN), which is a common secondary glomerulonephritis in pediatrics [167]. In HSPN, both plasma and urinary levels of LTB_4 and LTE_4 increase, while LXA_4 levels decrease, indicating that endogenous LXA_4 deficiency may be one of the causes of HSPN (which provides a basis for exploring new methods for the treatment of HSPN) [167]. Recent studies have shown that LXs inhibited the increase of renal/body weight ratio in diabetic animals and also reduced the glomerular dilatation and mesangial matrix deposition, in both high-fat diet-induced diabetes mouse model and unilateral ureteral obstruction (UUO) mouse model [168,169]. In addition, LXs can significantly reduce proteinuria and play an important role in reversing the CKD induced in diabetic $ApoE^{-/-}$ male mice [170]. In cultured human renal epithelial cells, treatment with LXs reduced TNF-α-driven Egr-1 activation, which may regulate the inflammation of kidney disease [170] [171,172]. As Egr-1 activity is elevated in renal tubular cells in patients with renal failure [173], this may be related to Egr-1, which mediates the TGF-β signaling pathway in the kidney, immune cell infiltration, and regulates the NF-κB activity and cytokine/chemokine expression in the kidney [173]. Brennan et al. had identified that Egr-1 as a downstream target for LXs, besides, they also confirmed the interaction between LXs and Egr-1 in studies of human renal tubular epithelial cells [170]. In summary, LXs have a significant positive effect on inhibiting kidney inflammation.

3.4. *EETs and Renal Inflammation*

It has been reported that 14,15-EET can alleviate the proteinuria and renal dysfunction caused by cyclosporine, which may be related to the inhibition of inflammatory cells infiltration into the kidney and reduction of renal fibrosis [174]. In the rat model of renal tubule-interstitial inflammation induced by unilateral ureteral obstruction (UUO), sEH deficiency has a beneficial effect on renal fibrosis and interstitial inflammation. The molecular mechanism may be associated with lack of sEH and the reduction of EETs degradation, which inhibited the transforming growth factor (TGF)-1/Smad3 signaling, diminished infiltration of neutrophils and macrophages, prevented expression levels of NF-κB target gene proteins (TNF-α and ICAM-1), decrease cell death caused by ROS, and causes PPAR inactivation [175]. Manhiani proved that soluble epoxide hydrolase gene deletion attenuated renal injury and inflammation with DOCA-salt hypertension [176]. In the kidney, EET has anti-inflammatory effects by blocking the activation of NF-kB and inhibiting the progression of renal inflammation by reducing renal macrophage infiltration [176]. Research also showed that, increased production of EET prevented microalbuminuria and kidney inflammation in the hyperglycemic overweight mice [177]. However, in the kidney, EET/DHET-ratios were increased in sEH knockout mice, but surprisingly, plasma creatinine concentration and IRI were higher than in the control group, which may be due to the formation of 20-HETE that eliminates the potentially beneficial effects of EET degradation [178]. In an I/R-induced AKI mouse model, the administration of 14,15-EET alleviated the dilated renal tubules, leading to an obvious reduction in plasma Cr, TNF-α and IL-6 [179]. These effects, discovered in I/R-caused AKI mice, may be due to the 14,15-EET reversing the I/R-induced declination of p-GSK3β expression, which induced the ratio of p-GSK3β/GSK3β back to a normal level [180]. In addition, the CYP450-derived eicosanoids could activate the eNOS and NO release. 14,15-EET can activate the endothelial cell NO synthase (eNOS) and NO release by blocking the Ca^{2+}-activated K^+, which eventually caused afferent arteries dilatation and reduces renal inflammation [181]. 5,6-EET, found in the kidneys of rabbits, is involved in the metabolism of two types of vasodilators, one being PGE_2/PGI_2 and the other being the adenosine analogue 5,6-epoxy-PGE [182]. In contrast, in the rat I/R kidney model, 5,6-EET caused COX-dependent renal vasoconstriction, whereas in isolated rat kidneys, 5,6-EET dilated blood vessels. In spontaneously hypertensive rats, 5,6-EET and 11,12-EET induced renal vasodilation more than 2 times greater than in Wistar Kyoto rats [183]. Stimulation of EETs activating adenosine 2A (A2A) may be an important mechanism for regulating microvascular tension in glomeruli [184]. It has been reported that 11,12-EET may represent an A2A-mediated mediator of glomerular microvascular expansion in rats. In rat glomerular pre-microvasculature, EET release was an important step in the activation of A2A receptors and adenylyl cyclase activation, and EETs mediated the activation of the Gs alpha protein by stimulating mono-ADP-ribosyltransferase [185]. The mechanism by which 11,12-EET dilates the afferent arterioles is possibly due to the phosphorylation of protein phosphatase 2A activity and Ca^{2+}-activated K^+ channels [186]. Recent research has proven that 11,12-EET is a major product of Cyp2c44 in mice, which is involved in regulating the excretion of epithelial sodium in the collecting duct. Cyp2c44 in the collecting duct can promote the excretion of Na^+ in the kidney under high salt or high K^+ environment by inhibiting epithelial Na^+ channel (ENaC), thus preventing excessive Na^+ absorption, suggesting that 11,12-EET may indirectly affect the renal inflammation through its role in regulation of blood pressure [187]. It is worth mentioning that 8,9-EET has a unique protective effect on the glomerulus [188]. Exogenous 8,9-EET (1–1000 nM) dose-dependently prevented a circulating permeability factor (FSPF)-induced increase in the glomerular albumin permeability [188]. The other three EET regioisomers, 8,9-EET metabolite, 8,9-dihydroxyeicosatrienoic acid and unrelated 11,14-eicosadienoic acid were ineffective, indicating the specificity of 8,9-EET for glomerular protection [188]. More importantly, a synthetic analog of 8,9-EET containing a double bond antagonized the effect of 8,9-EET on FSPF-induced increase in glomerular albumin permeability. These results indicate that the development of stable analogs of 8,9-EET may make sense to the effective management of glomerular dysfunction [188].

4. Treatments

A number of drugs for kidney inflammation based on the AA metabolic pathway are in the early stages of development for human disease treatment, and their study output is limited. The treatment of kidney disease based on AA is varied and many factors are involved, so here we only introduce strategies that are relevant to humans (Table 1).

Table 1. Drugs related to AA metabolism for kidney inflammation.

Compounds	Species	Targets	Kidney Disease	Outcome	Reference
Cyclosporine+ methylprednisolone	Human	Calcineurin and corticosteroid hormone receptor	IMN	Proteinuria ↓ PLA2R Ab ↓ Infiltration of defense cells ↓	[189]
Tacrolimus+corticosteroids, corticosteroids+cyclophosphamide, or corticosteroids alone.	Human	Peptidyl-prolyl isomerase and glucocorticoid receptors	IMN	Proteinuria ↓ Serum albumin ↑ Glomerular PLA2R ↓ Serum PLA2R-Ab ↓ Infiltration of defense cells ↑	[190]
Rituximab	Human	Pan-B-cell marker CD20	IMN/IgA Nephritis	Proteinuria ↓ GFR ↑ Serum albumin ↑ PLA2R Ab ↓ Infiltration of defense cells ↓	[191–193]
Prednisolone	Human	glucocorticoid receptors	IMN	GFR ↑ Proteinuria ↓ Serum albumin ↑ PLA2R Ab ↓ Infiltration of defense cells ↓	[194]
Cyclophosphamide or +corticosteroids	Human	glucocorticoid receptors (for corticosteroids)	IMN/IgA Nephritis	GFR ↑ Proteinuria ↓ Serum albumin ↑ PLA2R Ab ↓ Infiltration of defense cells ↓	[193,194]
Aspirin	Mouse and Human	COX-1/COX-2	AKI	GFR ↑ Serum creatinine ↓ Urinary output ↑ Proteinuria ↓	[195,196]
Ibuprofen	Human	COX-1/COX-2	ATIN	Pain control ↓	[197,198]
Nimesulide	Rats and Human	COX-1/COX-2	ATIN	Plasma renin activity ↓ Aldosterone level ↓ Urinary PTE2 level ↓	[199]
Indomethacin	Human	COX-1/COX-2	Renal failure	IL-6 ↓ IL-10 ↓	[199]
Carprofen	Human	COX-2	Renal failure	IL-1β ↓	[199]
Diclofenac acid	Rats and Human	COX1/COX2	Renal cancer	PGE2 level ↓	[200]
Zileuton	Human Mesangial Cells	LOX/COX-2	Renal cancer	Serum creatinine ↓ Interstitial fibrosis ↓	[201]
Licofelone	Mouse and Human	5-LOX/COX	Glomerulonephritis	IL-18 ↓ PGE2 ↓	[201]
Baicalein	Mouse	12/15-LOX	Diabetic nephropathy	12-HETE ↓ IL-6 ↓ Proteinuria ↓	[202]
PVPA	Rats	CYP450	Acute and chronic glomerulonephritis	Proteinuria ↓ Apoptosis in tubular epithelial cells ↓ Generation of reactive oxygen species ↓	[174]

4.1. *Phospholipase-Associated Therapy*

Current research has suggested that the M-type phospholipase A2 receptor (PLA_2R) is sensitive and specific for idiopathic membranous nephropathy (MN). Serum phospholipase A_2 receptor antibody (PLA_2R Ab) and circulating anti-phospholipase A_2 receptor antibodies (anti-PLA2R Abs) are now regarded as a valuable indicator of prognosis for patients with nephritis, especially in patients with idiopathic membranous nephropathy (IMN) [203,204]. IMN is one of the most common causes of adult primary NS. The KDIGO guidelines have recommend treatment with glucocorticoids and immunosuppressive agents for IMN [191,194]. Beck et al. reported that 35 patients with IMN were treated with rituximab (the anti- autoimmune disease drug), within whom 71% of patients were serum anti-PLA_2R -positive. After 12 months of rituximab therapy, serum anti-PLA_2R decreased or disappeared in 17 (68%) of these patients. After 12 months and 24 months of therapy, the rates of complete remission (CR) and partial response (PR) were 59% and 88%, respectively, and the decrease in antibody titer was earlier than the remission of proteinuria [189]. An earlier study of 37 biopsy confirmed IMN patients indicated that, after receiving standard immunosuppressive therapy (cyclosporine combined with methylprednisolone), the titer of PLA_2R-Ab positive patients gradually decreased with an ameliorated proteinuria [190]. A retrospective study that includes 113 IMN patients showed that, the tacrolimus (TAC) and corticosteroids, corticosteroids and cyclophosphamide (CYC) and corticosteroids alone respectively can decrease the serum PLA_2R-Ab titer and proteinuria in IMN patients [192]. As a conventional anti-tumor drug, rituximab seems to have a favorable result on MN [205]. 8 months after receiving rituximab, 22 patients with PLA_2R-related MN showed a decrease of proteinuria and PLA_2R Ab titer. At the meantime, renal function remained stable, and serum albumin increased [205]. Similar results were obtained in Beck's study, which suggested that rituximab can inhibit the progression of IMN by lowering the PLA_2R Ab titer [189]. Lowered PLA_2R Ab titer could also be achieved by oral administration of prednisolone or cyclical cyclophosphamide (CTX) or cyclophosphamide or mycophenolate mofetil (MMF) in combination with steroids in IMN patients, showing a beneficial result with elevated glomerular filtration rate (eGFR) [191,193]. A recent study showed that combination with corticosteroids and rituximab also decreases the serum creatinine and PLA_2R-Ab level [206]. However, one cannot ignore the fact that steroid treatment aggravated tubule-interstitial fibrosis in patients with acute interstitial nephritis [207]. A recent study also reported that corticosteroid treatment seems to increase the recurrence rate of TIN [208], suggesting that the PLA_2R-Ab therapy may only work in IMN patients. The data from this research seems contradictory, especially the small sample size, which makes it difficult to draw firm conclusions regarding their outcomes. Therefore, the prospect of corticosteroids for the anti- PLA_2R-Ab therapy needs more research and exploration.

4.2. COX-Associated Therapy

Nonsteroidal anti-inflammatory drugs (NSAIDs) are the main COX inhibitors. Their common mechanism of action is the inhibition of COX, and the most important result of this inhibition is the reduction of the production of PGs, thus playing anti-inflammatory, pain relieving and antipyretic roles [209]. COX inhibitors fall into two broad categories: non-specific COX inhibitors and specific COX-2 inhibitors. Among them, aspirin, ibuprofen, naproxen, etc. are usually used as non-specific COX inhibitors in the treatment of nephritis. Certain functional groups of COX-2 inhibitors (coxibs) can insert into the hydrophobic cavity formed by some amino acid residues of COX-2, causing the loss of their catalytic function [18]. In this case, AA cannot perform biological transformations under the catalysis of COX-2, thus blocking the synthesis of PGs as well as the inflammatory process [58]. Aspirin, also known as acetylsalicylic acid, is a well-known antipyretic analgesic that inhibits platelet aggregation and prevents thrombosis, which could also be used in kidney inflammatory diseases [210]. Aspirin is a non-specific COX inhibitor that inhibits both COX-1 and COX-2, which has a good effect on the prevention of primary and secondary thrombosis [211–213]. Aspirin treatment in MRL/MpJ-Fas^{lpr}/J (MRL/lpr) mouse could alleviate LN [195] and reduce the risk of platelet aggregation and micro-embolization, which may improve the GFR during renal perfusion, thereby improving kidney function [196]. At the same time, perioperative aspirin can reduce the thromboxane level in the urine, which is a powerful vasoconstrictor, and improve renal function [196]. A large prospective cohort study of more than 5000 patients undergoing cardiac surgery indicated that patients taking aspirin had a lower incidence of AKI than patients who did not take aspirin ($P < 0.001$) [214]. Above all, the incidence of renal failure was reduced by 74% in those who were taking aspirin [214]. However, according to a recent study, low-dose aspirin oral intake was shown to have no significant effect on kidney function during the 15 years after kidney transplantation [215]. This may be because aspirin can be rapidly hydrolyzed to salicylate immediately, a product that has an almost negligible effect on COX [210]. Further, the results found that aspirin increased the risk of massive hemorrhage and further increased the risk of subsequent AKI [197]. Since the findings in numerous studies are contradictory, additional research on the value of aspirin for kidney inflammation is essential.

As the most widely used NSAID, ibuprofen is the first choice for the treatment of inflammatory pain [198]. Compared with other NSAIDs and coxibs, ibuprofen has fewer side effects on the gastrointestinal tract and a relatively low incidence of liver and kidney damage [216]. However, the amount of urine was obviously reduced after the first day of treatment with ibuprofen in premature infants, and the serum creatinine concentration was significantly increased on the third day of treatment [217]. There seems to be a latent relationship between ibuprofen and acute tubule-interstitial nephritis (ATIN), which is a major factor contributing to the acute renal insufficiency that must be kept in mind when it is used for treatment [199,218,219].

Nimesulide, another NSAID, has selective inhibition of COX-2 and qualitative inhibition of COX-1, and the principal effect of nimesulide on kidney inflammation mainly involves renal hemodynamics and electrolyte excretion. The use of nimesulide in healthy volunteers during long-term use of furosemide causes a brief and acute decline in renal hemodynamics and attenuated the natriuretic, kaliuretic and diuretic effects of furosemide [220]. Nimesulide reduced the plasma renin activity, aldosterone levels, and urinary PTE_2 levels [220]. Meanwhile, diuretic-induced renin activity was attenuated by nimesulide. This suggests that nimesulide protects kidney function by allowing sodium and potassium retention [220]. However, it is interesting to remark that there was no significant change in serum creatinine and Tamm-Horsfall glycoprotein (THG) concentrations as well as no significant ffect on GFR after nimesulide in 16 healthy human volunteers [221]. The weak effect of nimesulide on renal toxicity may suggest that it has no strong inhibitory effect on renal COX at the therapeutic dose, which is similar to the results from Ceserani et al., who showed that nimesulide did not dramatically reduced urinary PTE_2 excretion in rats [222].

Several other NSAIDs also plays active role in the treatment of nephritis. Carprofen, an inhibitor of COX-mediated PG synthesis, increased the thick ascending limb of the loop of Henle at the tubular level and increased resorption of solute in the medullary segment of the upper extremity, thereby reducing sodium and chlorine excretion and potentially improving GFR or overall excretion of solute in the human kidney [200]. Diclofenac acid can reduce the recurrence survival rate and improve the survival rate of patients with renal cancer after surgery, which may be related to the fact that diclofenac acid inhibits the production of PGE_2, which in turn inhibited the process by which PGE_2 alters intracellular cyclic adenosine monophosphate levels to reduce the number and activity of natural killer cells [223–225].

However, as a COX-2 inhibitor, rofecoxib increases the risk of major cardiovascular events during treatment [226]. In addition, naproxen and celecoxib were related to the occurrence of AKI [227]. Studies have associated people who take naproxen, regardless of the dosage, with a higher risk of nephrotic syndrome and AIN [228]. Other NSAIDs may also have potential adverse effects on renal function [229], such as indomethacin, which can cause acute sodium retention in healthy adults and reduce GFR levels by inhibiting COX [230]. Studies have shown that live-donor nephrectomy patients that were treated with ketolic acid had significant increases of urinary albumin/creatinine ratio after 1 year and is an independent risk factor for reducing GFR (odds ratio 1.38) [231]. A study from *Lancet* indicated that NSAIDs, such as rofecoxib, celecoxib, ibuprofen, naproxen, and diclofenac, increase the risk of vascular events during treatment [232]. However, it has also been pointed out that all COX-2 inhibitors did not significantly promote renal events and arrhythmia events [233]. These findings provide insight for future research, and prospective clinical trials are needed to assess the curative effect and safety of NSAIDs for the treatment of renal inflammation.

4.3. LOX-Associated Therapy

The research related to LOX-associated therapy is mostly studied on experimental animals, and when it comes to human studies, zileuton is often mentioned. Zileuton blocks the conversion of AA to LTB_4 by inhibiting the 5-LOX activity and is often used for the prevention of inflammation-related diseases and for cancer treatment [234]. However, whether zileuton could be used to treat renal inflammation in humans still needs to be further confirmed by clinical trials. Licofelone is a novel dual anti-inflammatory drug that inhibits both COX and 5-LOX. A study has indicated that licofelone improved inflammation in human mesangial cells (HMCs) exposed to IL-18 in a dose-dependent manner, through inhibiting COX-2 enzyme activity and reducing PGE_2 release in HMCs [201]. Similarly, licofelone inhibited IL-18-induced 5-LOX enzyme activity and thereby reduces leukotriene release. In addition, licofelone blocked IL-18-induced phosphorylation of p38 proliferation protein kinase, inhibited the expression of monocyte chemoattractant protein 1 and interferon-γ. Licofelone also suppressed mesangial cell proliferation caused by IL-18 [201]. These results indicate that licofelone alleviates human glomerular inflammation by inhibiting IL-18-induced proinflammatory cytokine release and cell proliferation. A more exciting result was that licofelone inhibited IL-18-induced mesangial cell proliferation, and the results indicated that licofelone might be effective for the treatment of glomerulonephritis in children [201]. 2,3-diarylxanthones, dual inhibitors of COX and 5-LOX, are capable of preventing the production of LTB_4 in human neutrophils as well as decreasing PGE_2 production in human whole blood in a concentration-dependent manner [235]. According to the current results, the effect of lox-related drugs in regulating inflammation is still in the experimental study stage. Baicalein, a 12/15-LOX inhibitor, was demonstrated to prevent the elevation in renal 12-HETE production and reduce renal inflammation in strptozotocin-induced diabetic mice [202].

4.4. CYP450/sEH-Associated Therapy

There are two pharmacological approaches that have been used to chronically elevate endogenous levels of EETs in order to evaluate their renal and vascular protective effects in vivo. One approach is to increase the levels of EETs by inducing epoxygenases with fibric acid derivatives such as clofibrate, fenofibrate, and bezafibrate [236]. Fenofibrate has been shown to strongly induce renal protein expression of CYP2C23, a major CYP epoxygenase in the rat kidney, and increase the renal epoxygenase activity [236]. We have previously reported that a CYP450 inducer, gemfibrozil, has shown positive effects on CYP2C-related non-alcoholic steatotic hepatitis [237]. More importantly, the potential link between dyslipidemia and renal inflammation also reveals the potential values of fibric acid derivatives for the treatment of renal inflammation [238,239] among diabetic dyslipidemia patients [240–242]. However, some reports suggested that, the combined action of metamizole and gemfibrozil could synergistically affect the proximal tubule and increase the chances of renal damage [243]. Some studies have shown that the epoxyeicosatrienoic acid analog can effectively slow down the kidney damage associated with oxidative stress, inflammation, and endoplasmic reticulum stress [244,245]. For example, a new oral drug, PVPA, reduces the proteinuria and renal dysfunction caused by cyclosporine, inhibits the inflammatory cell infiltration in the kidney, and reduces the renal fibrosis [174]. Warfarin, an anticoagulant, is mainly metabolized by CYP2C [246–248], which can inhibit the proliferation of mesangial cells by interfering with the activation of Gas6, and plays an important role in the treatment of various human kidney diseases, such as acute and chronic glomerulonephritis and diabetic nephropathy [249].

Another approach to elevate EETs is to inhibit the conversion of EETs to their less active metabolites by soluble epoxide hydrolase (sEH) [250]. sEH plays a major role in several diseases, including hypertension, cardiac hypertrophy, arteriosclerosis [251]. Because of its possible role in cardiovascular and other diseases, sEH is being pursued as a pharmacological target, and potent small molecule inhibitors are available [252]. Such inhibitors, like UC1153 (AR9281) and GSK2256294, were taken to clinical trials for treatment of hypertension and chronic obstructive pulmonary disease respectively [252]. However, even with the promise of epoxygenase metabolites to protect the kidney and vasculature, further research in this area is necessary in view of the small number of trials on humans.

5. Conclusions

The present review aims to discuss the effect of AA metabolism on kidney inflammation, as well as to provide a theoretical basis for the treatment of kidney inflammation. AA metabolism and kidney inflammation are closely linked in multiple ways. Through a summary of previous studies, our conclusions help us to understand the effects of AA metabolism on the kidney in several ways and provide the therapeutical treatment for renal inflammation. However, the studies on the treatment of kidney inflammation based on AA metabolism require a large sample of randomized controlled trails to elucidate their efficacy.

Author Contributions: Z.W., and Z.G. conceived and designed the article; T.W., X.F., Z.G., Z.W., Q.C. and D.W. wrote the paper. J.K.P and D.W. edited the manuscript. All authors read and approved the manuscript.

References

1. Van Dorp, D.A. Essential fatty acid metabolism. *Proc. Nutr. Soc.* **1975**, *34*, 279–286. [CrossRef] [PubMed]
2. Sperling, R.I.; Benincaso, A.I.; Knoell, C.T.; Larkin, J.K.; Austen, K.F.; Robinson, D.R. Dietary omega-3 polyunsaturated fatty acids inhibit phosphoinositide formation and chemotaxis in neutrophils. *J. Clin. Investig.* **1993**, *91*, 651–660. [CrossRef] [PubMed]
3. De Jonge, H.W.; Dekkers, D.H.; Lamers, J.M. Polyunsaturated fatty acids and signalling via phospholipase C-beta and A2 in myocardium. *Mol. Cell. Biochem.* **1996**, *157*, 199–210. [CrossRef] [PubMed]
4. Calder, P.C. Marine omega-3 fatty acids and inflammatory processes: Effects, mechanisms and clinical relevance. *Biochim. Biophys. Acta* **2015**, *1851*, 469–484. [CrossRef] [PubMed]

5. Yates, C.M.; Calder, P.C.; Ed Rainger, G. Pharmacology and therapeutics of omega-3 polyunsaturated fatty acids in chronic inflammatory disease. *Pharmacol. Ther.* **2014**, *141*, 272–282. [CrossRef] [PubMed]
6. Rae, S.A.; Davidson, E.M.; Smith, M.J. Leukotriene B4, an inflammatory mediator in gout. *Lancet* **1982**, *2*, 1122–1124. [CrossRef]
7. Arachidonic acid, analgesics, and asthma. *Lancet* **1981**, *2*, 1266–1267.
8. Rand, A.A.; Barnych, B.; Morisseau, C.; Cajka, T.; Lee, K.S.S.; Panigrahy, D.; Hammock, B.D. Cyclooxygenase-derived proangiogenic metabolites of epoxyeicosatrienoic acids. *Proc. Natl. Acad. Sci. USA* **2017**, *114*, 4370–4375. [CrossRef]
9. Kopp, B.T.; Thompson, R.; Kim, J.; Konstan, R.; Diaz, A.; Smith, B.; Shrestha, C.; Rogers, L.K.; Hayes, D., Jr.; Tumin, D.; et al. Secondhand smoke alters arachidonic acid metabolism and inflammation in infants and children with cystic fibrosis. *Thorax* **2019**, *74*, 237–246. [CrossRef]
10. Chauhan, G.; Roy, K.; Kumar, G.; Kumari, P.; Alam, S.; Kishore, K.; Panjwani, U.; Ray, K. Distinct influence of COX-1 and COX-2 on neuroinflammatory response and associated cognitive deficits during high altitude hypoxia. *Neuropharmacology* **2019**, *146*, 138–148. [CrossRef]
11. Goldstein, A.R.; White, R.H.; Akuse, R.; Chantler, C. Long-term follow-up of childhood Henoch-Schonlein nephritis. *Lancet* **1992**, *339*, 280–282. [CrossRef]
12. Murakami, M.; Nakatani, Y.; Kuwata, H.; Kudo, I. Cellular components that functionally interact with signaling phospholipase A(2)s. *Biochim. Biophys. Acta* **2000**, *1488*, 159–166. [CrossRef]
13. Dubois, R.N.; Abramson, S.B.; Crofford, L.; Gupta, R.A.; Simon, L.S.; Van De Putte, L.B.; Lipsky, P.E. Cyclooxygenase in biology and disease. *FASEB J.* **1998**, *12*, 1063–1073. [CrossRef] [PubMed]
14. Lambert, I.H.; Hoffmann, E.K.; Christensen, P. Role of prostaglandins and leukotrienes in volume regulation by Ehrlich ascites tumor cells. *J. Membr. Biol.* **1987**, *98*, 247–256. [CrossRef] [PubMed]
15. Lipsky, P.E.; Brooks, P.; Crofford, L.J.; DuBois, R.; Graham, D.; Simon, L.S.; van de Putte, L.B.; Abramson, S.B. Unresolved issues in the role of cyclooxygenase-2 in normal physiologic processes and disease. *Arch. Intern. Med.* **2000**, *160*, 913–920. [CrossRef] [PubMed]
16. Ricciotti, E.; Yu, Y.; Grosser, T.; Fitzgerald, G.A. COX-2, the dominant source of prostacyclin. *Proc. Natl. Acad. Sci. USA* **2013**, *110*, E183. [CrossRef] [PubMed]
17. Thuresson, E.D.; Lakkides, K.M.; Rieke, C.J.; Sun, Y.; Wingerd, B.A.; Micielli, R.; Mulichak, A.M.; Malkowski, M.G.; Garavito, R.M.; Smith, W.L. Prostaglandin endoperoxide H synthase-1: The functions of cyclooxygenase active site residues in the binding, positioning, and oxygenation of arachidonic acid. *J. Biol. Chem.* **2001**, *276*, 10347–10357. [CrossRef]
18. Hawkey, C.J. COX-2 inhibitors. *Lancet* **1999**, *353*, 307–314. [CrossRef]
19. Kawahara, K.; Hohjoh, H.; Inazumi, T.; Tsuchiya, S.; Sugimoto, Y. Prostaglandin E2-induced inflammation: Relevance of prostaglandin E receptors. *Biochim. Biophys. Acta* **2015**, *1851*, 414–421. [CrossRef]
20. Smith, W.L.; Garavito, R.M.; DeWitt, D.L. Prostaglandin endoperoxide H synthases (cyclooxygenases)-1 and -2. *J. Biol. Chem.* **1996**, *271*, 33157–33160. [CrossRef]
21. Naraba, H.; Murakami, M.; Matsumoto, H.; Shimbara, S.; Ueno, A.; Kudo, I.; Oh-ishi, S. Segregated coupling of phospholipases A2, cyclooxygenases, and terminal prostanoid synthases in different phases of prostanoid biosynthesis in rat peritoneal macrophages. *J. Immunol.* **1998**, *160*, 2974–2982. [PubMed]
22. Smith, W.L.; Song, I. The enzymology of prostaglandin endoperoxide H synthases-1 and -2. *Prostaglandins Other Lipid Mediat.* **2002**, *68–69*, 115–128. [CrossRef]
23. Bahia, M.S.; Katare, Y.K.; Silakari, O.; Vyas, B.; Silakari, P. Inhibitors of microsomal prostaglandin E2 synthase-1 enzyme as emerging anti-inflammatory candidates. *Med. Res. Rev.* **2014**, *34*, 825–855. [CrossRef] [PubMed]
24. Hecker, M.; Haurand, M.; Ullrich, V.; Diczfalusy, U.; Hammarstrom, S. Products, kinetics, and substrate specificity of homogeneous thromboxane synthase from human platelets: Development of a novel enzyme assay. *Arch. Biochem. Biophys.* **1987**, *254*, 124–135. [CrossRef]
25. Goetzl, E.J.; An, S.; Smith, W.L. Specificity of expression and effects of eicosanoid mediators in normal physiology and human diseases. *FASEB J.* **1995**, *9*, 1051–1058. [CrossRef] [PubMed]
26. Stenson, W.F. The universe of arachidonic acid metabolites in inflammatory bowel disease: Can we tell the good from the bad? *Curr. Opin. Gastroenterol.* **2014**, *30*, 347–351. [CrossRef] [PubMed]
27. Alhouayek, M.; Muccioli, G.G. COX-2-derived endocannabinoid metabolites as novel inflammatory mediators. *Trends Pharmacol. Sci.* **2014**, *35*, 284–292. [CrossRef]

28. Li, H.S.; Hebda, P.A.; Kelly, L.A.; Ehrlich, G.D.; Whitcomb, D.C.; Dohar, J.E. Up-regulation of prostaglandin EP4 receptor messenger RNA in fetal rabbit skin wound. *Arch. Otolaryngol. Head Neck Surg.* **2000**, *126*, 1337–1343. [CrossRef]
29. Breyer, R.M.; Bagdassarian, C.K.; Myers, S.A.; Breyer, M.D. Prostanoid receptors: Subtypes and signaling. *Annu. Rev. Pharmacol. Toxicol.* **2001**, *41*, 661–690. [CrossRef]
30. Sandulache, V.C.; Chafin, J.B.; Li-Korotky, H.S.; Otteson, T.D.; Dohar, J.E.; Hebda, P.A. Elucidating the role of interleukin 1beta and prostaglandin E2 in upper airway mucosal wound healing. *Arch. Otolaryngol. Head Neck Surg.* **2007**, *133*, 365–374. [CrossRef]
31. Bauer, J.; Ripperger, A.; Frantz, S.; Ergun, S.; Schwedhelm, E.; Benndorf, R.A. Pathophysiology of isoprostanes in the cardiovascular system: Implications of isoprostane-mediated thromboxane A2 receptor activation. *Br. J. Pharmacol.* **2014**, *171*, 3115–3131. [CrossRef] [PubMed]
32. Ekambaram, P.; Lambiv, W.; Cazzolli, R.; Ashton, A.W.; Honn, K.V. The thromboxane synthase and receptor signaling pathway in cancer: An emerging paradigm in cancer progression and metastasis. *Cancer Metast. Rev.* **2011**, *30*, 397–408. [CrossRef] [PubMed]
33. Zhou, Z.; Sun, C.; Tilley, S.L.; Mustafa, S.J. Mechanisms underlying uridine adenosine tetraphosphate-induced vascular contraction in mouse aorta: Role of thromboxane and purinergic receptors. *Vasc. Pharmacol.* **2015**, *73*, 78–85. [CrossRef] [PubMed]
34. Smith, W.L.; DeWitt, D.L.; Garavito, R.M. Cyclooxygenases: Structural, cellular, and molecular biology. *Annu. Rev. Biochem.* **2000**, *69*, 145–182. [CrossRef] [PubMed]
35. Davies, N.M.; Good, R.L.; Roupe, K.A.; Yanez, J.A. Cyclooxygenase-3: Axiom, dogma, anomaly, enigma or splice error?—Not as easy as 1, 2, 3. *J. Pharm. Pharm. Sci.* **2004**, *7*, 217–226. [PubMed]
36. Chandrasekharan, N.V.; Dai, H.; Roos, K.L.; Evanson, N.K.; Tomsik, J.; Elton, T.S.; Simmons, D.L. COX-3, a cyclooxygenase-1 variant inhibited by acetaminophen and other analgesic/antipyretic drugs: Cloning, structure, and expression. *Proc. Natl. Acad. Sci. USA* **2002**, *99*, 13926–13931. [CrossRef] [PubMed]
37. Schwab, J.M.; Beiter, T.; Linder, J.U.; Laufer, S.; Schulz, J.E.; Meyermann, R.; Schluesener, H.J. COX-3—A virtual pain target in humans? *FASEB J.* **2003**, *17*, 2174–2175. [CrossRef] [PubMed]
38. Willoughby, D.A.; Moore, A.R.; Colville-Nash, P.R. COX-1, COX-2, and COX-3 and the future treatment of chronic inflammatory disease. *Lancet* **2000**, *355*, 646–648. [CrossRef]
39. Radmark, O.; Werz, O.; Steinhilber, D.; Samuelsson, B. 5-Lipoxygenase, a key enzyme for leukotriene biosynthesis in health and disease. *Biochim. Biophys. Acta* **2015**, *1851*, 331–339. [CrossRef]
40. Mittal, M.; Kumar, R.B.; Balagunaseelan, N.; Hamberg, M.; Jegerschold, C.; Radmark, O.; Haeggstrom, J.Z.; Rinaldo-Matthis, A. Kinetic investigation of human 5-lipoxygenase with arachidonic acid. *Bioorganic Med. Chem. Lett.* **2016**, *26*, 3547–3551. [CrossRef]
41. Powell, W.S.; Gravelle, F.; Gravel, S. Metabolism of 5(S)-hydroxy-6,8,11,14-eicosatetraenoic acid and other 5(S)-hydroxyeicosanoids by a specific dehydrogenase in human polymorphonuclear leukocytes. *J. Biol. Chem.* **1992**, *267*, 19233–19241. [PubMed]
42. Mastyugin, V.; Aversa, E.; Bonazzi, A.; Vafaes, C.; Mieyal, P.; Schwartzman, M.L. Hypoxia-induced production of 12-hydroxyeicosanoids in the corneal epithelium: Involvement of a cytochrome P-4504B1 isoform. *J. Pharmacol. Exp. Ther.* **1999**, *289*, 1611–1619. [PubMed]
43. Powell, W.S.; Rokach, J. Biosynthesis, biological effects, and receptors of hydroxyeicosatetraenoic acids (HETEs) and oxoeicosatetraenoic acids (oxo-ETEs) derived from arachidonic acid. *Biochim. Biophys. Acta* **2015**, *1851*, 340–355. [CrossRef] [PubMed]
44. Shimizu, T.; Radmark, O.; Samuelsson, B. Enzyme with dual lipoxygenase activities catalyzes leukotriene A4 synthesis from arachidonic acid. *Proc. Natl. Acad. Sci. USA* **1984**, *81*, 689–693. [CrossRef] [PubMed]
45. Green, A.R.; Freedman, C.; Tena, J.; Tourdot, B.E.; Liu, B.; Holinstat, M.; Holman, T.R. 5 S,15 S-Dihydroperoxyeicosatetraenoic Acid (5,15-diHpETE) as a Lipoxin Intermediate: Reactivity and Kinetics with Human Leukocyte 5-Lipoxygenase, Platelet 12-Lipoxygenase, and Reticulocyte 15-Lipoxygenase-1. *Biochemistry* **2018**, *57*, 6726–6734. [CrossRef] [PubMed]
46. Nakao, A.; Watanabe, T.; Ohishi, N.; Toda, A.; Asano, K.; Taniguchi, S.; Nosaka, K.; Noiri, E.; Suzuki, T.; Sakai, T.; et al. Ubiquitous localization of leukotriene A4 hydrolase in the rat nephron. *Kidney Int.* **1999**, *55*, 100–108. [CrossRef] [PubMed]
47. Baba, T.; Black, K.L.; Ikezaki, K.; Chen, K.N.; Becker, D.P. Intracarotid infusion of leukotriene C4 selectively increases blood-brain barrier permeability after focal ischemia in rats. *J. Cereb. Blood Flow Metab.* **1991**, *11*, 638–643. [CrossRef] [PubMed]

48. Porro, B.; Songia, P.; Squellerio, I.; Tremoli, E.; Cavalca, V. Analysis, physiological and clinical significance of 12-HETE: A neglected platelet-derived 12-lipoxygenase product. *J. Chromatogr. B* **2014**, *964*, 26–40. [CrossRef] [PubMed]
49. Witola, W.H.; Liu, S.R.; Montpetit, A.; Welti, R.; Hypolite, M.; Roth, M.; Zhou, Y.; Mui, E.; Cesbron-Delauw, M.F.; Fournie, G.J.; et al. ALOX12 in human toxoplasmosis. *Infect. Immun.* **2014**, *82*, 2670–2679. [CrossRef]
50. Serhan, C.N.; Sheppard, K.A. Lipoxin formation during human neutrophil-platelet interactions. Evidence for the transformation of leukotriene A4 by platelet 12-lipoxygenase in vitro. *J. Clin. Investig.* **1990**, *85*, 772–780. [CrossRef]
51. Fiore, S.; Ryeom, S.W.; Weller, P.F.; Serhan, C.N. Lipoxin recognition sites. Specific binding of labeled lipoxin A4 with human neutrophils. *J. Biol. Chem.* **1992**, *267*, 16168–16176. [PubMed]
52. Edenius, C.; Haeggstrom, J.; Lindgren, J.A. Transcellular conversion of endogenous arachidonic acid to lipoxins in mixed human platelet-granulocyte suspensions. *Biochem. Biophys. Res. Commun.* **1988**, *157*, 801–807. [CrossRef]
53. Sheppard, K.A.; Greenberg, S.M.; Funk, C.D.; Romano, M.; Serhan, C.N. Lipoxin generation by human megakaryocyte-induced 12-lipoxygenase. *Biochim. Biophys. Acta* **1992**, *1133*, 223–234. [CrossRef]
54. Moreno, J.J. New aspects of the role of hydroxyeicosatetraenoic acids in cell growth and cancer development. *Biochem. Pharmacol.* **2009**, *77*, 1–10. [CrossRef] [PubMed]
55. Medzhitov, R. Origin and physiological roles of inflammation. *Nature* **2008**, *454*, 428–435. [CrossRef] [PubMed]
56. Lasker, J.M.; Chen, W.B.; Wolf, I.; Bloswick, B.P.; Wilson, P.D.; Powell, P.K. Formation of 20-hydroxyeicosatetraenoic acid, a vasoactive and natriuretic eicosanoid, in human kidney. Role of Cyp4F2 and Cyp4A11. *J. Biol. Chem.* **2000**, *275*, 4118–4126. [CrossRef] [PubMed]
57. Wang, J.F.; Zhang, C.C.; Chou, K.C.; Wei, D.Q. Structure of cytochrome p450s and personalized drug. *Curr. Med. Chem.* **2009**, *16*, 232–244. [CrossRef]
58. Nebert, D.W.; Russell, D.W. Clinical importance of the cytochromes P450. *Lancet* **2002**, *360*, 1155–1162. [CrossRef]
59. Tacconelli, S.; Patrignani, P. Inside epoxyeicosatrienoic acids and cardiovascular disease. *Front. Pharmacol.* **2014**, *5*, 239. [CrossRef]
60. Aspromonte, N.; Monitillo, F.; Puzzovivo, A.; Valle, R.; Caldarola, P.; Iacoviello, M. Modulation of cardiac cytochrome P450 in patients with heart failure. *Expert Opin. Drug Metab. Toxicol.* **2014**, *10*, 327–339. [CrossRef]
61. Shahabi, P.; Siest, G.; Visvikis-siest, S. Influence of inflammation on cardiovascular protective effects of cytochrome P450 epoxygenase-derived epoxyeicosatrienoic acids. *Drug Metab. Rev.* **2014**, *46*, 33–56. [CrossRef]
62. Alsaad, A.M.; Zordoky, B.N.; Tse, M.M.; El-Kadi, A.O. Role of cytochrome P450-mediated arachidonic acid metabolites in the pathogenesis of cardiac hypertrophy. *Drug Metab. Rev.* **2013**, *45*, 173–195. [CrossRef]
63. Bellien, J.; Joannides, R. Epoxyeicosatrienoic acid pathway in human health and diseases. *J. Cardiovasc. Pharmacol.* **2013**, *61*, 188–196. [CrossRef] [PubMed]
64. Makita, K.; Falck, J.R.; Capdevila, J.H. Cytochrome P450, the arachidonic acid cascade, and hypertension: New vistas for an old enzyme system. *FASEB J.* **1996**, *10*, 1456–1463. [CrossRef] [PubMed]
65. Zeldin, D.C.; DuBois, R.N.; Falck, J.R.; Capdevila, J.H. Molecular cloning, expression and characterization of an endogenous human cytochrome P450 arachidonic acid epoxygenase isoform. *Arch. Biochem. Biophys.* **1995**, *322*, 76–86. [CrossRef] [PubMed]
66. Luo, G.; Zeldin, D.C.; Blaisdell, J.A.; Hodgson, E.; Goldstein, J.A. Cloning and expression of murine CYP2Cs and their ability to metabolize arachidonic acid. *Arch. Biochem. Biophys.* **1998**, *357*, 45–57. [CrossRef]
67. Wu, S.; Moomaw, C.R.; Tomer, K.B.; Falck, J.R.; Zeldin, D.C. Molecular cloning and expression of CYP2J2, a human cytochrome P450 arachidonic acid epoxygenase highly expressed in heart. *J. Biol. Chem.* **1996**, *271*, 3460–3468. [CrossRef]
68. Ma, J.; Qu, W.; Scarborough, P.E.; Tomer, K.B.; Moomaw, C.R.; Maronpot, R.; Davis, L.S.; Breyer, M.D.; Zeldin, D.C. Molecular cloning, enzymatic characterization, developmental expression, and cellular localization of a mouse cytochrome P450 highly expressed in kidney. *J. Biol. Chem.* **1999**, *274*, 17777–17788. [CrossRef]
69. Zhao, X.; Imig, J.D. Kidney CYP450 enzymes: Biological actions beyond drug metabolism. *Curr. Drug Metab.* **2003**, *4*, 73–84. [CrossRef]
70. Yu, Z.; Xu, F.; Huse, L.M.; Morisseau, C.; Draper, A.J.; Newman, J.W.; Parker, C.; Graham, L.; Engler, M.M.;

Hammock, B.D.; et al. Soluble epoxide hydrolase regulates hydrolysis of vasoactive epoxyeicosatrienoic acids. *Circ. Res.* **2000**, *87*, 992–998. [CrossRef]

71. Quigley, R.; Baum, M.; Reddy, K.M.; Griener, J.C.; Falck, J.R. Effects of 20-HETE and 19(S)-HETE on rabbit proximal straight tubule volume transport. *Am. J. Physiol. Ren. Physiol.* **2000**, *278*, F949–F953. [CrossRef] [PubMed]
72. Snider, N.T.; Kornilov, A.M.; Kent, U.M.; Hollenberg, P.F. Anandamide metabolism by human liver and kidney microsomal cytochrome p450 enzymes to form hydroxyeicosatetraenoic and epoxyeicosatrienoic acid ethanolamides. *J. Pharmacol. Exp. Ther.* **2007**, *321*, 590–597. [CrossRef] [PubMed]
73. Collins, X.H.; Harmon, S.D.; Kaduce, T.L.; Berst, K.B.; Fang, X.; Moore, S.A.; Raju, T.V.; Falck, J.R.; Weintraub, N.L.; Duester, G.; et al. Omega-oxidation of 20-hydroxyeicosatetraenoic acid (20-HETE) in cerebral microvascular smooth muscle and endothelium by alcohol dehydrogenase 4. *J. Biol. Chem.* **2005**, *280*, 33157–33164. [CrossRef] [PubMed]
74. Nguyen, X.; Wang, M.H.; Reddy, K.M.; Falck, J.R.; Schwartzman, M.L. Kinetic profile of the rat CYP4A isoforms: Arachidonic acid metabolism and isoform-specific inhibitors. *Am. J. Physiol.* **1999**, *276*, R1691–R1700. [CrossRef] [PubMed]
75. Gupta, R.; Yadav, A.; Misra, R.; Aggarwal, A. Urinary prostaglandin D synthase as biomarker in lupus nephritis: A longitudinal study. *Clin. Exp. Rheumatol.* **2015**, *33*, 694–698. [PubMed]
76. Somparn, P.; Hirankarn, N.; Leelahavanichkul, A.; Khovidhunkit, W.; Thongboonkerd, V.; Avihingsanon, Y. Urinary proteomics revealed prostaglandin H(2)D-isomerase, not Zn-alpha2-glycoprotein, as a biomarker for active lupus nephritis. *J. Proteom.* **2012**, *75*, 3240–3247. [CrossRef] [PubMed]
77. Smith, E.M.D.; Eleuteri, A.; Goilav, B.; Lewandowski, L.; Phuti, A.; Rubinstein, T.; Wahezi, D.; Jones, C.A.; Marks, S.D.; Corkhill, R.; et al. A Markov Multi-State model of lupus nephritis urine biomarker panel dynamics in children: Predicting changes in disease activity. *Clin. Immunol.* **2019**, *198*, 71–78. [CrossRef] [PubMed]
78. Pellefigues, C.; Dema, B.; Lamri, Y.; Saidoune, F.; Chavarot, N.; Loheac, C.; Pacreau, E.; Dussiot, M.; Bidault, C.; Marquet, F.; et al. Prostaglandin D2 amplifies lupus disease through basophil accumulation in lymphoid organs. *Nat. Commun.* **2018**, *9*, 725. [CrossRef]
79. Pettipher, R.; Hansel, T.T.; Armer, R. Antagonism of the prostaglandin D2 receptors DP1 and CRTH2 as an approach to treat allergic diseases. *Nat. Rev. Drug Discov.* **2007**, *6*, 313–325. [CrossRef]
80. Rajakariar, R.; Hilliard, M.; Lawrence, T.; Trivedi, S.; Colville-Nash, P.; Bellingan, G.; Fitzgerald, D.; Yaqoob, M.M.; Gilroy, D.W. Hematopoietic prostaglandin D2 synthase controls the onset and resolution of acute inflammation through PGD2 and 15-deoxyDelta12 14 PGJ2. *Proc. Natl. Acad. Sci. USA* **2007**, *104*, 20979–20984. [CrossRef]
81. Hirai, H.; Tanaka, K.; Yoshie, O.; Ogawa, K.; Kenmotsu, K.; Takamori, Y.; Ichimasa, M.; Sugamura, K.; Nakamura, M.; Takano, S.; et al. Prostaglandin D2 selectively induces chemotaxis in T helper type 2 cells, eosinophils, and basophils via seven-transmembrane receptor CRTH2. *J. Exp. Med.* **2001**, *193*, 255–261. [CrossRef] [PubMed]
82. Togel, F.; Isaac, J.; Hu, Z.; Weiss, K.; Westenfelder, C. Renal SDF-1 signals mobilization and homing of CXCR4-positive cells to the kidney after ischemic injury. *Kidney Int.* **2005**, *67*, 1772–1784. [CrossRef] [PubMed]
83. Devi, S.; Wang, Y.; Chew, W.K.; Lima, R.; Gonzalez, N.A.; Mattar, C.N.; Chong, S.Z.; Schlitzer, A.; Bakocevic, N.; Chew, S.; et al. Neutrophil mobilization via plerixafor-mediated CXCR4 inhibition arises from lung demargination and blockade of neutrophil homing to the bone marrow. *J. Exp. Med.* **2013**, *210*, 2321–2336. [CrossRef] [PubMed]
84. Daza, L.; Kornhauser, C.; Zamora, L.; Flores, J. Captopril effect on prostaglandin E2, thromboxane B2 and proteinuria in lupus nephritis patients. *Prostaglandins Other Lipid Mediat.* **2005**, *78*, 194–201. [CrossRef] [PubMed]
85. Ito, H.; Yan, X.; Nagata, N.; Aritake, K.; Katsumata, Y.; Matsuhashi, T.; Nakamura, M.; Hirai, H.; Urade, Y.; Asano, K.; et al. PGD2-CRTH2 pathway promotes tubulointerstitial fibrosis. *J. Am. Soc. Nephrol.* **2012**, *23*, 1797–1809. [CrossRef] [PubMed]
86. Lu, Y.; Zhou, Q.; Zhong, F.; Guo, S.; Hao, X.; Li, C.; Wang, W.; Chen, N. 15-Deoxy-Delta(12,14)-prostaglandin J(2) modulates lipopolysaccharide-induced chemokine expression by blocking nuclear factor-kappaB activation via peroxisome proliferator activated receptor-gamma-independent mechanism in renal tubular epithelial cells. *Nephron Exp. Nephrol.* **2013**, *123*, 1–10. [CrossRef] [PubMed]

87. Hart, D.; Lifschitz, M.D. Renal physiology of the prostaglandins and the effects of nonsteroidal anti-inflammatory agents on the kidney. *Am. J. Nephrol.* **1987**, *7*, 408–418. [CrossRef]
88. Dunn, M.J.; Hood, V.L. Prostaglandins and the kidney. *Am. J. Physiol.* **1977**, *233*, 169–184. [CrossRef]
89. Nasrallah, R.; Hassouneh, R.; Hebert, R.L. Chronic kidney disease: Targeting prostaglandin E2 receptors. *Am. J. Physiol. Ren. Physiol.* **2014**, *307*, F243–F250. [CrossRef]
90. Breyer, M.D.; Breyer, R.M. Prostaglandin E receptors and the kidney. *Am. J. Physiol. Ren. Physiol.* **2000**, *279*, F12–F23. [CrossRef]
91. Kotnik, P.; Nielsen, J.; Kwon, T.H.; Krzisnik, C.; Frokiaer, J.; Nielsen, S. Altered expression of COX-1, COX-2, and mPGES in rats with nephrogenic and central diabetes insipidus. *Am. J. Physiol. Ren. Physiol.* **2005**, *288*, F1053–F1068. [CrossRef] [PubMed]
92. Sanchez, T.; Moreno, J.J. Role of EP(1) and EP(4) PGE(2) subtype receptors in serum-induced 3T6 fibroblast cycle progression and proliferation. *Am. J. Physiol. Cell Physiol.* **2002**, *282*, C280–C288. [CrossRef] [PubMed]
93. Moore, B.B.; Ballinger, M.N.; White, E.S.; Green, M.E.; Herrygers, A.B.; Wilke, C.A.; Toews, G.B.; Peters-Golden, M. Bleomycin-induced E prostanoid receptor changes alter fibroblast responses to prostaglandin E2. *J. Immunol.* **2005**, *174*, 5644–5649. [CrossRef] [PubMed]
94. Yokoyama, U.; Iwatsubo, K.; Umemura, M.; Fujita, T.; Ishikawa, Y. The prostanoid EP4 receptor and its signaling pathway. *Pharmacol. Rev.* **2013**, *65*, 1010–1052. [CrossRef] [PubMed]
95. Breyer, M.D.; Davis, L.; Jacobson, H.R.; Breyer, R.M. Differential localization of prostaglandin E receptor subtypes in human kidney. *Am. J. Physiol.* **1996**, *270*, F912–F918. [CrossRef] [PubMed]
96. Thibodeau, J.F.; Nasrallah, R.; Carter, A.; He, Y.; Touyz, R.; Hebert, R.L.; Kennedy, C.R.J. PTGER1 deletion attenuates renal injury in diabetic mouse models. *Am. J. Pathol.* **2013**, *183*, 1789–1802. [CrossRef]
97. Rahal, S.; McVeigh, L.I.; Zhang, Y.; Guan, Y.; Breyer, M.D.; Kennedy, C.R. Increased severity of renal impairment in nephritic mice lacking the EP1 receptor. *Can. J. Physiol. Pharmacol.* **2006**, *84*, 877–885. [CrossRef]
98. Tang, L.; Loutzenhiser, K.; Loutzenhiser, R. Biphasic actions of prostaglandin E(2) on the renal afferent arteriole: Role of EP(3) and EP(4) receptors. *Circ. Res.* **2000**, *86*, 663–670. [CrossRef]
99. Srivastava, T.; Alon, U.S.; Cudmore, P.A.; Tarakji, B.; Kats, A.; Garola, R.E.; Duncan, R.S.; McCarthy, E.T.; Sharma, R.; Johnson, M.L.; et al. Cyclooxygenase-2, prostaglandin E2, and prostanoid receptor EP2 in fluid flow shear stress-mediated injury in the solitary kidney. *Am. J. Physiol. Ren. Physiol.* **2014**, *307*, F1323–F1333. [CrossRef]
100. Mohamed, R.; Jayakumar, C.; Ranganathan, P.V.; Ganapathy, V.; Ramesh, G. Kidney proximal tubular epithelial-specific overexpression of netrin-1 suppresses inflammation and albuminuria through suppression of COX-2-mediated PGE2 production in streptozotocin-induced diabetic mice. *Am. J. Pathol.* **2012**, *181*, 1991–2002. [CrossRef]
101. Hassouneh, R.; Nasrallah, R.; Zimpelmann, J.; Gutsol, A.; Eckert, D.; Ghossein, J.; Burns, K.D.; Hebert, R.L. PGE2 receptor EP3 inhibits water reabsorption and contributes to polyuria and kidney injury in a streptozotocin-induced mouse model of diabetes. *Diabetologia* **2016**, *59*, 1318–1328. [CrossRef] [PubMed]
102. Frolich, S.; Olliges, A.; Kern, N.; Schreiber, Y.; Narumiya, S.; Nusing, R.M. Temporal expression of the PGE2 synthetic system in the kidney is associated with the time frame of renal developmental vulnerability to cyclooxygenase-2 inhibition. *Am. J. Physiol. Ren. Physiol.* **2012**, *303*, F209–F219. [CrossRef] [PubMed]
103. Nakagawa, N.; Yuhki, K.; Kawabe, J.; Fujino, T.; Takahata, O.; Kabara, M.; Abe, K.; Kojima, F.; Kashiwagi, H.; Hasebe, N.; et al. The intrinsic prostaglandin E2-EP4 system of the renal tubular epithelium limits the development of tubulointerstitial fibrosis in mice. *Kidney Int.* **2012**, *82*, 158–171. [CrossRef] [PubMed]
104. Fujino, H.; Xu, W.; Regan, J.W. Prostaglandin E2 induced functional expression of early growth response factor-1 by EP4, but not EP2, prostanoid receptors via the phosphatidylinositol 3-kinase and extracellular signal-regulated kinases. *J. Biol. Chem.* **2003**, *278*, 12151–12156. [CrossRef] [PubMed]
105. Faour, W.H.; Gomi, K.; Kennedy, C.R. PGE(2) induces COX-2 expression in podocytes via the EP(4) receptor through a PKA-independent mechanism. *Cell Signal.* **2008**, *20*, 2156–2164. [CrossRef] [PubMed]
106. Jensen, B.L.; Mann, B.; Skott, O.; Kurtz, A. Differential regulation of renal prostaglandin receptor mRNAs by dietary salt intake in the rat. *Kidney Int.* **1999**, *56*, 528–537. [CrossRef] [PubMed]
107. Stitt-Cavanagh, E.M.; Faour, W.H.; Takami, K.; Carter, A.; Vanderhyden, B.; Guan, Y.; Schneider, A.; Breyer, M.D.; Kennedy, C.R. A maladaptive role for EP4 receptors in podocytes. *J. Am. Soc. Nephrol.* **2010**, *21* 1678–1690. [CrossRef] [PubMed]
108. Yamamoto, E.; Izawa, T.; Juniantito, V.; Kuwamura, M.; Sugiura, K.; Takeuchi, T.; Yamate, J. Involvement

of endogenous prostaglandin E2 in tubular epithelial regeneration through inhibition of apoptosis and epithelial-mesenchymal transition in cisplatin-induced rat renal lesions. *Histol. Histopathol.* **2010**, *25*, 995–1007. [CrossRef]

109. Vukicevic, S.; Simic, P.; Borovecki, F.; Grgurevic, L.; Rogic, D.; Orlic, I.; Grasser, W.A.; Thompson, D.D.; Paralkar, V.M. Role of EP2 and EP4 receptor-selective agonists of prostaglandin E(2) in acute and chronic kidney failure. *Kidney Int.* **2006**, *70*, 1099–1106. [CrossRef]
110. Mohamed, R.; Jayakumar, C.; Ramesh, G. Chronic administration of EP4-selective agonist exacerbates albuminuria and fibrosis of the kidney in streptozotocin-induced diabetic mice through IL-6. *Lab. Investig.* **2013**, *93*, 933–945. [CrossRef]
111. Chang, J.; Blazek, E.; Kreft, A.F.; Lewis, A.J. Inhibition of platelet and neutrophil phospholipase A2 by hydroxyeicosatetraenoic acids (HETES). A novel pharmacological mechanism for regulating free fatty acid release. *Biochem. Pharmacol.* **1985**, *34*, 1571–1575. [CrossRef]
112. Johnson, E.N.; Brass, L.F.; Funk, C.D. Increased platelet sensitivity to ADP in mice lacking platelet-type 12-lipoxygenase. *Proc. Natl. Acad. Sci. USA* **1998**, *95*, 3100–3105. [CrossRef] [PubMed]
113. Coulon, L.; Calzada, C.; Moulin, P.; Vericel, E.; Lagarde, M. Activation of p38 mitogen-activated protein kinase/cytosolic phospholipase A2 cascade in hydroperoxide-stressed platelets. *Free Radic. Biol. Med.* **2003**, *35*, 616–625. [CrossRef]
114. Jansen, M.P.; Emal, D.; Teske, G.J.; Dessing, M.C.; Florquin, S.; Roelofs, J.J. Release of extracellular DNA influences renal ischemia reperfusion injury by platelet activation and formation of neutrophil extracellular traps. *Kidney Int.* **2017**, *91*, 352–364. [CrossRef] [PubMed]
115. Fajas, L.; Auboeuf, D.; Raspe, E.; Schoonjans, K.; Lefebvre, A.M.; Saladin, R.; Najib, J.; Laville, M.; Fruchart, J.C.; Deeb, S.; et al. The organization, promoter analysis, and expression of the human PPARgamma gene. *J. Biol. Chem.* **1997**, *272*, 18779–18789. [CrossRef] [PubMed]
116. Berger, J.P.; Akiyama, T.E.; Meinke, P.T. PPARs: Therapeutic targets for metabolic disease. *Trends Pharmacol. Sci.* **2005**, *26*, 244–251. [CrossRef] [PubMed]
117. Platt, C.; Coward, R.J. Peroxisome proliferator activating receptor-gamma and the podocyte. *Nephrol. Dial. Transplant.* **2017**, *32*, 423–433. [CrossRef]
118. Nagy, L.; Tontonoz, P.; Alvarez, J.G.; Chen, H.; Evans, R.M. Oxidized LDL regulates macrophage gene expression through ligand activation of PPARgamma. *Cell* **1998**, *93*, 229–240. [CrossRef]
119. Huang, J.T.; Welch, J.S.; Ricote, M.; Binder, C.J.; Willson, T.M.; Kelly, C.; Witztum, J.L.; Funk, C.D.; Conrad, D.; Glass, C.K. Interleukin-4-dependent production of PPAR-gamma ligands in macrophages by 12/15-lipoxygenase. *Nature* **1999**, *400*, 378–382. [CrossRef]
120. Okamura, D.M.; Lopez-Guisa, J.M.; Koelsch, K.; Collins, S.; Eddy, A.A. Atherogenic scavenger receptor modulation in the tubulointerstitium in response to chronic renal injury. *Am. J. Physiol. Ren. Physiol.* **2007**, *293*, F575–F585. [CrossRef]
121. Fruchart, J.C. Peroxisome proliferator-activated receptor-alpha (PPARalpha): At the crossroads of obesity, diabetes and cardiovascular disease. *Atherosclerosis* **2009**, *205*, 1–8. [CrossRef] [PubMed]
122. Tanaka, Y.; Kume, S.; Araki, S.; Isshiki, K.; Chin-Kanasaki, M.; Sakaguchi, M.; Sugimoto, T.; Koya, D.; Haneda, M.; Kashiwagi, A.; et al. Fenofibrate, a PPARalpha agonist, has renoprotective effects in mice by enhancing renal lipolysis. *Kidney Int.* **2011**, *79*, 871–882. [CrossRef] [PubMed]
123. Stadler, K.; Goldberg, I.J.; Susztak, K. The evolving understanding of the contribution of lipid metabolism to diabetic kidney disease. *Curr. Diabetes Rep.* **2015**, *15*, 40. [CrossRef] [PubMed]
124. Fan, F.; Muroya, Y.; Roman, R.J. Cytochrome P450 eicosanoids in hypertension and renal disease. *Curr. Opin. Nephrol. Hypertens.* **2015**, *24*, 37–46. [CrossRef] [PubMed]
125. Croft, K.D.; McGiff, J.C.; Sanchez-Mendoza, A.; Carroll, M.A. Angiotensin II releases 20-HETE from rat renal microvessels. *Am. J. Physiol. Ren. Physiol.* **2000**, *279*, F544–F551. [CrossRef] [PubMed]
126. Parmentier, J.H.; Muthalif, M.M.; Saeed, A.E.; Malik, K.U. Phospholipase D activation by norepinephrine is mediated by 12(s)-, 15(s)-, and 20-hydroxyeicosatetraenoic acids generated by stimulation of cytosolic phospholipase a2. Tyrosine phosphorylation of phospholipase d2 in response to norepinephrine. *J. Biol. Chem.* **2001**, *276*, 15704–15711. [CrossRef] [PubMed]
127. Escalante, B.; Erlij, D.; Falck, J.R.; McGiff, J.C. Effect of cytochrome P450 arachidonate metabolites on ion transport in rabbit kidney loop of Henle. *Science* **1991**, *251*, 799–802. [CrossRef]
128. Capdevila, J.H.; Falck, J.R. The CYP P450 arachidonic acid monooxygenases: From cell signaling to blood pressure regulation. *Biochem. Biophys. Res. Commun.* **2001**, *285*, 571–576. [CrossRef]

129. Williams, J.M.; Fan, F.; Murphy, S.; Schreck, C.; Lazar, J.; Jacob, H.J.; Roman, R.J. Role of 20-HETE in the antihypertensive effect of transfer of chromosome 5 from Brown Norway to Dahl salt-sensitive rats. *Am. J. Physiol. Regul. Integr. Comp. Physiol.* **2012**, *302*, R1209–R1218. [CrossRef]
130. Williams, J.M.; Sarkis, A.; Hoagland, K.M.; Fredrich, K.; Ryan, R.P.; Moreno, C.; Lopez, B.; Lazar, J.; Fenoy, F.J.; Sharma, M.; et al. Transfer of the CYP4A region of chromosome 5 from Lewis to Dahl S rats attenuates renal injury. *Am. J. Physiol. Ren. Physiol.* **2008**, *295*, F1764–F1777. [CrossRef]
131. Dahly-Vernon, A.J.; Sharma, M.; McCarthy, E.T.; Savin, V.J.; Ledbetter, S.R.; Roman, R.J. Transforming growth factor-beta, 20-HETE interaction, and glomerular injury in Dahl salt-sensitive rats. *Hypertension* **2005**, *45*, 643–648. [CrossRef] [PubMed]
132. Roman, R.J.; Ma, Y.H.; Frohlich, B.; Markham, B. Clofibrate prevents the development of hypertension in Dahl salt-sensitive rats. *Hypertension* **1993**, *21*, 985–988. [CrossRef] [PubMed]
133. Ma, Y.H.; Schwartzman, M.L.; Roman, R.J. Altered renal P-450 metabolism of arachidonic acid in Dahl salt-sensitive rats. *Am. J. Physiol.* **1994**, *267*, R579–R589. [CrossRef] [PubMed]
134. Moreno, C.; Maier, K.G.; Hoagland, K.M.; Yu, M.; Roman, R.J. Abnormal pressure-natriuresis in hypertension: Role of cytochrome P450 metabolites of arachidonic acid. *Am. J. Hypertens.* **2001**, *14*, 90S–97S. [CrossRef]
135. Alonso-Galicia, M.; Maier, K.G.; Greene, A.S.; Cowley, A.W., Jr.; Roman, R.J. Role of 20-hydroxyeicosatetraenoic acid in the renal and vasoconstrictor actions of angiotensin II. *Am. J. Physiol. Regul. Integr. Comp. Physiol.* **2002**, *283*, R60–R68. [CrossRef] [PubMed]
136. McGiff, J.C.; Quilley, J. 20-HETE and the kidney: Resolution of old problems and new beginnings. *Am. J. Physiol.* **1999**, *277*, R607–R623. [CrossRef] [PubMed]
137. Roman, R.J. P-450 metabolites of arachidonic acid in the control of cardiovascular function. *Physiol. Rev.* **2002**, *82*, 131–185. [CrossRef]
138. Williams, J.M.; Sarkis, A.; Lopez, B.; Ryan, R.P.; Flasch, A.K.; Roman, R.J. Elevations in renal interstitial hydrostatic pressure and 20-hydroxyeicosatetraenoic acid contribute to pressure natriuresis. *Hypertension* **2007**, *49*, 687–694. [CrossRef]
139. Williams, J.M.; Murphy, S.; Burke, M.; Roman, R.J. 20-hydroxyeicosatetraeonic acid: A new target for the treatment of hypertension. *J. Cardiovasc. Pharmacol.* **2010**, *56*, 336–344. [CrossRef]
140. Nilakantan, V.; Maenpaa, C.; Jia, G.; Roman, R.J.; Park, F. 20-HETE-mediated cytotoxicity and apoptosis in ischemic kidney epithelial cells. *Am. J. Physiol. Ren. Physiol.* **2008**, *294*, F562–F570. [CrossRef]
141. Lameire, N.; Vanholder, R. Pathophysiologic features and prevention of human and experimental acute tubular necrosis. *J. Am. Soc. Nephrol.* **2001**, *12* (Suppl. 17), S20–S32.
142. Fan, F.; Ge, Y.; Lv, W.; Elliott, M.R.; Muroya, Y.; Hirata, T.; Booz, G.W.; Roman, R.J. Molecular mechanisms and cell signaling of 20-hydroxyeicosatetraenoic acid in vascular pathophysiology. *Front. Biosci.* **2016**, *21*, 1427–1463.
143. Regner, K.R.; Zuk, A.; Van Why, S.K.; Shames, B.D.; Ryan, R.P.; Falck, J.R.; Manthati, V.L.; McMullen, M.E.; Ledbetter, S.R.; Roman, R.J. Protective effect of 20-HETE analogues in experimental renal ischemia reperfusion injury. *Kidney Int.* **2009**, *75*, 511–517. [CrossRef] [PubMed]
144. Roman, R.J.; Akbulut, T.; Park, F.; Regner, K.R. 20-HETE in acute kidney injury. *Kidney Int.* **2011**, *79*, 10–13. [CrossRef]
145. Eid, A.A.; Gorin, Y.; Fagg, B.M.; Maalouf, R.; Barnes, J.L.; Block, K.; Abboud, H.E. Mechanisms of podocyte injury in diabetes: Role of cytochrome P450 and NADPH oxidases. *Diabetes* **2009**, *58*, 1201–1211. [CrossRef] [PubMed]
146. Eid, S.; Maalouf, R.; Jaffa, A.A.; Nassif, J.; Hamdy, A.; Rashid, A.; Ziyadeh, F.N.; Eid, A.A. 20-HETE and EETs in diabetic nephropathy: A novel mechanistic pathway. *PLoS ONE* **2013**, *8*, e70029. [CrossRef] [PubMed]
147. Roshanravan, H.; Kim, E.Y.; Dryer, S.E. 20-Hydroxyeicosatetraenoic Acid (20-HETE) Modulates Canonical Transient Receptor Potential-6 (TRPC6) Channels in Podocytes. *Front. Physiol.* **2016**, *7*, 351. [CrossRef]
148. Kriz, W.; Lemley, K.V. A potential role for mechanical forces in the detachment of podocytes and the progression of CKD. *J. Am. Soc. Nephrol.* **2015**, *26*, 258–269. [CrossRef]
149. Omata, K.; Tsutsumi, E.; Sheu, H.L.; Utsumi, Y.; Abe, K. Effect of aging on renal cytochrome P450-dependent arachidonic acid metabolism in Dahl rats. *J. Lipid Mediat.* **1993**, *6*, 369–373. [PubMed]
150. Moore, K.P.; Wood, J.; Gove, C.; Tan, K.C.; Eason, J.; Taylor, G.W.; Williams, R. Synthesis and metabolism of cysteinyl leukotrienes by the isolated pig kidney. *Adv. Prostaglandin Thromboxane Leukot. Res.* **1991**, *21B*, 697–700. [CrossRef] [PubMed]

151. Klausner, J.M.; Paterson, I.S.; Goldman, G.; Kobzik, L.; Rodzen, C.; Lawrence, R.; Valeri, C.R.; Shepro, D.; Hechtman, H.B. Postischemic renal injury is mediated by neutrophils and leukotrienes. *Am. J. Physiol.* **1989**, *256*, F794–F802. [CrossRef] [PubMed]
152. Sener, G.; Sakarcan, A.; Sehirli, O.; Eksioglu-Demiralp, E.; Sener, E.; Ercan, F.; Gedik, N.; Yegen, B.C. Chronic renal failure-induced multiple-organ injury in rats is alleviated by the selective CysLT1 receptor antagonist montelukast. *Prostaglandins Other Lipid Mediat.* **2007**, *83*, 257–267. [CrossRef] [PubMed]
153. Noiri, E.; Yokomizo, T.; Nakao, A.; Izumi, T.; Fujita, T.; Kimura, S.; Shimizu, T. An in vivo approach showing the chemotactic activity of leukotriene B(4) in acute renal ischemic-reperfusion injury. *Proc. Natl. Acad. Sci. USA* **2000**, *97*, 823–828. [CrossRef] [PubMed]
154. Landgraf, S.S.; Silva, L.S.; Peruchetti, D.B.; Sirtoli, G.M.; Moraes-Santos, F.; Portella, V.G.; Silva-Filho, J.L.; Pinheiro, C.S.; Abreu, T.P.; Takiya, C.M.; et al. 5-Lypoxygenase products are involved in renal tubulointerstitial injury induced by albumin overload in proximal tubules in mice. *PLoS ONE* **2014**, *9*, e107549. [CrossRef] [PubMed]
155. Zimmerman, G.A.; McIntyre, T.M. Neutrophil adherence to human endothelium in vitro occurs by CDw18 (Mo1, MAC-1/LFA-1/GP 150,95) glycoprotein-dependent and -independent mechanisms. *J. Clin. Investig.* **1988**, *81*, 531–537. [CrossRef] [PubMed]
156. Yared, A.; Albrightson-Winslow, C.; Griswold, D.; Takahashi, K.; Fogo, A.; Badr, K.F. Functional significance of leukotriene B4 in normal and glomerulonephritic kidneys. *J. Am. Soc. Nephrol.* **1991**, *2*, 45–56. [PubMed]
157. Zedan, M.M.; El-Refaey, A.; Zaghloul, H.; Abdelrahim, M.E.; Osman, A.; Zedan, M.M.; Eltantawy, N. Montelukast as an add-on treatment in steroid dependant nephrotic syndrome, randomised-controlled trial. *J. Nephrol.* **2016**, *29*, 585–592. [CrossRef]
158. Planaguma, A.; Kazani, S.; Marigowda, G.; Haworth, O.; Mariani, T.J.; Israel, E.; Bleecker, E.R.; Curran-Everett, D.; Erzurum, S.C.; Calhoun, W.J.; et al. Airway lipoxin A4 generation and lipoxin A4 receptor expression are decreased in severe asthma. *Am. J. Respir. Crit. Care Med.* **2008**, *178*, 574–582. [CrossRef]
159. Cheng, X.; He, S.; Yuan, J.; Miao, S.; Gao, H.; Zhang, J.; Li, Y.; Peng, W.; Wu, P. Lipoxin A4 attenuates LPS-induced mouse acute lung injury via Nrf2-mediated E-cadherin expression in airway epithelial cells. *Free Radic. Biol. Med.* **2016**, *93*, 52–66. [CrossRef]
160. Kieran, N.E.; Maderna, P.; Godson, C. Lipoxins: Potential anti-inflammatory, proresolution, and antifibrotic mediators in renal disease. *Kidney Int.* **2004**, *65*, 1145–1154. [CrossRef]
161. Christie, P.E.; Spur, B.W.; Lee, T.H. The effects of lipoxin A4 on airway responses in asthmatic subjects. *Am. Rev. Respir. Dis.* **1992**, *145*, 1281–1284. [CrossRef] [PubMed]
162. Dahlen, S.E.; Franzen, L.; Raud, J.; Serhan, C.N.; Westlund, P.; Wikstrom, E.; Bjorck, T.; Matsuda, H.; Webber, S.E.; Veale, C.A.; et al. Actions of lipoxin A4 and related compounds in smooth muscle preparations and on the microcirculation in vivo. *Adv. Exp. Med. Biol.* **1988**, *229*, 107–130. [PubMed]
163. Wu, S.H.; Liao, P.Y.; Yin, P.L.; Zhang, Y.M.; Dong, L. Elevated expressions of 15-lipoxygenase and lipoxin A4 in children with acute poststreptococcal glomerulonephritis. *Am. J. Pathol.* **2009**, *174*, 115–122. [CrossRef] [PubMed]
164. Rodgers, K.; McMahon, B.; Mitchell, D.; Sadlier, D.; Godson, C. Lipoxin A4 modifies platelet-derived growth factor-induced pro-fibrotic gene expression in human renal mesangial cells. *Am. J. Pathol.* **2005**, *167*, 683–694. [CrossRef]
165. O'Meara, Y.M.; Brady, H.R. Lipoxins, leukocyte recruitment and the resolution phase of acute glomerulonephritis. *Kidney Int. Suppl.* **1997**, *58*, S56–S61. [PubMed]
166. Munger, K.A.; Montero, A.; Fukunaga, M.; Uda, S.; Yura, T.; Imai, E.; Kaneda, Y.; Valdivielso, J.M.; Badr, K.F. Transfection of rat kidney with human 15-lipoxygenase suppresses inflammation and preserves function in experimental glomerulonephritis. *Proc. Natl. Acad. Sci. USA* **1999**, *96*, 13375–13380. [CrossRef] [PubMed]
167. Davin, J.C.; Coppo, R. Henoch-Schonlein purpura nephritis in children. *Nat. Rev. Nephrol.* **2014**, *10*, 563–573. [CrossRef] [PubMed]
168. Borgeson, E.; Docherty, N.G.; Murphy, M.; Rodgers, K.; Ryan, A.; O'Sullivan, T.P.; Guiry, P.J.; Goldschmeding, R.; Higgins, D.F.; Godson, C. Lipoxin A(4) and benzo-lipoxin A(4) attenuate experimental renal fibrosis. *FASEB J.* **2011**, *25*, 2967–2979. [CrossRef]
169. Borgeson, E.; Johnson, A.M.; Lee, Y.S.; Till, A.; Syed, G.H.; Ali-Shah, S.T.; Guiry, P.J.; Dalli, J.; Colas, R.A.; Serhan, C.N.; et al. Lipoxin A4 Attenuates Obesity-Induced Adipose Inflammation and Associated Liver and Kidney Disease. *Cell Metab.* **2015**, *22*, 125–137. [CrossRef]

170. Brennan, E.P.; Mohan, M.; McClelland, A.; Tikellis, C.; Ziemann, M.; Kaspi, A.; Gray, S.P.; Pickering, R.; Tan, S.M.; Ali-Shah, S.T.; et al. Lipoxins Regulate the Early Growth Response-1 Network and Reverse Diabetic Kidney Disease. *J. Am. Soc. Nephrol.* **2018**, *29*, 1437–1448. [CrossRef]
171. Sun, S.; Ning, X.; Zhai, Y.; Du, R.; Lu, Y.; He, L.; Li, R.; Wu, W.; Sun, W.; Wang, H. Egr-1 mediates chronic hypoxia-induced renal interstitial fibrosis via the PKC/ERK pathway. *Am. J. Nephrol.* **2014**, *39*, 436–448. [CrossRef] [PubMed]
172. McMahon, B.; Stenson, C.; McPhillips, F.; Fanning, A.; Brady, H.R.; Godson, C. Lipoxin A4 antagonizes the mitogenic effects of leukotriene D4 in human renal mesangial cells. Differential activation of MAP kinases through distinct receptors. *J. Biol. Chem.* **2000**, *275*, 27566–27575. [CrossRef] [PubMed]
173. Ho, L.C.; Sung, J.M.; Shen, Y.T.; Jheng, H.F.; Chen, S.H.; Tsai, P.J.; Tsai, Y.S. Egr-1 deficiency protects from renal inflammation and fibrosis. *J. Mol. Med.* **2016**, *94*, 933–942. [CrossRef] [PubMed]
174. Yeboah, M.M.; Hye Khan, M.A.; Chesnik, M.A.; Sharma, A.; Paudyal, M.P.; Falck, J.R.; Imig, J.D. The epoxyeicosatrienoic acid analog PVPA ameliorates cyclosporine-induced hypertension and renal injury in rats. *Am. J. Physiol. Ren. Physiol.* **2016**, *311*, F576–F585. [CrossRef] [PubMed]
175. Kim, J.; Imig, J.D.; Yang, J.; Hammock, B.D.; Padanilam, B.J. Inhibition of soluble epoxide hydrolase prevents renal interstitial fibrosis and inflammation. *Am. J. Physiol. Ren. Physiol.* **2014**, *307*, F971–F980. [CrossRef]
176. Manhiani, M.; Quigley, J.E.; Knight, S.F.; Tasoobshirazi, S.; Moore, T.; Brands, M.W.; Hammock, B.D.; Imig, J.D. Soluble epoxide hydrolase gene deletion attenuates renal injury and inflammation with DOCA-salt hypertension. *Am. J. Physiol. Ren. Physiol.* **2009**, *297*, F740–F748. [CrossRef] [PubMed]
177. Roche, C.; Guerrot, D.; Harouki, N.; Duflot, T.; Besnier, M.; Remy-Jouet, I.; Renet, S.; Dumesnil, A.; Lejeune, A.; Morisseau, C.; et al. Impact of soluble epoxide hydrolase inhibition on early kidney damage in hyperglycemic overweight mice. *Prostaglandins Other Lipid Mediat.* **2015**, *120*, 148–154. [CrossRef]
178. Zhu, Y.; Blum, M.; Hoff, U.; Wesser, T.; Fechner, M.; Westphal, C.; Gurgen, D.; Catar, R.A.; Philippe, A.; Wu, K.; et al. Renal Ischemia/Reperfusion Injury in Soluble Epoxide Hydrolase-Deficient Mice. *PLoS ONE* **2016**, *11*, e0145645. [CrossRef]
179. Hercule, H.C.; Schunck, W.H.; Gross, V.; Seringer, J.; Leung, F.P.; Weldon, S.M.; da Costa Goncalves, A.; Huang, Y.; Luft, F.C.; Gollasch, M. Interaction between P450 eicosanoids and nitric oxide in the control of arterial tone in mice. *Arterioscler. Thromb. Vasc. Biol.* **2009**, *29*, 54–60. [CrossRef]
180. Deng, B.Q.; Luo, Y.; Kang, X.; Li, C.B.; Morisseau, C.; Yang, J.; Lee, K.S.S.; Huang, J.; Hu, D.Y.; Wu, M.Y.; et al. Epoxide metabolites of arachidonate and docosahexaenoate function conversely in acute kidney injury involved in GSK3beta signaling. *Proc. Natl. Acad. Sci. USA* **2017**, *114*, 12608–12613. [CrossRef]
181. Wang, D.; Borrego-Conde, L.J.; Falck, J.R.; Sharma, K.K.; Wilcox, C.S.; Umans, J.G. Contributions of nitric oxide, EDHF, and EETs to endothelium-dependent relaxation in renal afferent arterioles. *Kidney Int.* **2003**, *63*, 2187–2193. [CrossRef] [PubMed]
182. Ma, S.K.; Wang, Y.; Chen, J.; Zhang, M.Z.; Harris, R.C.; Chen, J.K. Overexpression of G-protein-coupled receptor 40 enhances the mitogenic response to epoxyeicosatrienoic acids. *PLoS ONE* **2015**, *10*, e0113130. [CrossRef] [PubMed]
183. Pomposiello, S.I.; Quilley, J.; Carroll, M.A.; Falck, J.R.; McGiff, J.C. 5,6-epoxyeicosatrienoic acid mediates the enhanced renal vasodilation to arachidonic acid in the SHR. *Hypertension* **2003**, *42*, 548–554. [CrossRef] [PubMed]
184. Cheng, M.K.; Doumad, A.B.; Jiang, H.; Falck, J.R.; McGiff, J.C.; Carroll, M.A. Epoxyeicosatrienoic acids mediate adenosine-induced vasodilation in rat preglomerular microvessels (PGMV) via A2A receptors. *Br. J. Pharmacol.* **2004**, *141*, 441–448. [CrossRef] [PubMed]
185. Carroll, M.A.; Doumad, A.B.; Li, J.; Cheng, M.K.; Falck, J.R.; McGiff, J.C. Adenosine2A receptor vasodilation of rat preglomerular microvessels is mediated by EETs that activate the cAMP/PKA pathway. *Am. J. Physiol. Ren. Physiol.* **2006**, *291*, F155–F161. [CrossRef] [PubMed]
186. Imig, J.D.; Dimitropoulou, C.; Reddy, D.S.; White, R.E.; Falck, J.R. Afferent arteriolar dilation to 11, 12-EET analogs involves PP2A activity and Ca2+-activated K+ Channels. *Microcirculation* **2008**, *15*, 137–150. [CrossRef] [PubMed]
187. Wang, W.H.; Zhang, C.; Lin, D.H.; Wang, L.; Graves, J.P.; Zeldin, D.C.; Capdevila, J.H. Cyp2c44 epoxygenase in the collecting duct is essential for the high K+ intake-induced antihypertensive effect. *Am. J. Physiol. Ren. Physiol.* **2014**, *307*, F453–F460. [CrossRef]
188. Sharma, M.; McCarthy, E.T.; Reddy, D.S.; Patel, P.K.; Savin, V.J.; Medhora, M.; Falck, J.R. 8,9-Epoxyeicosatrienoic acid protects the glomerular filtration barrier. *Prostaglandins Other Lipid Mediat.* **2009**,

89, 43–51. [CrossRef]

189. Beck, L.H., Jr.; Fervenza, F.C.; Beck, D.M.; Bonegio, R.G.; Malik, F.A.; Erickson, S.B.; Cosio, F.G.; Cattran, D.C.; Salant, D.J. Rituximab-induced depletion of anti-PLA2R autoantibodies predicts response in membranous nephropathy. *J. Am. Soc. Nephrol.* **2011**, *22*, 1543–1550. [CrossRef]
190. Thokhonelidze, I.; Maglakelidze, N.; Sarishvili, N.; Kasradze, T.; Dalakishvili, K. Association of anti-phospholipasea2-receptor antibodies with clinical course of idiopathic membranous nephropathy. *Georgian Med News* **2015**, 49–53.
191. Ramachandran, R.; Hn, H.K.; Kumar, V.; Nada, R.; Yadav, A.K.; Goyal, A.; Kumar, V.; Rathi, M.; Jha, V.; Gupta, K.L.; et al. Tacrolimus combined with corticosteroids versus Modified Ponticelli regimen in treatment of idiopathic membranous nephropathy: Randomized control trial. *Nephrology* **2016**, *21*, 139–146. [CrossRef] [PubMed]
192. Wei, S.Y.; Wang, Y.X.; Li, J.S.; Zhao, S.L.; Diao, T.T.; Wang, Y.; Wang, C.; Qin, Y.; Cao, Y.; Wei, Q.; et al. Serum Anti-PLA2R Antibody Predicts Treatment Outcome in Idiopathic Membranous Nephropathy. *Am. J. Nephrol.* **2016**, *43*, 129–140. [CrossRef] [PubMed]
193. Bech, A.P.; Hofstra, J.M.; Brenchley, P.E.; Wetzels, J.F. Association of anti-PLA(2)R antibodies with outcomes after immunosuppressive therapy in idiopathic membranous nephropathy. *Clin. J. Am. Soc. Nephrol.* **2014**, *9*, 1386–1392. [CrossRef] [PubMed]
194. Radhakrishnan, J.; Cattran, D.C. The KDIGO practice guideline on glomerulonephritis: Reading between the (guide)lines–application to the individual patient. *Kidney Int.* **2012**, *82*, 840–856. [CrossRef] [PubMed]
195. Gonzalo-Gil, E.; Garcia-Herrero, C.; Toldos, O.; Usategui, A.; Criado, G.; Perez-Yague, S.; Barber, D.F.; Pablos, J.L.; Galindo, M. Microthrombotic Renal Vascular Lesions Are Associated to Increased Renal Inflammatory Infiltration in Murine Lupus Nephritis. *Front. Immunol.* **2018**, *9*, 1948. [CrossRef] [PubMed]
196. Gerrah, R.; Ehrlich, S.; Tshori, S.; Sahar, G. Beneficial effect of aspirin on renal function in patients with renal insufficiency postcardiac surgery. *J. Cardiovasc. Surg.* **2004**, *45*, 545–550.
197. Garg, A.X.; Kurz, A.; Sessler, D.I.; Cuerden, M.; Robinson, A.; Mrkobrada, M.; Parikh, C.R.; Mizera, R.; Jones, P.M.; Tiboni, M.; et al. Perioperative aspirin and clonidine and risk of acute kidney injury: A randomized clinical trial. *JAMA* **2014**, *312*, 2254–2264. [CrossRef] [PubMed]
198. De Martino, M.; Chiarugi, A.; Boner, A.; Montini, G.; De' Angelis, G.L. Working towards an Appropriate Use of Ibuprofen in Children: An Evidence-Based Appraisal. *Drugs* **2017**, *77*, 1295–1311. [CrossRef]
199. Lipman, G.S.; Shea, K.; Christensen, M.; Phillips, C.; Burns, P.; Higbee, R.; Koskenoja, V.; Eifling, K.; Krabak, B.J. Ibuprofen versus placebo effect on acute kidney injury in ultramarathons: A randomised controlled trial. *Emerg. Med. J.* **2017**, *34*, 637–642. [CrossRef] [PubMed]
200. Kaojarern, S.; Chennavasin, P.; Anderson, S.; Brater, D.C. Nephron site of effect of nonsteroidal anti-inflammatory drugs on solute excretion in humans. *Am. J. Physiol.* **1983**, *244*, F134–F139. [CrossRef]
201. Wu, Y.J.; Xue, M.; Chen, H. Licofelone inhibits interleukin-18-induced pro-inflammatory cytokine release and cellular proliferation in human mesangial cells. *Basic Clin. Pharmacol. Toxicol.* **2012**, *111*, 166–172. [CrossRef] [PubMed]
202. Faulkner, J.; Pye, C.; Al-Shabrawey, M.; Elmarakby, A.A. Inhibition of 12/15-Lipoxygenase Reduces Renal Inflammation and Injury in Streptozotocin-Induced Diabetic Mice. *J. Diabetes Metab.* **2015**, *6*. [CrossRef]
203. Hofstra, J.M.; Beck, L.H., Jr.; Beck, D.M.; Wetzels, J.F.; Salant, D.J. Anti-phospholipase A(2) receptor antibodies correlate with clinical status in idiopathic membranous nephropathy. *Clin. J. Am. Soc. Nephrol.* **2011**, *6*, 1286–1291. [CrossRef] [PubMed]
204. Debiec, H.; Ronco, P. PLA2R autoantibodies and PLA2R glomerular deposits in membranous nephropathy. *N. Engl. J. Med.* **2011**, *364*, 689–690. [CrossRef] [PubMed]
205. Pourcine, F.; Dahan, K.; Mihout, F.; Cachanado, M.; Brocheriou, I.; Debiec, H.; Ronco, P. Prognostic value of PLA2R autoimmunity detected by measurement of anti-PLA2R antibodies combined with detection of PLA2R antigen in membranous nephropathy: A single-centre study over 14 years. *PLoS ONE* **2017**, *12*, e0173201. [CrossRef] [PubMed]
206. Jullien, P.; Seitz Polski, B.; Maillard, N.; Thibaudin, D.; Laurent, B.; Ollier, E.; Alamartine, E.; Lambeau, G.; Mariat, C. Anti-phospholipase A2 receptor antibody levels at diagnosis predicts spontaneous remission of idiopathic membranous nephropathy. *Clin. Kidney J.* **2017**, *10*, 209–214. [CrossRef] [PubMed]
207. Buysen, J.G.; Houthoff, H.J.; Krediet, R.T.; Arisz, L. Acute interstitial nephritis: A clinical and morphological study in 27 patients. *Nephrol. Dial. Transplant.* **1990**, *5*, 94–99. [CrossRef] [PubMed]

208. Eddy, A.A. Drug-induced tubulointerstitial nephritis: Hypersensitivity and necroinflammatory pathways. *Pediatric Nephrol.* **2019**, 1–8. [CrossRef] [PubMed]
209. Di Rosa, M.; Giroud, J.P.; Willoughby, D.A. Studies on the mediators of the acute inflammatory response induced in rats in different sites by carrageenan and turpentine. *J. Pathol.* **1971**, *104*, 15–29. [CrossRef] [PubMed]
210. De Gaetano, G.; Bucchi, F.; Gambino, M.C.; Cerletti, C. Does oral aspirin spare the kidney? *Lancet* **1986**, *1*, 736. [CrossRef]
211. Berger, J.S.; Brown, D.L.; Becker, R.C. Low-dose aspirin in patients with stable cardiovascular disease: A meta-analysis. *Am. J. Med.* **2008**, *121*, 43–49. [CrossRef] [PubMed]
212. Antithrombotic Trialists, C.; Baigent, C.; Blackwell, L.; Collins, R.; Emberson, J.; Godwin, J.; Peto, R.; Buring, J.; Hennekens, C.; Kearney, P.; et al. Aspirin in the primary and secondary prevention of vascular disease: Collaborative meta-analysis of individual participant data from randomised trials. *Lancet* **2009**, *373*, 1849–1860. [CrossRef]
213. Vandvik, P.O.; Lincoff, A.M.; Gore, J.M.; Gutterman, D.D.; Sonnenberg, F.A.; Alonso-Coello, P.; Akl, E.A.; Lansberg, M.G.; Guyatt, G.H.; Spencer, F.A. Primary and secondary prevention of cardiovascular disease: Antithrombotic Therapy and Prevention of Thrombosis, 9th ed: American College of Chest Physicians Evidence-Based Clinical Practice Guidelines. *Chest* **2012**, *141*, e637S–e668S. [CrossRef] [PubMed]
214. Karzai, W.; Priebe, H.J. Aspirin and mortality from coronary bypass surgery. *N. Engl. J. Med.* **2003**, *348*, 1057–1059. [PubMed]
215. Ali, H.; Shaaban, A.; Murtaza, A.; Howell, L.E.; Ahmed, A. Effect of Long-Term, Low-Dose Aspirin Therapy on Renal Graft Function. *Exp. Clin. Transplant.* **2017**, *15*, 400–404. [CrossRef] [PubMed]
216. Rainsford, K.D. Ibuprofen: Pharmacology, efficacy and safety. *Inflammopharmacology* **2009**, *17*, 275–342. [CrossRef] [PubMed]
217. Van Overmeire, B.; Allegaert, K.; Casaer, A.; Debauche, C.; Decaluwe, W.; Jespers, A.; Weyler, J.; Harrewijn, I.; Langhendries, J.P. Prophylactic ibuprofen in premature infants: A multicentre, randomised, double-blind, placebo-controlled trial. *Lancet* **2004**, *364*, 1945–1949. [CrossRef]
218. Haas, M.; Spargo, B.H.; Wit, E.J.; Meehan, S.M. Etiologies and outcome of acute renal insufficiency in older adults: A renal biopsy study of 259 cases. *Am. J. Kidney Dis.* **2000**, *35*, 433–447. [CrossRef]
219. Martinez Lopez, A.B.; Alvarez Blanco, O.; De Pablos, A.L.; San-Jose, M.D.M.; De La Blanca, A.R.S. Ibuprofen-induced acute interstitial nephritis in the paediatric population. *Nefrologia* **2016**, *36*, 69–71. [CrossRef]
220. Steinhauslin, F.; Munafo, A.; Buclin, T.; Macciocchi, A.; Biollaz, J. Renal effects of nimesulide in furosemide-treated subjects. *Drugs* **1993**, *46* (Suppl. 1), 257–262. [CrossRef]
221. Warrington, S.J.; Ravic, M.; Dawnay, A. Renal and general tolerability of repeated doses of nimesulide in normal subjects. *Drugs* **1993**, *46* (Suppl. 1), 263–269. [CrossRef]
222. Ceserani, R.; Casciarri, I.; Cavalletti, E.; Cazzulani, P. Action of Nimesulide on Rat Gastric Prostaglandins and Renal Function. *Drug Investig.* **1991**, *3*, 14–21. [CrossRef]
223. Forget, P.; Machiels, J.P.; Coulie, P.G.; Berliere, M.; Poncelet, A.J.; Tombal, B.; Stainier, A.; Legrand, C.; Canon, J.L.; Kremer, Y.; et al. Neutrophil: Lymphocyte ratio and intraoperative use of ketorolac or diclofenac are prognostic factors in different cohorts of patients undergoing breast, lung, and kidney cancer surgery. *Ann. Surg. Oncol.* **2013**, *20* (Suppl. 3), S650–S660. [CrossRef]
224. Yakar, I.; Melamed, R.; Shakhar, G.; Shakhar, K.; Rosenne, E.; Abudarham, N.; Page, G.G.; Ben-Eliyahu, S. Prostaglandin e(2) suppresses NK activity in vivo and promotes postoperative tumor metastasis in rats. *Ann. Surg. Oncol.* **2003**, *10*, 469–479. [CrossRef] [PubMed]
225. Ostrand-Rosenberg, S.; Sinha, P. Myeloid-derived suppressor cells: Linking inflammation and cancer. *J. Immunol.* **2009**, *182*, 4499–4506. [CrossRef] [PubMed]
226. Bombardier, C.; Laine, L.; Reicin, A.; Shapiro, D.; Burgos-Vargas, R.; Davis, B.; Day, R.; Ferraz, M.B.; Hawkey, C.J.; Hochberg, M.C.; et al. Comparison of upper gastrointestinal toxicity of rofecoxib and naproxen in patients with rheumatoid arthritis. VIGOR Study Group. *N. Engl. J. Med.* **2000**, *343*, 1520–1528. [CrossRef]
227. Ungprasert, P.; Cheungpasitporn, W.; Crowson, C.S.; Matteson, E.L. Individual non-steroidal anti-inflammatory drugs and risk of acute kidney injury: A systematic review and meta-analysis of observational studies. *Eur. J. Intern. Med.* **2015** *26*, 285–291. [CrossRef] [PubMed]
228. Colebatch, A.N.; Marks, J.L.; van der Heijde, D.M.; Edwards, C.J. Safety of nonsteroidal antiinflammatory drugs and/or paracetamol in people receiving methotrexate for inflammatory arthritis: A Cochrane systematic

review. *J. Rheumatol. Suppl.* **2012**, *90*, 62–73. [CrossRef] [PubMed]
229. Nawaz, F.A.; Larsen, C.P.; Troxell, M.L. Membranous nephropathy and nonsteroidal anti-inflammatory agents. *Am. J. Kidney Dis.* **2013**, *62*, 1012–1017. [CrossRef] [PubMed]
230. Catella-Lawson, F.; McAdam, B.; Morrison, B.W.; Kapoor, S.; Kujubu, D.; Antes, L.; Lasseter, K.C.; Quan, H.; Gertz, B.J.; FitzGerald, G.A. Effects of specific inhibition of cyclooxygenase-2 on sodium balance, hemodynamics, and vasoactive eicosanoids. *J. Pharmacol. Exp. Ther.* **1999**, *289*, 735–741. [PubMed]
231. Takahashi, K.; Patel, A.K.; Nagai, S.; Safwan, M.; Putchakayala, K.G.; Kane, W.J.; Malinzak, L.E.; Denny, J.E.; Yoshida, A.; Kim, D.Y. Perioperative Ketorolac Use: A Potential Risk Factor for Renal Dysfunction After Live-Donor Nephrectomy. *Ann. Transplant.* **2017**, *22*, 563–569. [CrossRef] [PubMed]
232. Griffin, M.R. High-dose non-steroidal anti-inflammatories: Painful choices. *Lancet* **2013**, *382*, 746–748. [CrossRef]
233. Zhang, J.; Ding, E.L.; Song, Y. Adverse effects of cyclooxygenase 2 inhibitors on renal and arrhythmia events: Meta-analysis of randomized trials. *JAMA* **2006**, *296*, 1619–1632. [CrossRef] [PubMed]
234. Gounaris, E.; Heiferman, M.J.; Heiferman, J.R.; Shrivastav, M.; Vitello, D.; Blatner, N.R.; Knab, L.M.; Phillips, J.D.; Cheon, E.C.; Grippo, P.J.; et al. Zileuton, 5-lipoxygenase inhibitor, acts as a chemopreventive agent in intestinal polyposis, by modulating polyp and systemic inflammation. *PLoS ONE* **2015**, *10*, e0121402. [CrossRef] [PubMed]
235. Santos, C.M.M.; Ribeiro, D.; Silva, A.M.S.; Fernandes, E. 2,3-Diarylxanthones as Potential Inhibitors of Arachidonic Acid Metabolic Pathways. *Inflammation* **2017**, *40*, 956–964. [CrossRef] [PubMed]
236. Muller, D.N.; Theuer, J.; Shagdarsuren, E.; Kaergel, E.; Honeck, H.; Park, J.K.; Markovic, M.; Barbosa-Sicard, E.; Dechend, R.; Wellner, M.; et al. A peroxisome proliferator-activated receptor-alpha activator induces renal CYP2C23 activity and protects from angiotensin II-induced renal injury. *Am. J. Pathol.* **2004**, *164*, 521–532. [CrossRef]
237. Gai, Z.; Visentin, M.; Gui, T.; Zhao, L.; Thasler, W.E.; Hausler, S.; Hartling, I.; Cremonesi, A.; Hiller, C.; Kullak-Ublick, G.A. Effects of Farnesoid X Receptor Activation on Arachidonic Acid Metabolism, NF-kB Signaling, and Hepatic Inflammation. *Mol. Pharmacol.* **2018**, *94*, 802–811. [CrossRef]
238. Shlipak, M.G.; Fried, L.F.; Cushman, M.; Manolio, T.A.; Peterson, D.; Stehman-Breen, C.; Bleyer, A.; Newman, A.; Siscovick, D.; Psaty, B. Cardiovascular mortality risk in chronic kidney disease: Comparison of traditional and novel risk factors. *JAMA* **2005**, *293*, 1737–1745. [CrossRef]
239. Muntner, P.; He, J.; Astor, B.C.; Folsom, A.R.; Coresh, J. Traditional and nontraditional risk factors predict coronary heart disease in chronic kidney disease: Results from the atherosclerosis risk in communities study. *J. Am. Soc. Nephrol.* **2005**, *16*, 529–538. [CrossRef]
240. Garg, A.; Grundy, S.M. Management of dyslipidemia in NIDDM. *Diabetes Care* **1990**, *13*, 153–169. [CrossRef]
241. Garg, A.; Grundy, S.M. Gemfibrozil alone and in combination with lovastatin for treatment of hypertriglyceridemia in NIDDM. *Diabetes* **1989**, *38*, 364–372. [CrossRef] [PubMed]
242. Siavash, M.; Amini, M. Vitamin C may have similar beneficial effects to Gemfibrozil on serum high-density lipoprotein-cholesterol in type 2 diabetic patients. *J. Res. Pharm. Pract.* **2014**, *3*, 77–82. [CrossRef] [PubMed]
243. Martin-Navarro, J.A.; Petkov-Stoyanov, V.; Gutierrez-Sanchez, M.J.; Pedraza-Cezon, L. Acute renal failure secondary to interstitial acute nephritis and Fanconi syndrome for metamizole and gemfibrozil. *Nefrologia* **2016**, *36*, 321–323. [CrossRef] [PubMed]
244. Khan, M.A.; Liu, J.; Kumar, G.; Skapek, S.X.; Falck, J.R.; Imig, J.D. Novel orally active epoxyeicosatrienoic acid (EET) analogs attenuate cisplatin nephrotoxicity. *FASEB J.* **2013**, *27*, 2946–2956. [CrossRef] [PubMed]
245. Node, K.; Huo, Y.; Ruan, X.; Yang, B.; Spiecker, M.; Ley, K.; Zeldin, D.C.; Liao, J.K. Anti-inflammatory properties of cytochrome P450 epoxygenase-derived eicosanoids. *Science* **1999**, *285*, 1276–1279. [CrossRef] [PubMed]
246. Farzamikia, N.; Sakhinia, E.; Afrasiabirad, A. Pharmacogenetics-Based Warfarin Dosing in Patients with Cardiac Valve Replacement: The Effects of CYP2C9 and VKORC1 Gene Polymorphisms. *Lab. Med.* **2017**, *49*, 25–34. [CrossRef]
247. Pei, L.; Tian, X.; Long, Y.; Nan, W.; Jia, M.; Qiao, R.; Zhang, J. Establishment of a Han Chinese-specific pharmacogenetic-guided warfarin dosing algorithm. *Medicine* **2018**, *97*, e12178. [CrossRef]
248. Spatzenegger, M.; Jaeger, W. Clinical importance of hepatic cytochrome P450 in drug metabolism. *Drug Metab. Rev.* **1995**, *27*, 397–417. [CrossRef]
249. Yanagita, M. Gas6, warfarin, and kidney diseases. *Clin. Exp. Nephrol.* **2004**, *8*, 304–309. [CrossRef]
250. Zeldin, D.C.; Wei, S.; Falck, J.R.; Hammock, B.D.; Snapper, J.R.; Capdevila, J.H. Metabolism of

epoxyeicosatrienoic acids by cytosolic epoxide hydrolase: Substrate structural determinants of asymmetric catalysis. *Arch. Biochem. Biophys.* **1995**, *316*, 443–451. [CrossRef]

251. Imig, J.D.; Hammock, B.D. Soluble epoxide hydrolase as a therapeutic target for cardiovascular diseases. *Nat. Rev. Drug Discov.* **2009**, *8*, 794–805. [CrossRef] [PubMed]

252. Shen, H.C.; Hammock, B.D. Discovery of inhibitors of soluble epoxide hydrolase: A target with multiple potential therapeutic indications. *J. Med. Chem.* **2012**, *55*, 1789–1808. [CrossRef] [PubMed]

4

Targeting ROS and cPLA2/COX2 Expressions Ameliorated Renal Damage in Obese Mice with Endotoxemia

Jia-Feng Chang [1,2,3,4,5,†], Jih-Chen Yeh [2,6,†], Chun-Ta Ho [2], Shih-Hao Liu [7], Chih-Yu Hsieh [1,2], Ting-Ming Wang [8,9], Shu-Wei Chang [10], I-Ta Lee [11], Kuo-Yang Huang [12], Jen-Yu Wang [4] and Wei-Ning Lin [4,*]

1 Division of Nephrology, Department of Internal Medicine, En Chu Kong Hospital, New Taipei City 237, Taiwan
2 Renal Care Joint Foundation, New Taipei City 220, Taiwan
3 Department of Nursing, Yuanpei University of Medical Technology, Hsinchu 300, Taiwan
4 Graduate Institution of Biomedical and Pharmaceutical Science, College of Medicine, Fu Jen Catholic University, New Taipei City 242, Taiwan
5 Division of Nephrology, Department of Internal Medicine, Shuang Ho Hospital, Taipei Medical University, New Taipei City 235, Taiwan
6 Department of Dentistry, Far Eastern Memorial Hospital, New Taipei City 220, Taiwan
7 Division of Pathology, En-Chu-Kong Hospital, New Taipei City 237, Taiwan
8 Department of Orthopaedic Surgery, School of Medicine, National Taiwan University, Taipei 106, Taiwan
9 Department of Orthopaedic Surgery, National Taiwan University Hospital, Taipei 106, Taiwan
10 Department of Civil Engineering, National Taiwan University, Taipei 106, Taiwan
11 School of Dentistry, College of Oral Medicine, Taipei Medical University, Taipei 110, Taiwan
12 Graduate Institute of Pathology and Parasitology, National Defense Medical Center, Taipei 114, Taiwan
* Correspondence: 081551@mail.fju.edu.tw
† These authors contributed equally to this work.

Abstract: Obesity is associated with metabolic endotoxemia, reactive oxygen species (ROS), chronic inflammation, and obese kidney fibrosis. Although the fat–intestine–kidney axis has been documented, the pathomechanism and therapeutic targets of obese kidney fibrosis remain unelucidated. To mimic obese humans with metabolic endotoxemia, high-fat-diet-fed mice (HF group) were injected with lipopolysaccharide (LPS) to yield the obese kidney fibrosis–metabolic endotoxemia mouse model (HL group). Therapeutic effects of ROS, cytosolic phospholipases A2 (cPLA2) and cyclooxygenase-2 (COX-2) inhibitors were analyzed with a quantitative comparison of immunohistochemistry stains and morphometric approach in the tubulointerstitium of different groups. Compared with basal and HF groups, the HL group exhibited the most prominent obese kidney fibrosis, tubular epithelial lipid vacuoles, and lymphocyte infiltration in the tubulointerstitium. Furthermore, inhibitors of nonspecific ROS, cPLA2 and COX-2 ameliorated the above renal damages. Notably, the ROS-inhibitor-treated group ameliorated not only oxidative injury but also the expression of cPLA2 and COX-2, indicating that ROS functions as the upstream signaling molecule in the inflammatory cascade of obese kidney fibrosis. ROS acts as a key messenger in the signaling transduction of obese kidney fibrosis, activating downstream cPLA2 and COX-2. The given antioxidant treatment ameliorates obese kidney fibrosis resulting from a combined high-fat diet and LPS—ROS could serve as a potential therapeutic target of obese kidney fibrosis with metabolic endotoxemia.

Keywords: obese kidney fibrosis; endotoxemia; ROS; cPLA2 and COX-2

1. Introduction

The worldwide increase in the prevalence of obesity has occurred in parallel with an increasing prevalence of chronic diseases, including diabetes mellitus, hypertension, cardiovascular diseases and chronic kidney disease (CKD) [1]. In light of this, the focus of World Kidney Day 2017 is kidney disease and obesity. It is found that the increase of BMI positively related to the presence and development of low estimated glomerular filtration rate and the incidence of end-stage renal disease [2]. Even metabolically healthy obesity is not a harmless condition—the phenotype of obese humans, no matter the abnormalities of metabolism, is reversely correlated with renal function [3]. In addition, the fat–intestine–kidney axis has a pivotal position in the mechanism of obese kidney disease, involving metabolic endotoxemia (ME) from intestinal dysbiosis, reactive oxygen species (ROS), systemic inflammation, and progressive renal fibrosis [4]. The rupture of the epithelial barrier results in the translocation of endotoxin and changes in the microbiome, which correlate to the occurrence of inflammation [5]. The evaluation of blood bacterial DNA shows that *Proteobacteria phylum*, *Gammaproteobacteria* class, and *Enterobacteriaceae* and *Pseudomonadaceae* families are more abundant in the CKD group compared with healthy controls [6]. Furthermore, there is elevated plasma lipopolysaccharide (LPS)-binding protein in hemodialysis patients with metabolic syndrome and obesity [7]. These studies suggested that LPS, also called endotoxin, functioned as a linker between the gut microbiome and CKD.

Emerging evidence indicates that prostaglandin (PG) pathways intricately interact with diabetes, metabolic syndrome, CKD progression, and cardiovascular events [8]. In a fatty rat model, renal cyclooxygenase-2 (COX-2) protein expression was accentuated and correlated with metabolic abnormalities [9]. Furthermore, a myriad of studies showed inhibition of cytoplasmic phospholipase A2 (cPLA2) and downstream signals attenuate renal injury [10–13]. Initiation of the PG signaling pathway usually occurs with the release of arachidonic acids from phospholipids within membranes by cPLA2. The subsequent conversion of arachidonic acid into PG is facilitated by COX-2, leading to inflammation and fibrosis in the kidney. Indeed, compared with healthy controls, renal tissues in CKD groups exhibit higher expressions of fibroblasts and the *COX-2* gene [14]. Although cPLA2 and eicosanoids contributed to renal oxidative stress, inflammation, and end-organ damage [15], eradication of bone-marrow-derived cPLA2 attenuated the eicosanoid storm and renal fibrosis [16].

Intracellular redox imbalance plays important roles in the pathogenesis of CKD. Plasma cells of CKD patients show activation of NF-κB and up-regulated expression of pro-inflammatory and pro-oxidant genes, as well as down-regulation of Nrf2-associated antioxidant gene expression [14]. Similarly, the nephrotoxic agent, aristolochic acid I, increases protein abundance of the NADPH oxidase subunits NOX4, $p47^{phox}$, $p22^{phox}$ and 3-nitrotyrosine in rats within 8 to 24 weeks [17]. Moreover, upregulation of intracellular ROS promotes the expression of inflammatory genes, including *cPLA2* and *COX-2* [18,19]. In fact, ameliorating oxidative stress via modulating forkhead box class O1 (FOXO1) expression attenuated high glucose-induced renal proximal tubular cell injury [20].

Despite previously documented implications, the pathomechanism and therapeutic targets of obese kidney fibrosis (OKF) remain unelucidated. To mimic obese humans with ME, we developed a combined high-fat-diet-fed (HF) and lipopolysaccharide (LPS)-treated mouse model to explore inflammatory signaling pathways of OKF. We hypothesized that OKF is involved in ROS generations, activating downstream cPLA2 and COX-2, resulting in progressive tubulointerstitial fibrosis. Thus, ROS could serve as a potential therapeutic target of OKF. Quantitative comparison of immunohistochemical (IHC) staining and morphometric approach were used to test this hypothesis.

2. Results

2.1. HF Mice with ME Exhibit the Most Prominent Renal Fibrosis, Depositions of Lipid Vacuoles in Tubular Epithelium, and Lymphocyte Infiltration in Tubulointerstitium

Recent evidence indicates that adipose tissue inflammation in obesity and metabolic syndrome is not strictly a macrophage-dependent phenomenon. Lymphocytes, especially T cells, infiltrate the adipose tissue and mediate the inflammatory response. The infiltration of T effector cells precedes the accumulation of macrophages in adipose tissue and reducing regulatory T cells during obesity are thought to contribute to the development of adipose tissue inflammation [21]. Deposition of lipid vacuoles (LV) in proximal tubular epithelial cells are the typical features of fatty kidneys [22,23], and renal fibrosis is a hallmark and common outcome across all kinds of progressive CKD [24]. To investigate human obese kidney fibrosis with metabolic endotoxemia, we used an experimental rodent model, fed a high-fat diet with LPS injection (called the OKF-ME model) (Figure 1). In accordance with previous studies [22,23], our high-fat diet course induced shedding of renal tubule epithelial cells, tubular LV deposition and increased lymphocyte infiltration in renal tubulointerstitium with or without LPS treatment at week 15 (Figure 2A). Compared with the basal group and HF mice, the HL group exhibited the most prominent fibrosis (Figure 2B), tubular LV accumulation (Figure 2C), and lymphocyte infiltration in tubulointerstitium (Figure 2D). Current data demonstrate that HF and ME result in not only renal tubule injury but also tubulointerstitial inflammation and fibrosis.

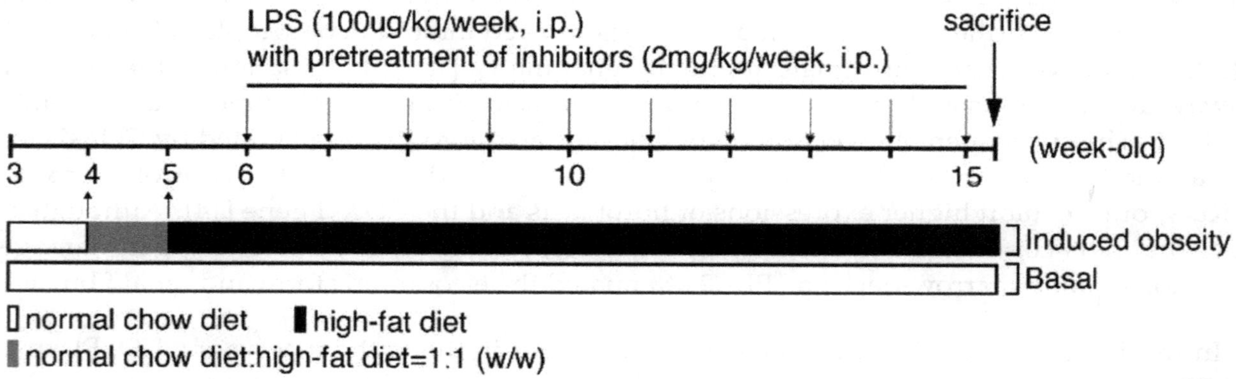

Figure 1. Model of obese kidney fibrosis with metabolic endotoxemia (OKF-ME). Mice were randomized into three groups: normal chow-fed control group (basal group), high-fat diet-fed group (HF group), and high-fat diet-fed group with lipopolysaccharides (LPS) treatment (HL group). The HL group was induced with LPS (100 μg/kg/week intraperitoneal (i.p.) injection) as the working model of OKF-ME.

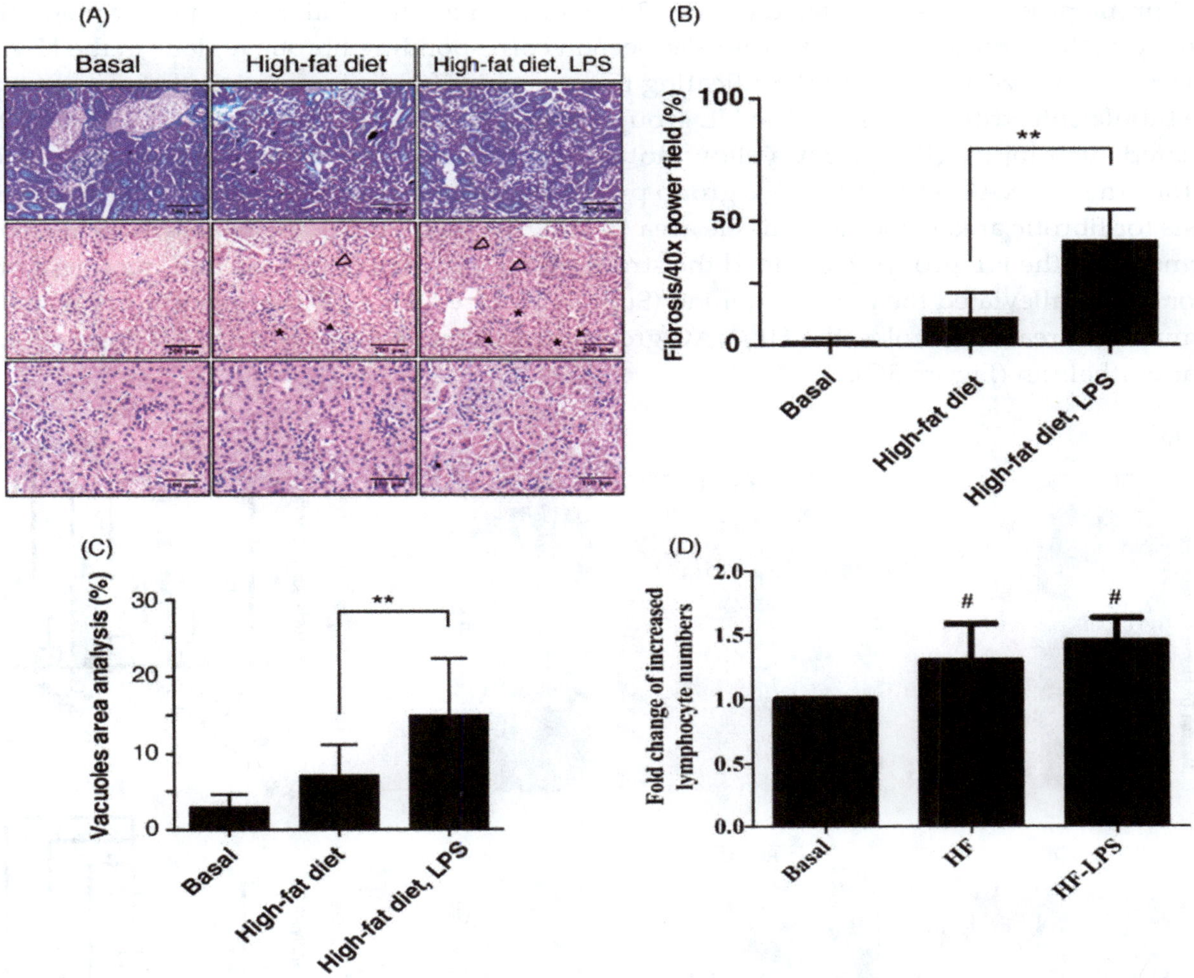

Figure 2. HF mice with ME exhibit the most prominent renal fibrosis, depositions of lipid vacuoles in tubular epithelium, and lymphocyte infiltration in tubulointerstitium. (**A**) Mice were scarified at the end of treatment, and kidney tissues were extracted for histological staining (Haematoxylin and Eosin and Masson's trichrome staining). Compared with the basal group and HF mice, the HL group exhibited the most prominent renal fibrosis, depositions of lipid vacuoles in tubular epithelium, and lymphocyte infiltration in the tubulointerstitium. Black hollow triangles indicate shedding of tubules. Black arrows indicate infiltration of lymphocytes. Stars indicate lipid vacuoles. Scale bars in the panels are 200 μm or 100 μm as indicated. Quantification analyses were performed by ImageJ software for (**B**) fibrosis area (**C**) lipid vacuoles and (**D**) lymphocyte number. Data are expressed as mean ± SD ($n = 8$); ** $p < 0.01$, to compare the differences between the two indicated groups. # $p < 0.05$, compared with the basal group.

2.2. *Inhibitors of ROS, cPLA2, and COX-2 Attenuate the Tubulointerstitial Fibrosis in HF Mice with ME*

As we had already proven that HF and ME result in tubulointerstitial fibrosis, we aimed to investigate the underlying mechanism and inflammatory signaling pathways of OKF. Our previous research has contributed a mechanistic insight of uremic lung injury in a CKD mouse model, showing that ROS activates downstream PG pathways and recruits leukocytes to injured sites [25]. Furthermore, recent studies reported inhibitions of ROS and cPLA2/COX-2 ameliorates renal damages [10–13]. Nonetheless, therapeutic effects of the above inhibitors on OKF remain unclear. To investigate which factor mediated the progression of OKF, N-acetylcysteine (NAC; ROS scavenger), AACOCF3 (AAC; cPLA2 inhibitor), and NS-398 (COX-2 inhibitor) were used. Our results demonstrate significant fibrosis was found in juxtamedullary to medullar regions of HF and HL groups (Figure 3A). In corresponding fibrotic regions, the HL/NAC group exhibited residual renal tubular structures, suggesting that the above fibrotic process was attenuated (Figure 3A, zoom-in region). Under high-power magnification, evident epithelioid tubular-like cells were also seen in corresponding fibrotic regions in the HL/NS-398 group (Figure 3A, zoom-in region), indicating tissue repair after inflammation. In contrast with the severe tubularinterstitial fibrosis in the HL group, inhibitor-treated groups of NAC, AAC and NS-398 attenuated such injury (Figure 3A, yellow dotted line regions). To compare therapeutic effects of inhibitors, the HL/NAC and HL/NS-398 group presented the lowest degree of OKF after quantification analysis for fibrotic area verses total tissue area (%) (Figure 3B). Indeed, the results of Sirius Red stain confirmed that the HL groups contained the strongest red staining of fibrosis and treatment of NAC, AAC or NS398 alleviated the fibrotic staining (Supplementary Data 1). After quantification analysis to determine the area of vacuoles, the HL/NAC group exerted the lowest degree of LV deposition in the tubular epithelium (Figure 3C).

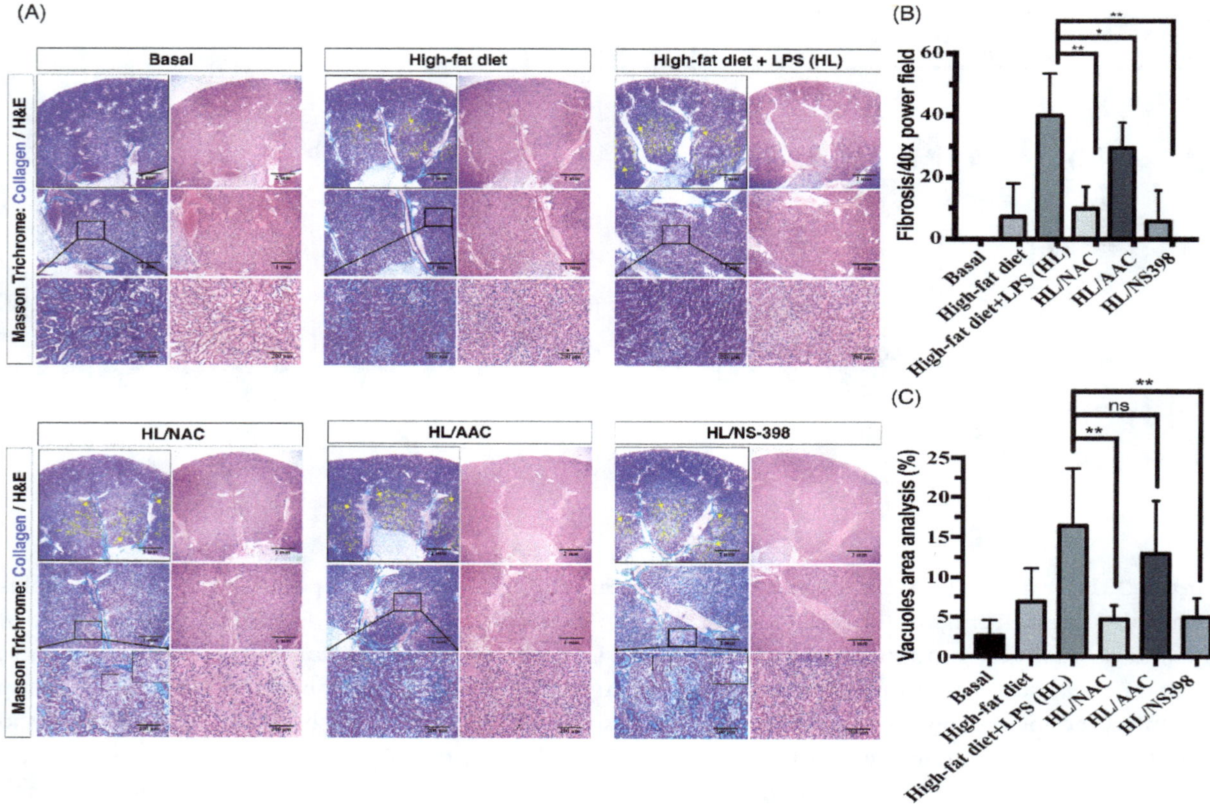

Figure 3. Inhibitors of reactive oxygen species (ROS), cPLA2, and COX-2 attenuate the tubulointerstitial fibrosis in HF mice with ME. (**A**) The HL group exerts the most significant collagen deposition and tubulointerstitial fibrosis in the juxtamedullary to medullar regions. In corresponding fibrotic regions, the HL/N-acetylcysteine (NAC) group exhibited residual renal tubular structures, suggesting that the above fibrotic process was attenuated (zoom-in region). Under high-power magnification, evident epithelioid tubular-like cells were also visible in corresponding fibrotic regions in the HL/NS-398 group (zoom-in region), indicating tissue repair after inflammation. In contrast with the profound tubularinterstitial fibrosis in HL group, inhibitor-treated groups of NAC, AACOCF3 (AAC) and NS-398 attenuated such injury (yellow dotted line regions). The fibrosis area was marked by yellow dotted lines. Yellow arrows indicated the borderline of the fibrosis area. Scale bars are 2 mm, 1mm and 200 μm in the panels. (**B**) To compare the therapeutic effects of inhibitors, the HL/NAC and HL/NS-398 group presented the lowest degree of OKF after quantification analysis for the fibrotic area verses total tissue area (%). (**C**) After quantification analysis for the area of vacuoles, the HL/NAC group exerted the lowest degree of lipid vacuole deposition in the tubular epithelium. Quantification analysis was performed by image J. Data are expressed as mean ± SD ($n = 8$); * $p < 0.05$; and ** $p < 0.01$ to compare the differences between the two indicated groups. ns, not significant.

2.3. *Scavengers of Non-Specific ROS Attenuate Not Only Oxidative Injury But Also Downstream Pathways of cPLA2 and COX-2 in Obese Kidney Fibrosis with Metabolic Endotoxemia*

As we have proven, ROS, cPLA2 and COX-2 were involved in OKF with ME, the key messenger of signal transduction pathways in the OKF mechanism remain unclear. Given that ROS could function as a short-lived intracellular second messenger in signaling transduction [25–27], we hypothesized that ROS could function as an upstream signal transducer in cPLA2 and COX-2-mediated inflammatory pathways. To investigate it further, expressions of 8-hydroxy-2′-deoxyguanosine (8-OHdG), a derivative of oxidized deoxyguanosine, was evaluated as an indicator of oxidative damages. Results of IHC assay showed that there is an increased expression of 8-OHdG in the HL group (HF mice with ME) and treatment of NAC (scavenger of ROS) reduced the stain density of 8-OHdG in the HL/NAC group (Figure 4A,B). On the aspects of cPLA2 and COX-2 expression, as expected, the HL group (HF mice with ME) exerted the highest expression of cPLA2 and COX-2, which were ameliorated by AACOCF3 (AAC, inhibitor of cPLA2) and NS-398 (inhibitor of COX-2), respectively (Figure 5). Notably, the NAC-treated group ameliorated not only oxidative injury but also expressions of cPLA2 and COX-2 after the quantification analysis (Figure 5C,D), indicating that ROS acts as the upstream signal in the inflammatory cascades of OKF. Western blot was further used to confirm the results of IHC. As shown in the Supplementary Data 2, HL-induced expression of cPLA2 and COX-2 were attenuated by treatment of AAC, NAC or NS-398, separately. Collectively, ROS serves as a key pro-inflammatory signal to activate PG pathways, and ultimately, leads to OKF.

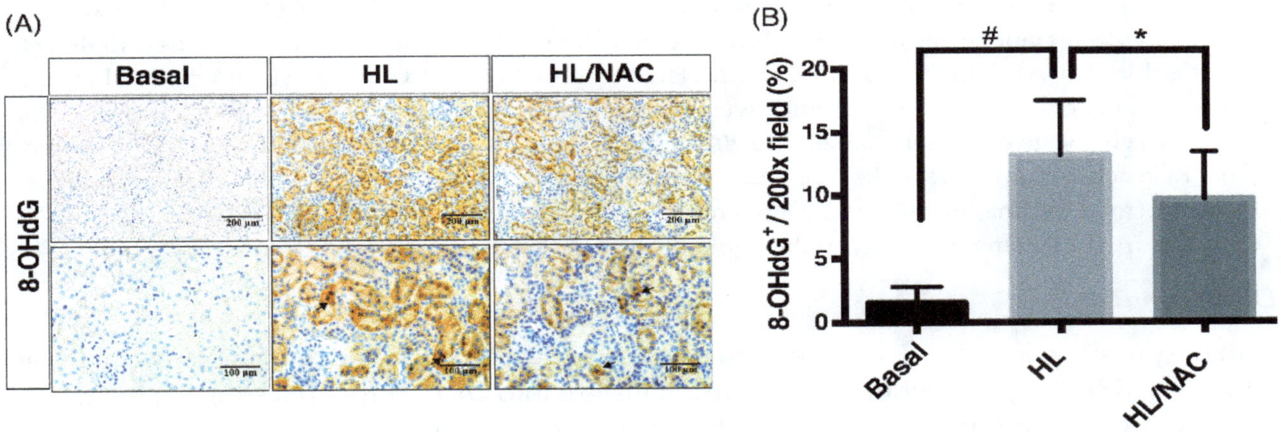

Figure 4. Scavengers of non-specific ROS attenuate oxidative injury in obese kidney fibrosis with metabolic endotoxemia. (**A**) Immunohistochemical staining methods were used to detect expressions of 8-OHdG. The HL group (HF mice with ME) exerts the highest expression of 8-OHdG, which was ameliorated by NAC. Scale bars are 200 µm or 100 µm in the panels. (**B**) Quantification analysis was performed by imageJ software. Data are expressed as mean ± SD ($n = 8$); * $p < 0.05$, # $p < 0.01$, to compare the differences between the two indicated groups.

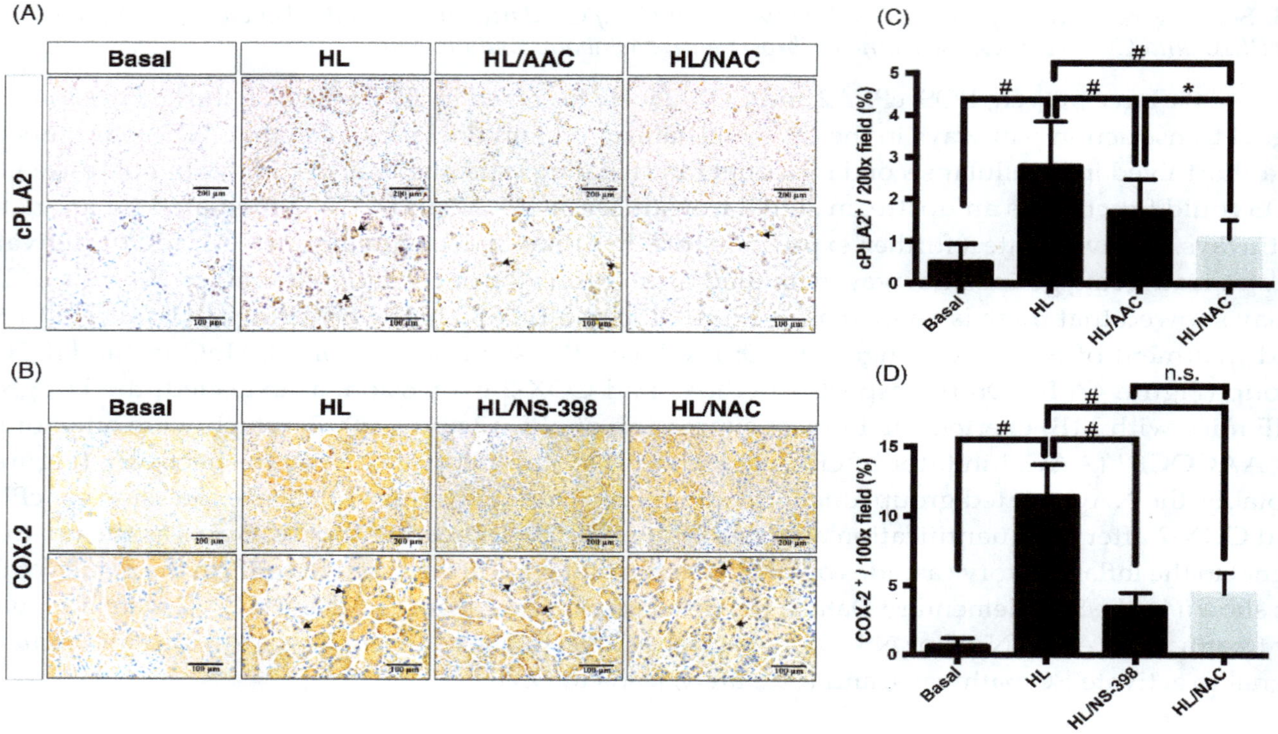

Figure 5. Scavengers of non-specific ROS reduced expression of cPLA2 and COX-2 in obese kidney fibrosis with metabolic endotoxemia. Immunohistochemical staining methods were used to detect expressions of (**A**) cPLA2, and (**B**) COX-2. The HL group (HF mice with ME) exerts the highest expression of cPLA2 and COX-2, which were ameliorated by NAC, AACCOCFS (AAC), and NS-398, respectively. Scale bars in the panels are 200 μm or 100 μm. (**C**,**D**) Quantification analysis indicated that ROS acts as the upstream key signal in the inflammatory cascades of OKF. Quantification analysis as performed by ImageJ software. Data are expressed as mean ± SD (n = 8); * $p < 0.05$, # $p < 0.01$, to compare the differences between the two indicated groups. n.s., not significant.

3. Discussion

In the present study, an OKF-ME mouse model was developed to demonstrate how a high-fat diet and LPS impair kidneys, providing a mechanical insight into OKF. Through testing the effects of ROS and cPLA2/COX-2 inhibitors, major breakthroughs were achieved, and the new findings markedly advance our understanding of OKF process.

3.1. The Fat–Intestine–Kidney Axis

The fat–intestine–kidney axis is the foundation stone of OKF, and underlying mechanisms are increasingly recognized through both human and animal models [4]. The role of an HF diet in promoting an obesogenic gut microbiota is undergoing confirmation, and gut dysbiosis can direct host storage of lipids in adipose tissue [28]. It has become more evident that the gut microbiota is altered in obesity, leading to activation of the LPS-toll-like receptor 4 (TLR4) axis and modulation of the intestinal barrier integrity [29]. Thus, intestinal dysbiosis in obesity has recently been recognized as a key environmental factor driving metabolic diseases, and ME via the increased paracellular transport of LPS is believed to contribute to chronic high-grade inflammation [30,31]. Studies in mice demonstrated that a HF diet or LPS infusion induced a two- to threefold increase in circulating LPS levels, contributing to the development of obesity and increased insulin resistance [32,33], and vice versa, LPS and TLR4 initiate a well-characterized signaling cascade that elicits intricate pro-oxidant and pro-inflammatory pathways in obesity [34]. A high LPS concentration is found in patients with type 2 diabetes [35], which is termed ME and reduced by the administration of hypoglycemic agents with potential anti-inflammatory effects [36]. Continuous administration of LPS resulted in recruiting inflammatory cells, activating mTOR signaling, tubular injury and collagen deposition in mice kidneys [37]. By contrast, the administration of antioxidants protects renal blood flow in LPS-treated animal models [38]. Recently, adipose-specific PLA2 have received attention for potential anti-obesity and anti-diabetic roles. Both genetic and pharmacological inhibition of particular PLA2s has resulted in obesity-resistant mouse models, suggesting a potential to develop new drugs [39]. In addition, COX-2 has long been believed to play a role in the inflammatory process as a result of obesity with an HF diet [9,40]. Given the role of PG pathways and oxidative stress in the etiology of obesity-induced renal injuries, the fat–intestine–kidney axis may intricately interact with ROS, cPLA2 and COX-2 in OKF progression. Current data suggest a healthy lifestyle—including antioxidant foods and the avoidance of excessive dietary fat intake—may ensure a friendly gut microbiota and positively affect prevention and treatment of various metabolic disorders.

3.2. Therapeutic Targets of ROS, cPLA2 and COX-2 in Kidney Diseases

Renal tubules are the main structure of the kidney and can be subjected to a variety of damage, including hypoxia, proteinuria, toxins, metabolic disorders, inflammation and oxidative stress [41]. Thus, tubular epithelial damage plays a pivotal role in renal fibrinogenesis [42,43], and PG pathways are crucial homeostatic modulators of kidney function [3]. Through the effects of cPLA2 in the initial stage, membrane phospholipids release arachidonic acid. In the following stepwise conversion of arachidonic acid by COX enzymes and PGE synthase, the major product of PGE2 is elevated and responsible for not only cardiovascular risks but also renal diseases [8]. Recent studies have shown that cPLA2 enhances proliferation and de-differentiation in human renal tubular epithelial cells [44], and silencing cPLA2 expression in knock-out (KO) mice is able to ameliorate pro-inflammatory eicosanoids production, inflammatory cell recruitment, and severity of fibrosis [16]. In another mouse model of high-carbohydrate high-fat-diet-induced obesity, the cPLA2 inhibitor treatment attenuated visceral adiposity and improved most features of metabolic syndrome, including insulin sensitivity, glucose intolerance, and cardiovascular abnormalities [10]. A considerable amount of literature reported that cPLA2 is a useful therapeutic target for diverse diseases. There are a number of concerns in using cPLA2 as a therapeutic target, especially because most of the studies are based on disease models comparing cPLA2 wild type (WT) and KO mice, which may not accurately reflect processes contributing to human diseases. This is apparent from the differences between mice and humans as a consequence of cPLA2 deficiency, e.g., cPLA2 is the first regulatory enzyme in the pathway for the production of numerous lipid mediators. Although, targeting cPLA2 may be beneficial in some diseases where COX metabolites contribute to diseases, such as asthma and arthritis [45]. However, PGs regulate labor and birth in humans, and an important source of PGs is amnion fibroblasts in fetal membranes [46,47]. Considering the essential roles of cPLA2 in human health, particularly for maintenance of the small intestine and female reproduction, is also a concern for targeting cPLA2 in OKF. Moreover, selective COX-2 inhibitors used in the rat model of an HF diet improved insulin sensitivity and TNFα mRNA expression [40]. Nonetheless, the nephrotoxic effect of COX-2 inhibitor for CKD patients is another concern in clinical practice.

Our research indicates ROS serve as a predisposition factor of OKF and thus a therapeutic target, activating downstream PG pathways and tubulointerstitial fibrosis. In contrast with PG inhibitors, NAC can easily be applied to a clinical therapeutic strategy, because a large oral dose of antioxidant is well tolerated without systemic side effects. Notably, the origin, the kinetics, and the localization of ROS generation all influence responses of T lymphocytes and inflammatory cells [48]. Shen Y et al. reported that the administration of NAC significantly mitigated oxidative and fibrotic responses resulting from angiotensin-II upregulation in the obstructed kidneys of mice, including expressions of fibronectin, collagen I, α-SMA and TGF-β [13].

We recognize several limitations of our study. In the first place, endogenous plasma creatinine levels and creatinine clearance as a tool to evaluate renal function were not evaluated in our mouse model. Difficulties have included the lack of an accurate, reproducible method to estimate renal function in conscious mice, problems obtaining sufficient blood volume and precisely timed urine collections repeatedly. Next, further parameters of tubulointerstitial injury in our OKF mouse models were not provided, e.g., neutrophil gelatinase-associated lipocalin, transforming growth factor beta, and alpha-smooth muscle actin. From the perspectives of nephrologists and pathologists, whereas the single method of Masson's trichrome staining can easily and convincingly diagnose tubulointerstitial fibrosis in routine clinical practice of human renal biopsies.

In conclusion, our research has contributed a mechanistic insight into OKF-ME, showing that a high-fat diet and ME impair kidneys through lipid deposition in the tubular epithelium, recruiting lymphocytes, triggering ROS to activate downstream PG pathways, and ultimately, tubulointerstitial fibrosis (Figure 6). ROS may serve as a predisposition factor of PG inflammatory pathways and OKF. We also elucidate that non-specific antioxidant NAC attenuates a high-fat diet and ME-induced renal inflammation and fibrosis. The protective effects are superior to cPLA2 and COX-2 inhibitors. This potential therapeutic target can easily be applied to clinical practice, because a large oral dose of NAC is well tolerated without systemic side effects. In light of the growing prevalence of obesity worldwide with an increasing trend in total medicare expenditures, the organ-protective effects of NAC should be tested in OKF patients who are in urgent need of new therapeutics. Several important issues in this research merit further discussion.

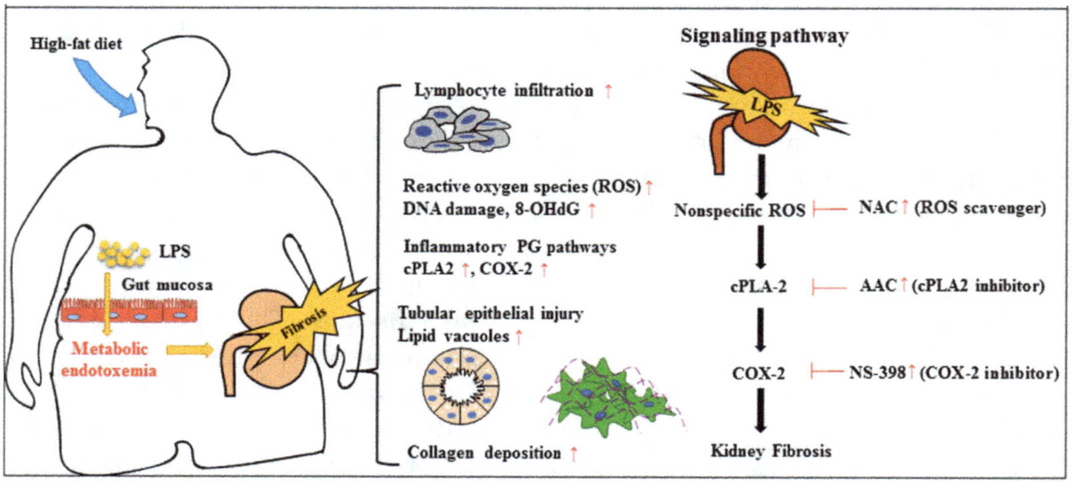

Figure 6. Potential mechanisms of obese kidney fibrosis induced by the fat–intestine–kidney axis. The schematic diagram has contributed a mechanistic insight into obese kidney fibrosis (OKF) with metabolic endotoxemia (ME). A high-fat diet leads to intestinal dysbiosis and hyperpermeability, favoring translocation of microbiome-derived lipopolysaccharide (LPS) to the bloodstream. A high-fat diet and ME impair kidneys through lipid deposition in the tubular epithelium, recruiting lymphocytes, triggering ROS to activate downstream prostaglandin pathways, and ultimately tubulointerstitial fibrosis. ROS may serve as predisposition factors and thus therapeutic targets in the prevention of OKF-ME. Different levels of the inhibitors' activity are indicated as red arrows.

4. Materials and Methods

4.1. Materials

Most materials and methods were previously described [25]. Other materials utilized in this study can be purchased from Santa Cruz Biotechnology (Santa Cruz, CA, USA) or Sigma (St. Louis, MO, USA), including the inhibitor of cPLA2 (AACOCF3 (AAC)/Arachidonyltrifluoromethane), COX-2 (NS-398/N-[2-(cyclohexyloxy)-4-nitrophenyl] methanesulfonamide), and nonspecific ROS (NAC/N-Acetyl L-Cysteine).

4.2. Creating Animal Models to Mimic Obese Kidney Fibrosis (OKF) in Humans

A WT C57BL/6NCrlBltw mouse was provided by BioLASCO Taiwan Co., Ltd. (Taipei, Taiwan). The study was approved by the Animal Care and Use Committee of the Fu Jen Laboratory Animal Center (IACUC number: A10603; 1, March, 2017). All animals were handled according to the guidelines of the Animal Care Committee of Fu Jen Catholic University and NIH Guides for the Care and Use of Laboratory Animals. Animals were maintained in a temperature-controlled room (22 °C) under 12 h light–dark cycles. One week after arrival, four-week-old mice were divided into different groups. The control group received continuous feeding of a normal chow (Lactamin, Stockholm, Sweden). The HF group was first fed with a mix of a high-fat diet (#D12492, Research Diets, New Brunswick, NJ) and normal chow (w:w = 1:1) for diet adaptation for one week, then a complete high-fat diet course was given for the next 10 weeks. To create the animal model of OKF with ME, six-week-old mice that were fed with a high-fat diet were injected with LPS (10 μg/kg/week, intraperitoneal (i.p.) injection) as the HL group. If inhibitors were used, various inhibitors (2 mg/kg/week, i.p.) were injected one hour before LPS injection as inhibitor-treated groups. Mice were then sacrificed at the age of fifteen weeks, and kidneys were quickly removed and preserved in formalin for paraffin embedment for further analyses.

4.3. Tissue Preparation for Histopathological Evaluation of H&E Stain

Mice were anaesthetized via the inhalation of isoflurane and euthanized by cervical dislocation. Kidneys were removed and fixed in 10% formalin. Specimens were embedded in paraffin and sliced into 2–3 μm in thickness. Subsequently, the kidney tissues were stained with Hematoxylin-eosin (H&E stain). The images were captured using a Nikon Digital Camera Microscope (Nikon, Tokyo, Japan).

4.4. Masson's Trichrome Staining Method

Masson's trichrome staining method was used to determine the extent of collagen deposition and fibrosis in mouse kidney tissues. In the corresponding area, H&E staining of the adjacent paraffin section was performed for comparisons of tissue morphology. The experiments were conducted as follows: sections were first deparaffinized and rehydrated in ethanol/water solutions then post-fixed with Bouin's solution for 1 h at room temperature. The fixation buffer was removed, and slides were stained with iron hematoxylin, Biebrich scarlet-acid fuchsin, and phosphomolybdic-phosphotungstic acid sequentially for 10 min per stain. Slides were then stained with Aniline blue. Finally, slides were washed in 10% acetate solution for 3–5 min and mounted in the mounting medium for observations to be made.

4.5. Immunohistochemistry Staining Method

Immunohistochemistry (IHC) was performed manually or automatically with an autostainer (BenchMark XT, Ventana Medical Systems Inc., Tucson, AZ, USA). For the manual protocol, paraffin sections were first deparaffinized and rehydrated in ethanol/water solutions. Epitopes on tissue were then retrieved with Heat-Induced Epitope Retrieval (HIER) in citrate buffer (0.01 M, pH 6.0). For blocking endogenous peroxidase activity, sections were treated with 3% hydrogen peroxide for 30 min in the dark. To reduce non-specific primary antibody binding, Blocking Buffer (DAKO) was used for one hour at room temperature. Sections were then incubated with primary antibodies at 4 °C overnight. Rabbit anti-mouse COX-2, anti-human cPLA2, and anti-8-OHdG polyclonal antibodies were purchased from Santa Cruz Biotechnology (SC-1747-R, SC-7891, and SC-139586, Santa Cruz, CA, USA). Afterward, staining was detected with a DAKO polymer system. For image acquisitions, three random high-power magnification fields were obtained in each sample by a Nikon Digital Camera Microscope (Nikon, Tokyo, Japan). All slides were reviewed by a blinded pathologist (Dr. Shih-Hao Liu), and the area percentage of staining in a 200× power magnification field were analyzed by NIH ImageJ software (Version 1.47, Bethesda, MD, USA).

4.6. Statistical Analysis of Data

All data are expressed as the mean ± SD using the GraphPad Prism Program (GraphPad, San Diego, CA, USA). Quantitative data were analyzed with a non-paired Student's t-test. The significance threshold was set at 5% ($p < 0.05$). All of the experiments were performed at least three times.

Author Contributions: J.-F.C. and W.-N.L. were responsible for study design, data interpretation, study supervision, and manuscript draft. C.-T.H., S.-H.L. and C.-Y.H. assisted with digital analysis for immunohistochemistry staining and morphometric analysis in histopathology. J.-Y.W. assisted the protein extraction. J.-C.Y., S.-W.C., T.-M.W., I.-T.L., and K.-Y.H. were responsible for writing and revision of the manuscript.

Abbreviations

CKD	chronic kidney disease
COX-2	cyclooxygenase-2
cPLA2	cytosolic phospholipases A2
HF group	high-fat diet-fed group injected with lipopolysaccharide
IHC	immunohistochemistry
LPS	lipopolysaccharide
ME	metabolic endotoxemia
OKF	obese kidney fibrosis
PG	prostaglandin
ROS	reactive oxygen species

References

1. Stenvinkel, P.; Zoccali, C.; Ikizler, T.A. Obesity in CKD—What should nephrologists know? *J. Am. Soc. Nephrol.* **2013**, *24*, 1727–1736. [CrossRef]
2. Kovesdy, C.P.; Furth, S.L.; Zoccali, C.; on Behalf of the World Kidney Day Steering Committee. Obesity and Kidney Disease: Hidden Consequences of the Epidemic. *Am. J. Hypertens.* **2017**, *30*, 328–336. [CrossRef]
3. Jung, C.H.; Lee, M.J.; Kang, Y.M.; Hwang, J.Y.; Kim, E.H.; Park, J.Y.; Kim, H.K.; Lee, W.J. The risk of chronic kidney disease in a metabolically healthy obese population. *Kidney Int.* **2015**, *88*, 843–850. [CrossRef]
4. Câmara, N.O.S.; Iseki, K.; Kramer, H.; Liu, Z.-H.; Sharma, K. Kidney disease and obesity: Epidemiology, mechanisms and treatment. *Nat. Rev. Nephrol.* **2017**, *13*, 181. [CrossRef]
5. Hobby, G.P.; Karaduta, O.; Dusio, G.F.; Singh, M.; Zybailov, B.L.; Arthur, J.M. Chronic Kidney Disease and the Gut Microbiome. *Am. J. Physiol. Renal Physiol.* **2019**. [CrossRef]
6. Shah, N.B.; Allegretti, A.S.; Nigwekar, S.U.; Kalim, S.; Zhao, S.; Lelouvier, B.; Servant, F.; Serena, G.; Thadhani, R.I.; Raj, D.S.; et al. Blood Microbiome Profile in CKD: A Pilot Study. *Clin. J. Am. Soc. Nephrol. CJASN* **2019**. [CrossRef]
7. Lim, P.S.; Chang, Y.K.; Wu, T.K. Serum Lipopolysaccharide-Binding Protein is Associated with Chronic Inflammation and Metabolic Syndrome in Hemodialysis Patients. *Blood Purif.* **2019**, *47*, 28–36. [CrossRef]
8. Nasrallah, R.; Hassouneh, R.; Hébert, R.L. PGE2, kidney disease, and cardiovascular risk: Beyond hypertension and diabetes. *J. Am. Soc. Nephrol.* **2016**, *27*, 666–676. [CrossRef]
9. Komers, R.; Zdychova, J.; Cahova, M.; Kazdova, L.; Lindsley, J.N.; Anderson, S. Renal cyclooxygenase-2 in obese Zucker (fatty) rats. *Kidney Int.* **2005**, *67*, 2151–2158. [CrossRef]
10. Iyer, A.; Lim, J.; Poudyal, H.; Reid, R.C.; Suen, J.Y.; Webster, J.; Prins, J.B.; Whitehead, J.P.; Fairlie, D.P.; Brown, L. An inhibitor of phospholipase A2 group IIA modulates adipocyte signaling and protects against diet-induced metabolic syndrome in rats. *Diabetes* **2012**, *61*, 2320–2329. [CrossRef]
11. Jia, Z.; Zhang, Y.; Ding, G.; Heiney, K.M.; Huang, S.; Zhang, A. Role of COX-2/mPGES-1/prostaglandin E2 cascade in kidney injury. *Mediat. Inflamm.* **2015**, *2015*, 147894. [CrossRef]

12. Câmara, N.O.; Martins, J.O.; Landgraf, R.G. Emerging roles for eicosanoids in renal diseases. *Curr. Opin. Nephrol. Hypertens.* **2009**, *18*, 21–27. [CrossRef]
13. Shen, Y.; Miao, N.-J.; Xu, J.-L.; Gan, X.-X.; Xu, D.; Zhou, L.; Xue, H.; Zhang, W.; Lu, L.-M. *N*-acetylcysteine alleviates angiotensin II-mediated renal fibrosis in mouse obstructed kidneys. *Acta Pharmacol. Sin.* **2016**, *37*, 637. [CrossRef]
14. Chen, D.Q.; Cao, G.; Chen, H.; Liu, D.; Su, W.; Yu, X.Y.; Vaziri, N.D.; Liu, X.H.; Bai, X.; Zhang, L.; et al. Gene and protein expressions and metabolomics exhibit activated redox signaling and wnt/beta-catenin pathway are associated with metabolite dysfunction in patients with chronic kidney disease. *Redox Biol.* **2017**, *12*, 505–521. [CrossRef]
15. Khan, N.S.; Song, C.Y.; Thirunavukkarasu, S.; Fang, X.R.; Bonventre, J.V.; Malik, K.U. Cytosolic Phospholipase A2alpha Is Essential for Renal Dysfunction and End-Organ Damage Associated with Angiotensin II-Induced Hypertension. *Am. J. Hypertens.* **2016**, *29*, 258–265. [CrossRef]
16. Montford, J.R.; Lehman, A.M.B.; Bauer, C.D.; Klawitter, J.; Klawitter, J.; Poczobutt, J.M.; Scobey, M.; Weiser-Evans, M.; Nemenoff, R.A.; Furgeson, S.B. Bone marrow-derived cPLA2α contributes to renal fibrosis progression. *J. Lipid Res.* **2018**, *59*, 380–390. [CrossRef]
17. Zhao, Y.Y.; Wang, H.L.; Cheng, X.L.; Wei, F.; Bai, X.; Lin, R.C.; Vaziri, N.D. Metabolomics analysis reveals the association between lipid abnormalities and oxidative stress, inflammation, fibrosis, and Nrf2 dysfunction in aristolochic acid-induced nephropathy. *Sci. Rep.* **2015**, *5*, 12936. [CrossRef]
18. Chen, H.M.; Yang, C.M.; Chang, J.F.; Wu, C.S.; Sia, K.C.; Lin, W.N. AdipoR-increased intracellular ROS promotes cPLA2 and COX-2 expressions via activation of PKC and p300 in adiponectin-stimulated human alveolar type II cells. *Am. J. Physiol. Lung Cell Mol. Physiol.* **2016**, *311*, L255–L269. [CrossRef]
19. Hsu, P.S.; Lin, C.M.; Chang, J.F.; Wu, C.S.; Sia, K.C.; Lee, I.T.; Huang, K.Y.; Lin, W.N. Participation of NADPH Oxidase-Related Reactive Oxygen Species in Leptin-Promoted Pulmonary Inflammation: Regulation of cPLA2alpha and COX-2 Expression. *Int. J. Mol. Sci.* **2019**, *20*, 1078. [CrossRef]
20. Ji, L.; Wang, Q.; Huang, F.; An, T.; Guo, F.; Zhao, Y.; Liu, Y.; He, Y.; Song, Y.; Qin, G. FOXO1 Overexpression Attenuates Tubulointerstitial Fibrosis and Apoptosis in Diabetic Kidneys by Ameliorating Oxidative Injury via TXNIP-TRX. *Oxidative Med. Cell. Longev.* **2019**, *2019*, 3286928. [CrossRef]
21. Reilly, S.M.; Saltiel, A.R. Adapting to obesity with adipose tissue inflammation. *Nat. Rev. Endocrinol.* **2017**, *13*, 633. [CrossRef]
22. De Vries, A.P.; Ruggenenti, P.; Ruan, X.Z.; Praga, M.; Cruzado, J.M.; Bajema, I.M.; D'Agati, V.; Lamb, H.J.; Barlovic, D.P.; Hojs, R. Fatty kidney: Emerging role of ectopic lipid in obesity-related renal disease. *Lancet Diabetes Endocrinol.* **2014**, *2*, 417–426. [CrossRef]
23. Jiang, T.; Wang, Z.; Proctor, G.; Moskowitz, S.; Liebman, S.E.; Rogers, T.; Lucia, M.S.; Li, J.; Levi, M. Diet-induced obesity in C57BL/6J mice causes increased renal lipid accumulation and glomerulosclerosis via a sterol regulatory element-binding protein-1c-dependent pathway. *J. Biol. Chem.* **2005**, *280*, 32317–32325. [CrossRef]
24. Zhou, D.; Liu, Y. Renal fibrosis in 2015: Understanding the mechanisms of kidney fibrosis. *Nat. Rev. Nephrol.* **2016**, *12*, 68. [CrossRef]
25. Chang, J.-F.; Liang, S.-S.; Thanasekaran, P.; Chang, H.-W.; Wen, L.-L.; Chen, C.-H.; Liou, J.-C.; Yeh, J.-C.; Liu, S.-H.; Dai, H.-M. Translational Medicine in Pulmonary-Renal Crosstalk: Therapeutic Targeting of p-Cresyl Sulfate Triggered Nonspecific ROS and Chemoattractants in Dyspneic Patients with Uremic Lung Injury. *J. Clin. Med.* **2018**, *7*, 266. [CrossRef]
26. Droge, W. Free radicals in the physiological control of cell function. *Physiol. Rev.* **2002**, *82*, 47–95. [CrossRef]
27. Finkel, T. Signal transduction by reactive oxygen species in non-phagocytic cells. *J. Leukoc. Biol.* **1999**, *65*, 337–340. [CrossRef]
28. Wong, A.C.; Vanhove, A.S.; Watnick, P.I. The interplay between intestinal bacteria and host metabolism in health and disease: Lessons from Drosophila melanogaster. *Dis. Models Mech.* **2016**, *9*, 271–281. [CrossRef]
29. Musso, G.; Gambino, R.; Cassader, M. Obesity, diabetes, and gut microbiota: The hygiene hypothesis expanded? *Diabetes Care* **2010**, *33*, 2277–2284. [CrossRef]
30. Marchesi, J.R.; Adams, D.H.; Fava, F.; Hermes, G.D.; Hirschfield, G.M.; Hold, G.; Quraishi, M.N.; Kinross, J.; Smidt, H.; Tuohy, K.M. The gut microbiota and host health: A new clinical frontier. *Gut* **2016**, *65*, 330–339. [CrossRef]
31. Rosas-Villegas, A.; Sánchez-Tapia, M.; Avila-Nava, A.; Ramírez, V.; Tovar, A.; Torres, N. Differential effect of sucrose and fructose in combination with a high fat diet on intestinal microbiota and kidney oxidative stress.

Nutrients **2017**, *9*, 393. [CrossRef]

32. Cani, P.D.; Amar, J.; Iglesias, M.A.; Poggi, M.; Knauf, C.; Bastelica, D.; Neyrinck, A.M.; Fava, F.; Tuohy, K.M.; Chabo, C. Metabolic endotoxemia initiates obesity and insulin resistance. *Diabetes* **2007**, *56*, 1761–1772. [CrossRef]
33. Cani, P.D.; Bibiloni, R.; Knauf, C.; Waget, A.; Neyrinck, A.M.; Delzenne, N.M.; Burcelin, R. Changes in gut microbiota control metabolic endotoxemia-induced inflammation in high-fat diet–induced obesity and diabetes in mice. *Diabetes* **2008**, *57*, 1470–1481. [CrossRef]
34. Boutagy, N.E.; McMillan, R.P.; Frisard, M.I.; Hulver, M.W. Metabolic endotoxemia with obesity: Is it real and is it relevant? *Biochimie* **2016**, *124*, 11–20. [CrossRef]
35. Creely, S.J.; McTernan, P.G.; Kusminski, C.M.; Khanolkar, M.; Evans, M.; Louise Harte, A.; Kumar, S. Lipopolysaccharide activates an innate immune system response in human adipose tissue in obesity and type 2 diabetes. *Am. J. Physiol.-Endocrinol. Metabol.* **2007**, *292*, E740–E747. [CrossRef]
36. Mohanty, P.; Aljada, A.; Ghanim, H.; Hofmeyer, D.; Tripathy, D.; Syed, T.; Al-Haddad, W.; Dhindsa, S.; Dandona, P. Evidence for a potent antiinflammatory effect of rosiglitazone. *J. Clin. Endocrinol. Metab.* **2004**, *89*, 2728–2735. [CrossRef]
37. Chen, H.; Zhu, J.; Liu, Y.; Dong, Z.; Liu, H.; Liu, Y.; Zhou, X.; Liu, F.; Chen, G. Lipopolysaccharide induces chronic kidney injury and fibrosis through activation of mTOR signaling in macrophages. *Am. J. Nephrol.* **2015**, *42*, 305–317. [CrossRef]
38. Magder, S.; Parthenis, D.; Ghouleh, I. Preservation of Renal Blood Flow by the Antioxidant EUK-134 in LPS-Treated Pigs. *Int. J. Mol. Sci.* **2015**, *16*, 6801–6817. [CrossRef]
39. Abbott, M.J.; Tang, T.; Sul, H.S. The role of phospholipase A2-derived mediators in obesity. *Drug Discov. Today Disease Mech.* **2010**, *7*, e213–e218. [CrossRef]
40. Hsieh, P.S.; Jin, J.S.; Chiang, C.F.; Chan, P.C.; Chen, C.H.; Shih, K.C. COX-2-mediated inflammation in fat is crucial for obesity-linked insulin resistance and fatty liver. *Obesity* **2009**, *17*, 1150–1157. [CrossRef]
41. Liu, B.-C.; Tang, T.-T.; Lv, L.-L.; Lan, H.-Y. Renal tubule injury: A driving force toward chronic kidney disease. *Kidney Int.* **2018**, *93*, 568–579. [CrossRef]
42. Grande, M.T.; Sánchez-Laorden, B.; López-Blau, C.; De Frutos, C.A.; Boutet, A.; Arévalo, M.; Rowe, R.G.; Weiss, S.J.; López-Novoa, J.M.; Nieto, M.A. Snail1-induced partial epithelial-to-mesenchymal transition drives renal fibrosis in mice and can be targeted to reverse established disease. *Nat. Med.* **2015**, *21*, 989. [CrossRef]
43. Lovisa, S.; LeBleu, V.S.; Tampe, B.; Sugimoto, H.; Vadnagara, K.; Carstens, J.L.; Wu, C.-C.; Hagos, Y.; Burckhardt, B.C.; Pentcheva-Hoang, T. Epithelial-to-mesenchymal transition induces cell cycle arrest and parenchymal damage in renal fibrosis. *Nat. Med.* **2015**, *21*, 998. [CrossRef]
44. Montford, J.R.; Lehman, A.M.; Scobey, M.S.; Weiser-Evans, M.C.; Nemenoff, R.A.; Furgeson, S.B. Cytosolic phospholipase A2α increases proliferation and de-differentiation of human renal tubular epithelial cells. *Prostaglandins Lipid Mediat.* **2016**, *126*, 1–8. [CrossRef]
45. Hegen, M.; Sun, L.; Uozumi, N.; Kume, K.; Goad, M.E.; Nickerson-Nutter, C.L.; Shimizu, T.; Clark, J.D. Cytosolic phospholipase A2α–deficient mice are resistant to collagen-induced arthritis. *J. Exp. Med.* **2003**, *197*, 1297–1302. [CrossRef]
46. Challis, J.R.; Matthews, S.G.; Gibb, W.; Lye, S.J. Endocrine and paracrine regulation of birth at term and preterm. *Endocr. Rev.* **2000**, *21*, 514–550. [CrossRef]
47. Challis, J.R.; Sloboda, D.M.; Alfaidy, N.; Lye, S.J.; Gibb, W.; Patel, F.A.; Whittle, W.L.; Newnham, J.P. Prostaglandins and mechanisms of preterm birth. *Reprod. Camb.* **2002**, *124*, 1–17. [CrossRef]
48. Belikov, A.V.; Schraven, B.; Simeoni, L. T cells and reactive oxygen species. *J. Biomed. Sci.* **2015**, *22*, 85. [CrossRef]

5

Renal Regenerative Potential of Extracellular Vesicles Derived from miRNA-Engineered Mesenchymal Stromal Cells

Marta Tapparo [1,†], Stefania Bruno [1,†], Federica Collino [2], Gabriele Togliatto [1], Maria Chiara Deregibus [3], Paolo Provero [4], Sicheng Wen [5], Peter J. Quesenberry [5] and Giovanni Camussi [1,*]

1 Department of Medical Sciences and Molecular Biotechnology Center, University of Torino, 10126 Torino, Italy; marta.tapparo@unito.it (M.T.); stefania.bruno@unito.it (S.B.); gabriele.togliatto@unito.it (G.T.)

2 Department of Biomedical Sciences and Paediatric Research Institute "Citta della Speranza", University of Padova, 35129 Padova, Italy; federica.collino@unipd.it

3 2i3T Società per la gestione dell'incubatore di imprese e per il trasferimento tecnologico Scarl, University of Torino, 10126 Torino, Italy; mariachiara.deregibus@unito.it

4 Department of Molecular Biotechnology and Health Sciences and Molecular Biotechnology Center, University of Torino, 10126 Torino, Italy; paolo.provero@unito.it

5 Division of Hematology/Oncology, Brown University, Rhode Island Hospital, Providence, Rhode Island, RI 02912, USA; swen@lifespan.org (S.W.); PQuesenberry@lifespan.org (P.J.Q.)

* Correspondence: giovanni.camussi@unito.it

† These authors contributed equally to this work.

Abstract: Extracellular vesicles (EVs) derived from mesenchymal stromal cells (MSCs) possess pro-regenerative potential in different animal models with renal injury. EVs contain different molecules, including proteins, lipids and nucleic acids. Among the shuttled molecules, miRNAs have a relevant role in the pro-regenerative effects of EVs and are a promising target for therapeutic interventions. The aim of this study was to increase the content of specific miRNAs in EVs that are known to be involved in the pro-regenerative effect of EVs, and to assess the capacity of modified EVs to contribute to renal regeneration in in vivo models with acute kidney injuries. To this purpose, MSCs were transiently transfected with specific miRNA mimics by electroporation. Molecular analyses showed that, after transfection, MSCs and derived EVs were efficiently enriched in the selected miRNAs. In vitro and in vivo experiments indicated that EVs engineered with miRNAs maintained their pro-regenerative effects. Of relevance, engineered EVs were more effective than EVs derived from naïve MSCs when used at suboptimal doses. This suggests the potential use of a low amount of EVs (82.5×10^6) to obtain the renal regenerative effect.

Keywords: mesenchymal stromal cells; extracellular vesicles; acute kidney injury; modified-MSCs; microRNA

---

1. Introduction

Mesenchymal stromal cells (MSCs) are one of the most studied adult stem cells and have been extensively applied in the field of regenerative medicine. In the last years, many studies have demonstrated that their therapeutic effects are mainly mediated by the secretion of bioactive molecules (such as RNAs, proteins, and lipids) that can be directly released in the local microenvironment or packaged in extracellular vesicles (EVs) [1]. Paracrine factors released by MSCs, including EVs, induce the recovery of injured tissue and modulate the immune response and inflammation [2,3]. Many reports have demonstrated the application of MSCs and of their derived EVs in the recovery of renal dysfunction [4]. Different preclinical models of acute and chronic kidney injuries have been used to demonstrate the efficacy of EVs from MSCs in the amelioration of acute kidney injury (AKI) and in preventing progression at the chronic stage [5]. Recently, we tested different subpopulations of MSC-derived EVs in renal regeneration. Most of the effects observed in the recovery from AKI were ascribed to the exosomal fraction, which carried mRNA, miRNAs and proteins that induced the proliferation of tubular cells. Despite the inefficiency of the non-exosomal fraction, we observed that the effect of the exosomal fraction and the total-EVs was not significantly different in terms of pro-regenerative potential, suggesting that the ineffective fraction did not interfere with the exosomal fraction activity [6]. Moreover, MSCs may be manipulated in culture by transferring specific miRNA to EV-producing cells to obtain modified-EVs with potentiated pro-regenerative or reparative effects [7–11]. In this work, we set up a method to increase—in MSCs and in their total-EVs—the content of specific miRNAs involved in renal regeneration. To assess the capacities of modified-EVs to contribute to AKI recovery, we tested them in vitro on murine renal tubular epithelial cells and in vivo in a model of AKI induced by glycerol injection.

2. Results

2.1. Identification of Pro-Regenerative miRNAs Carried by EVs

In our previous study, we performed RNA sequencing (RNA-Seq) analysis to detect the molecular changes that occurred in the kidneys of AKI mice treated with MSC-derived EVs (EV-CTRL) vs. untreated AKI mice (AKI) (Gene Expression Omnibus accession number GSE59958) [12]. In this study, the potential healing miRNAs were selected from among known human miRNAs that were predicted to significantly down-regulate RNAs modulated in our treatments with a bio-informatic approach, as described in the Methods section. The obtained miRNA families (Table 1) were posteriorly cross-matched with a list of 50 miRNAs with increased expression in the MSC-derived EVs [6]. The following miRNAs were identified: miR-10a-5p, miR-127-3p, miR-29a-3p, let-7a and miR-30a-5p. miR-486-5p was also selected because it was the most enriched miRNA in the exosomal fraction, which was the more effective fraction in promoting AKI recovery [6].

Table 1. List of miRNA families for which targets were significantly modulated by extracellular vesicle (EV) administration in acute kidney injury (AKI) mice.

	FC Non-Targets	FC Targets	p	Rank
miR-10abc/10a-5p	0.03	0.06	0.0313	1
let-7/98/4458/4500	0.03	0.06	0.0476	2
miR-127/127-3p	0.03	0.25	0.0431	12
miR-30abcdef/30abe-5p/384-5p	0.03	0.07	0.0003	13
miR-29abcd	0.03	0.07	0.0047	24
miR-192/215	0.03	0.14	0.0035	50
miR-140/140-5p/876-3p/1244	0.03	0.10	0.0177	72
miR-377	0.03	0.08	0.0203	96
miR-202-3p	0.03	0.08	0.0060	124

miRNAs with targets that showed significant down-regulation in EV treated-vs. untreated-AKI mice were listed and correlated with their enrichment in EVs isolated at 100,000 g (p value < 0.05). Non-targets: Median fold change (FC, logarithmic treated vs. untreated) of the genes that are not miRNA targets. Targets: Median FC of the genes that are miRNA targets. p: p-value generated by Mann–Whitney test, comparing the FC of targets vs. non-target miRNAs. Rank: List of the expressed miRNAs based on their abundance inside EVs.

To evaluate the potential of selected miRNAs to promote tubular cell proliferation, murine tubular epithelial cells (mTECs) were treated with miRNA mimics and submitted to hypoxia/reoxygenation conditions. mTECs treated with miR-10a-5p (miR10a), miR-127-3p (miR127), miR-29a-3p (miR29a) and miR-486-5p (miR486) were able to proliferate to some degree in the hypoxia/reoxygenation culture, even if the obtained results did not reach statistical significance, unlike let-7b- and miR-30a-5p-

(miR30a-)treated tubular cells (Figure 1), which only supported the beneficial effects of selected EV-miRNAs in AKI.

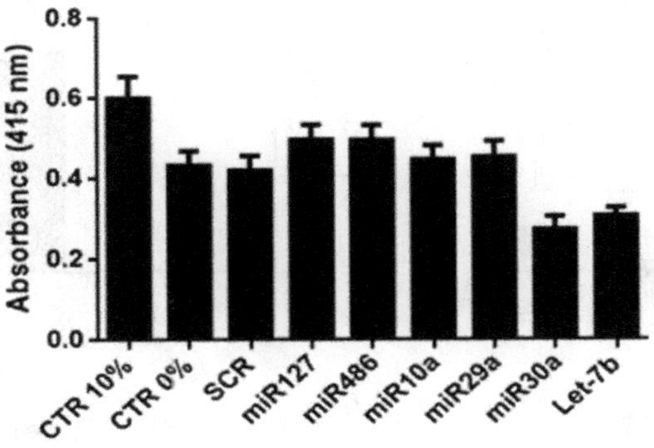

Figure 1. In vitro effect of selected miRNA mimics. Different miRNA mimics (miR127, miR486, miR10a, miR29a, miR30a and let-7b-100 nM) were added to murine tubular epithelial cells (mTECs) maintained in hypoxia for 48 h, after which proliferation was evaluated following 24 h of re-oxygenation. mTECs were maintained in medium supplemented with 10% fetal calf serum (FCS) or 0% FCS, used respectively as the positive (CTR 10%) and negative (CTR 0%) controls. Data are reported as mean ± SEM for three different experiments performed in quadruplicate.

2.2. Generation of MSCs and Derived EVs Engineered with miRNAs

MSCs were subjected to electroporation (MSC-EP) in order to enrich their content of the selected miRNAs. Different electroporation protocols were tested (EP1-3, Table 2, Materials and Methods section) and transfection efficiency was evaluated by qRT-PCR. The EP1 protocol (990 V, 40 msec, 1 pulse) was selected because of the enhanced expression of the control miRNA mimic observed in the MSCs and the maintained cell viability (Figure 2A). We also set up the optimal dose of miRNA mimic to transfect MSCs. As seen in Figure 2B, 25 pmol/4 × 10^4 cells was the lowest dose tested that increased the expression of the control miRNA. Expression of the selected miRNAs was then assessed using the transfection condition identified during setting. We detected an increased expression of the selected miRNAs in MSC-EP after 24 h (Figure 2C) that remained stable until day 7. Of notice, we observed a higher expression for miR-127 and miR-486 with respect to the other two miRNAs, suggesting a different efficiency of transfection.

EVs from MSC-EP (EV-EP), enriched with different miRNA mimics (Figure 3), were isolated 24 h after transfection and subsequently characterized for size distribution and particle number by NanoSight. EVs derived from MSC-EP showed similar size profiles to naïve MSC EVs. No differences were observed among EV-EP that were simply electroporated or transfected with scramble (SCR) mimic (EV-SCR) or with different miRNAs mimics (EV-miR127, EV-miR486, EV-miR10a, EV-miR29a) (Figure 4A). Moreover, evaluation of particle number did not show any variation between the different mimic-enriched EV-EP.

Additionally, typical MSC marker expression on EV-EP was maintained, suggesting that electroporation did not affect surface molecule expression. As described in Reference [6], EVs derived from naïve MSCs or MSC-EP in the presence of different miRNA mimics expressed the typical exosomal marker (CD63) and MSC markers (CD73, CD44 and CD29) (Figure 4B). Electron microscopy confirmed that EV-EP maintained the same morphology as EV-CTRL (Figure 4C).

miRNA enrichment was then evaluated by real-time PCR for the different EV-EP. The expression of miR-127, miR-10a, miR-29a and miR-486 was increased in MSC-EP-derived EVs with respect to MSC-EVs derived from cells that were only electroporated or from SCR-transfected MSC-EP (Figure 2D). As seen in the MSC-EP and their respective EVs, the efficiency of enrichment was slightly different according to the mimic used. For instance, miR-29a was less enriched in EVs with respect to the other mimics. Instead, we observed a higher increase in the expression for miR-127 and miR-486.

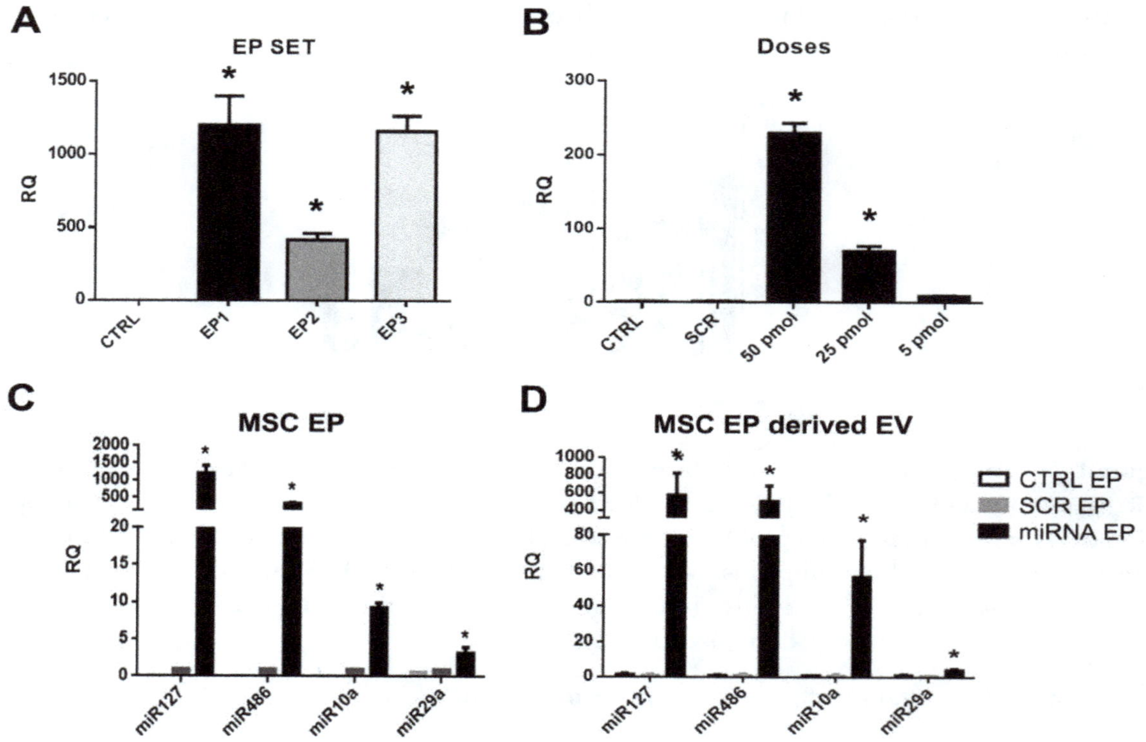

Figure 2. miRNA enrichment evaluation in mesenchymal stromal cells subjected to electroporation (MSC-EP) and derived EVs. (**A**) Representative real-time PCR showing the efficiency of transfection for different electroporation protocols (EP1-3). ANOVA with Dunnett's multiple comparison test was performed. * $p < 0.05$ EP protocol vs. CTRL (non elecroporated cells); (**B**) representative real-time PCR showing the efficiency of transfection for different doses of control miRNA mimic obtained with EP1 electroporation conditions. ANOVA with Dunnett's multiple comparison test was performed. $p < 0.05$ different control miRNA doses vs. scramble (SCR); (**C**) representative real-time PCR showing the increased expression of the selected miRNAs (miR10a, miR29a, miR127, miR486) 24 h after transfection in MSC-EP and (**D**) in derived EVs collected 24 h after transfection. Data were normalized in respect to MSC transfected with the SCR. Data are represented as relative quantification (RQ) ± SEM. * $p < 0.05$ MSC-EP SCR vs. MSC-EP transfected with mimics and * $p < 0.05$ EV-SCR vs. EV transfected with mimics. Multiple *t* test with Holm–Sidak method correction was performed.

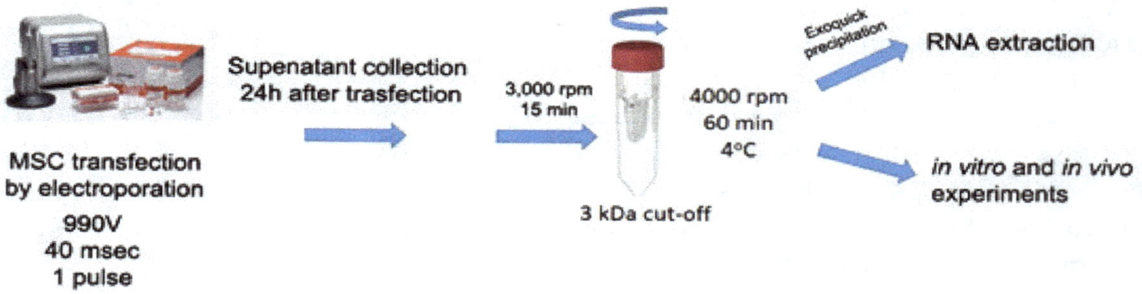

Figure 3. Schematic illustration of the engineering method used to transiently transfect MSCs. MSCs were transfected via a neon electroporation system with different miRNA mimics. EVs were collected after 24 h and supernatant, previously centrifuged at 2000 *g* to eliminate cell debris, was concentrated by 3 kDa filter tube. EVs were then used for in vitro and in vivo experiments or precipitated by Exoquick and used for RNA extraction.

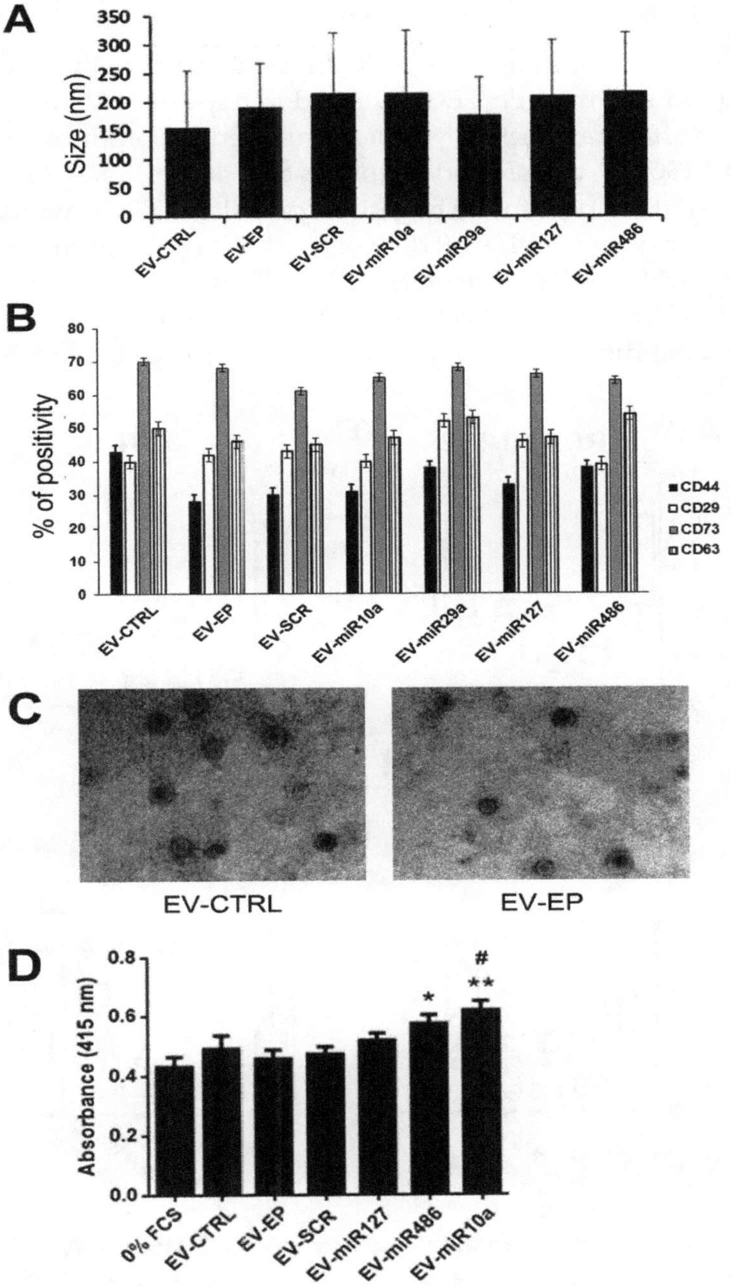

Figure 4. Characterization of EVs derived from naïve MSCs and from EP MSCs. (**A**) Size of EVs obtained from naïve MSC (EV-CTRL), from electroporated MSC (EV-EP) and transfected with scramble (EV-SCR) or with different miRNA mimics (EV-mir10a, EV-miR29a, EV-miR127, EV-miR486), evaluated by nanoparticle tracking analysis (NTA). Data reported are mean ± SD for three different experiments. No statistically significant differences were observed among the different types of EVs; (**B**) cytofluorimetric analysis of the expression of MSC (CD44, CD29 and CD73) and exosomal (CD63) markers, in different EV populations. Data reported are the mean ± SD for three different experiments. No statistically significant differences were observed in marker expression among the different types of EVs; (**C**) representative micrographs of transmission electron microscopy of EV-CTRL (left) and EV-EP (right). EVs negatively stained with NanoVan (magnification ×100,000); and (**D**) different types of EVs (1000/cells) were added to mTECs maintained for 48 h in hypoxia, after which proliferation was evaluated following 24 h of reoxygenation. Data are reported as mean ± SEM for three different experiments in quadruplicate. ANOVA with Dunnett's multiple comparison test was performed. ** $p < 0.01$ and * $p < 0.05$ mTEC stimulated with EV-mimic vs. mTEC maintained in 0% FCS, # $p < 0.05$ EV-miR10a vs. mTEC stimulated with EV-EP.

2.3. In Vitro and In Vivo Effects of EVs

EVs obtained from naïve MSCs and from MSC-EP transfected with SCR or with 10a, 127 and 486 miRNA mimics were tested in vitro on mTECs cultured in hypoxia. EV-miR29a was not further tested since the miR-29a in EVs after transfection was less enriched in comparison with the other miRNAs considered. EVs from MSC-EP transfected with 10a and 486 miRNA mimics induced significant proliferation of mTECs with respect to the negative controls (mTECs maintained with 0% fetal calf serum [FCS]). Only EVs enriched with miR10a induced a significant increase in proliferation with respect to EVs obtained by MSC-EP (Figure 4D).

MSC electroporation did not interfere with the renal pro-regenerative capacity of EVs; EV-EP significantly improved renal function and morphology similarly to naïve MSC-EVs (Figure 5).

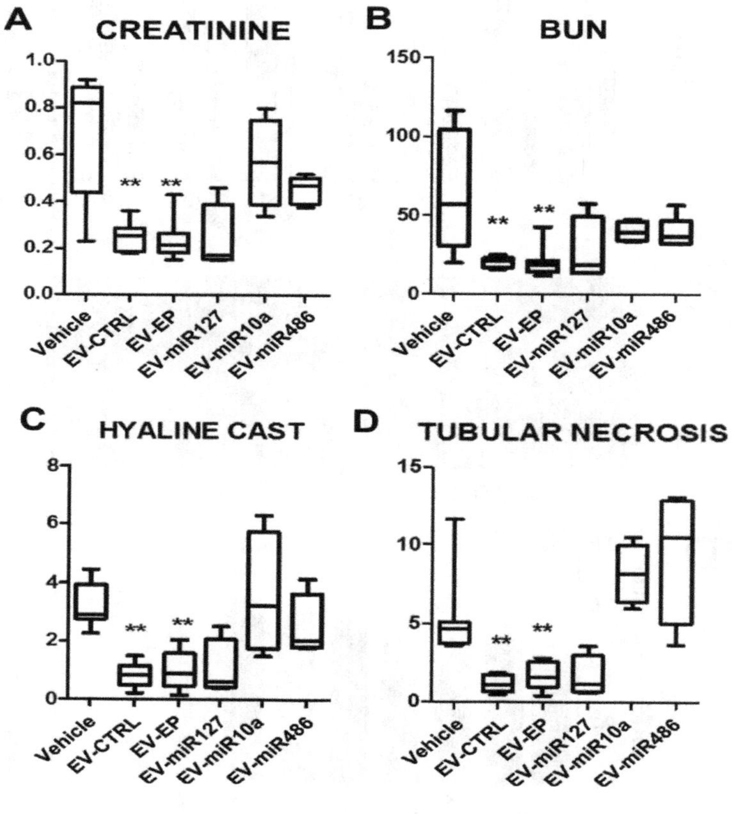

Figure 5. Effect of EVs derived from naïve or electroporated MSC in AKI mice: Functional and morphological evaluation. (**A**) Creatinine and (**B**) blood urea nitrogen (BUN) values in AKI mice injected with vehicle alone (Vehicle) or with 165×10^6 EVs derived from naïve MSCs (EV-CTRL) or from electroporated MSCs (EV-EP) transfected with different miRNA mimics (EV-miR127, EV-miR10a, EV-miR486). EVs were injected at day 3 and mice were sacrificed at day 5 after glycerol administration. Results are expressed as mean ± SD; ANOVA with Dunnett's multiple comparison test was performed. ** $p < 0.01$ EV-CTRL and EV-EP vs. Vehicle. Morphometric evaluation of (**C**) hyaline casts and (**D**) tubular necrosis in AKI mice treated with vehicle alone (Vehicle) or injected with 165×10^6 EVs derived from naïve MSCs (EV-CTRL) or from electroporated MSCs (EV-EP) transfected with different miRNA mimics (EV-miR127, EV-miR10a, EV-miR486). Results are expressed as mean ± SD; ANOVA with Dunnett's multiple comparison test was performed. ** $p < 0.01$ EV-CTRL and EV-EP vs. Vehicle.

Treatment of AKI mice with a dose of miRNA-enriched EVs comparable to the effective dose of EV-CTRL (165×10^6 EV/mouse) did not show any significant improvement. In fact, in some experimental conditions (EV-miR10a and EV-miR486), a worsening was even observed, suggesting that changing the composition of miRNAs content in MSC-EVs altered their pro-regenerative properties

(Figure 5). The administration of EV-miR127 did not show a worsening of kidney function and morphology, nor an amelioration of kidney function (Figure 5).

To better understand whether miRNA-enriched EVs could improve the biological activities of EVs, we treated AKI mice with an ineffective dose of unmodified EVs. A half-dose of these EVs (82.5×10^6 EV/mouse) did not induce significant functional or morphological improvements (Figure 6). In contrast, half-doses of EVs obtained from MSC-EP transfected with miRNA mimic-486 or -10a induced a significant amelioration of renal function and morphology (Figure 6). These findings suggest that the regenerative effect of MSC-derived EVs is related to a balanced composition of miRNAs and, therefore, modification in miRNA content may increase the effectiveness of EVs at lower doses, but not improve the effective dose of naïve EVs.

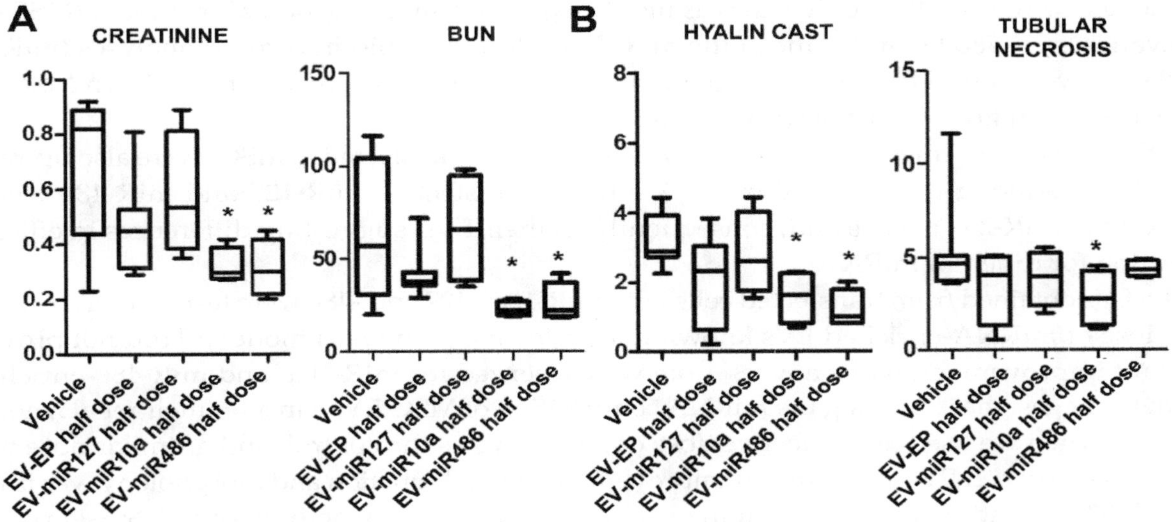

Figure 6. Effect of EVs derived from naïve or miRNA-enriched MSC in AKI mice: Functional and morphological evaluation. (**A**) Creatinine and BUN values in AKI mice injected with vehicle alone (Vehicle) or with 82.5×10^6 EVs derived from electroporated MSCs (EV-EP) and transfected with different miRNA mimics (EV-miR127, EV-miR10a, EV-miR486). EVs were injected at day 3 and mice were sacrificed at day 5 after glycerol administration. Results are expressed as mean ± SD; ANOVA with Dunnett's multiple comparison test was performed. * $p < 0.05$ EV-miR10a half-dose and EV-miR486 half-dose vs. Vehicle. (**B**) Morphometric evaluation of hyaline casts and tubular necrosis in AKI mice treated with vehicle alone (Vehicle) or with 82.5×10^6 EVs derived from electroporated MSCs (EV-EP) and transfected with different miRNA mimics (EV-miR127, EV-miR10a, EV-miR486). Results are expressed as mean ± SD; ANOVA with Dunnett's multiple comparison test was performed. * $p < 0.05$ EV-miR10a half-dose and EV-miR486 half-dose vs. Vehicle for hyaline cast; * $p < 0.05$ EV-miR10a half-dose vs. Vehicle, for tubular necrosis.

3. Discussion

Recent studies have shown that paracrine mechanisms, including EVs, are responsible for stem/progenitor cell-mediated renal regenerative effect [5]. EVs derived from MSCs shuttle different molecules (proteins, lipids, and nucleic acids) that may contribute to their pro-regenerative potential. Among the different shuttled molecules, miRNAs have been reported to be one of the factors involved in the pro-regenerative effects of MSC-EVs. Indeed, miRNA deregulation by Drosha-knockdown in MSCs has been reported to inhibit the regenerative potential of MSCs and of their derived EVs in a murine model of AKI [12]. This suggests a critical role of miRNA content in MSCs and MSC-EVs in the recovery following an AKI.

The idea of using EVs as carriers for selected miRNA cargo became very attractive in the last decades. EVs overcome many problems related to stability and preservation of their cargo from degradation in circulation. Different approaches were developed in order to modify EV content to enhance their homing capacity (proteins) or their effect (miRNAs, mRNAs and drugs) [13]. Direct manipulation of EVs implies the temporary disruption of EV membranes by different techniques, such as electroporation, sonication or chemical transfection [14]. Another technique used to enhance miRNA content in EVs is engineering of the parental cells. Some recent works demonstrated that is possible to load miRNA mimic or antimiR into MSCs by transfection, as well as to increase the pro-regenerative properties of EVs in different tissue injuries [7–11,15] or to potentiate their anti-tumor effect [16,17].

In this study, we set up a method to increase the content of specific miRNAs involved in renal regeneration in MSCs and their respective EVs. Potentially regenerative miRNAs were selected using a bio-informatic approach based on predicted interactions between the miRNAs present inside the MSC-EVs with genes modulated during AKI treatment with MSC-EVs. Moreover, this list was implemented with miR-486-5p, which was highly expressed in the exosomal fraction of MSC-EVs [6]. Of relevance, miR-486-5p and some of the miRNAs selected by bio-informatic analyses (miR-10a-5p, miR-29a-3p) were found to be down-regulated in EVs obtained by Drosha knock-down MSCs, which were ineffective in glycerol induced AKI [12].

In this work, we demonstrated that the miRNA mimics transfected in MSCs were also up-regulated in their EVs. Among the different miRNA mimics transfected, miR-127 and miR-486 were more enriched than miR-29a in cells and, consequently, in their EVs, suggesting differences in efficiency of transfection for different miRNAs.

The EVs obtained from transfected cells with miR-10a, -127 and -486 were tested in vivo. Treatment with a dose of miRNA-enriched EVs known to be effective in the AKI model [6] did not provide any significant improvement, while a worsening was observed for miR-10a- and miR-486-enriched EVs. These data suggest that changing the miRNA composition of MSC-EVs can alter their renal regenerative capacities. When we used an ineffective dose of naïve-EVs as the control, and a similar dose miR-10a- and miR-486-enriched EVs, a significant improvement of renal function and morphology was invariably observed. These findings indicate that in order to detect biological activity of miRNA-enriched EVs, low doses of EV should be studied. Moreover, these data highlight the important role of miR-10a and of miR-486 in the pro-regenerative effect exerted by MSC-EVs in AKI. Interestingly, miR-486 is also in exosomes derived from human endothelial progenitor cells, which have been shown to possess renal regenerative capacity in ischemia-reperfusion injury models [18].

In conclusion, our study has demonstrated that it is possible to modify the miRNA content of MSCs and their EVs. Changing the amount of pro-regenerative miRNAs in EVs was found to modify the window of biological activity of these EVs. Therefore, this may be a strategy to reduce the amount of EVs used in therapy. We previously showed that EVs derived from MSCs accumulated specifically in the kidneys of mice with AKI compared to healthy controls [19]. Since in the present study the bio-distribution of miRNA-enriched EVs was not evaluated, we cannot rule out the possibility that miRNA-enriched EVs have a different bio-distribution.

4. Materials and Methods

4.1. Cell Cultures and EV-CTRL Isolation

Bone marrow MSCs were purchased from Lonza (Basel, Switzerland) and cultured in a mesenchymal stem cells basal medium bullet kit (Lonza). MSCs were used for the different experiments until passage 6 and expressed the typical MSC markers (CD105, CD29, CD73, CD44 and CD90).

MSC-EVs, used as control (EV-CTRL), were obtained by ultracentrifugation, as described in Reference [6]. Briefly, EVs were obtained from supernatants of MSCs cultured overnight in (Roswell Park Memorial Institute (RPMI) medium. After removal of cell debris and apoptotic bodies by centrifugation at 3000× g for 20 min, EVs were purified by 2 h ultracentrifugation at 100,000× g at 4 °C. EVs from control MSCs or from modified MSCs were used freshly or stored at −80 °C after resuspension in RPMI supplemented with 1% dimethyl sulfoxide (DMSO, Sigma, St. Louis, MO, USA).

Murine renal tubular epithelial cells (mTECs) were obtained as previously described [20] and cultured in Dulbecco's Modified Eagle Medium (DMEM) low glucose (Euroclone, Pero, Italy) supplemented with 10% fetal calf serum (FCS, Euroclone), penicillin (50 IU/mL), and streptomycin (50 μg/mL) (Sigma). Murine TECs were characterized for positive staining to cytokeratin, alkaline phosphatase and aminopeptidase A, and for negative staining for endothelial (von Willebrand factor), hematopoietic (CD45) and glomerular (nephrin) markers.

4.2. MSC Transfection and Collection of Engineered MSC-EVs

To obtain miRNA-enriched MSCs, cells were transiently transfected by electroporation (MSC-EP) (neon transfection system) using a 100 μl tip (Thermo Fisher Scientific, Waltham, MA, USA), according to the manufacturer's protocol. Different electroporation conditions with a control miRNA mimic (100 nM) were tested in order to find the optimal protocol (Table 2 and Figure 2A). The electroporation conditions were set to 990 V, 40 msec and 1 pulse (EP1 protocol).

Table 2. Electroporation protocols tested to transfect MSCs.

	EP1	EP2	EP3
Voltage	990	1100	990
msec	40	30	30
Pulse	1	1	2

Three different doses (5, 25 and 50 nmol /4 × 10^4 cells) of a control miRNA mimic were evaluated to find the optimal dose to transfect MSCs (Figure 2B). The dose 25 nmol/4 × 10^4 cells was selected for subsequent experiments. The transfection efficiency was evaluated by qRT-PCR with the miScript PCR system (Qiagen, Venlo, The Netherlands), following the manufacturer's protocol.

These electroporation conditions did not affect cell viability.

Selected miRNA mimics (hsa-miR-10a-5p, hsa-miR-29a-3p, hsa-miR-127-3p, hsa-miR-486-5p) (Qiagen) were used to enrich MSCs (600 pmol/10^6 cells). As a control, MSCs were transfected with AllStars Negative Control siRNA (SCR-Qiagen) and used for normalization of transfection with different mimics. For modified MSCs, EV collection was carried out starting from a four sub-confluent flask (T75, Euroclone S.p.A) 24 h after the electroporation, starving MSCs over-night in RPMI (Euroclone). The collected medium was centrifuged at 2000 *g* for 20 min to eliminate cell debris. Supernatant was then micro-filtrated and concentrated by an Amicon® Ultra 15 mL 3 kDa cut off filter (Merck-Millipore, Darnstadt, Germany) at 4000 rpm 60 min at 4 °C. EV samples were stored at −80 °C, with addition of 1% DMSO (Sigma).

4.3. EV Characterization

Analysis of size distribution and enumeration of EVs from naïve MSCs and from MSC-EP (enriched or not with specific miRNA mimics) were performed using NanoSight NS300 (NanoSight Ltd., Amesbury, UK) equipped with a 405 nm laser and nanoparticle tracking analysis (NTA) 3.2 software, as described in Reference [6]. Using a laser light source, particles in the sample are illuminated and the scattered light is captured by the camera and displayed on a connected computer running NTA. Using NTA, the particles are automatically tracked and sized based on Brownian motion and the diffusion coefficient. Three videos of 30 s were recorded to perform the analyses.

EV-surface expression markers were analyzed by Guava easyCyte™ Flow Cytometer (Millipore), as previously described [21]. FITC-, PE- or APC-conjugated antibodies against CD44, CD29, CD73 and CD63 (all from Miltenyi Biotec GmbH, Bergisch Gladbach, Germany) were employed. Isotopic IgG was used as the negative control. Briefly, EVs were incubated at 4 °C for 15 min with the antibodies, then diluted 1:3 and acquired immediately. Samples were acquired using a Guava easyCyte Flow Cytometer (Millipore) and analyzed with InCyte software.

Transmission electron microscopy was performed on CTRL-EVs and EV-EP placed on 200 mesh nickel formvar carbon-coated grids (Electron Microscopy Science, Hatfield, PA, USA) and left to adhere for 20 min, as described in Reference [22]. The grids were then incubated with 2.5% glutaraldehyde containing 2% sucrose and, after washings in distilled water, the EVs were negatively stained with NanoVan (Nanoprobes, Yaphank, NK, USA) and observed using a Jeol JEM 1010 electron microscope (Jeol, Tokyo, Japan).

4.4. RNA Analysis

RNA from MSC-EP was extracted by TRIzol™ (Ambion, Thermo Fisher Scientific, Waltham, MA, USA) according to the manufacturer's protocol.

Only for RNA analysis, Exoquick (System Biosciences, LLC, Palo Alto, CA, USA) was used to precipitate EVs obtained from MSC-EP (EV-EP), MSC transfected with scrambled siRNA (EV-SCR) or with the selected mimics (EV-miR127, EV-miR10a, EV-miR486, EV-miR29a). RNA was extracted with RNA/DNA/Protein Purification Plus Kit (Norgen Biotek Corp, Thorold, ON, Canada), following the manufacturer's protocol.

RNA concentration was spectroscopically determined by NanoDrop2000 (Thermo Fisher Scientific). cDNA was synthetized and RT-PCR was performed by using miRCURY™ LNA™ Universal RT microRNA PCR (Exiqon-Qiagen, Vedbaek, Denmark). Specific primers set for hsa-miR-127-3p, hsa-miR-10a-5p, hsa-miR-29a-3p, hsa-miR-486-5 were used. U6 spike-in was used for housekeeping (Exiqon-Qiagen). Data were normalized with respect to MSC transfected with the SCR and were represented as relative quantification (RQ) ± SEM.

4.5. Integrating miRNA Expression in MSC EVs and RNA Analysis in AKI Animals

To identify potentially relevant miRNAs carried by MSC EVs and involved in the positive readout associated with EVs treatment, we proceeded as follows: For each miRNA family listed in TargetScan we generated a list of predicted targets. We then compared the fold-change in expression of these targets with the fold-change in expression of all the genes that were predicted targets of miRNAs but not of the miRNA families under analysis. The miRNA families selected were those for which the targets showed significant down-regulation in the kidneys of AKI mice treated with MSC-derived EVs vs. untreated AKI mice (AKI), as detected in Reference [12]. The obtained miRNA families were then matched with the list of miRNAs detected inside the total extracellular vesicle population (100K TOT) in Reference [6].

4.6. mTEC Proliferation Assay

mTEC were seeded in 96-well plates at a density of 1000 cells/well and maintained in a hypoxia chamber (Stem Cell Technology, Vancouver)) for 48 h with 1% O_2 in DMEM + 10% FCS (positive control), DMEM + 0% FCS (negative control). During the reoxygenation step, mTEC were treated for 24 h with mimics of selected miRNAs (100 nM) or 500 EV/mTEC. Cell proliferation was assessed by a 5-bromo-2'-deoxy-uridine (BrdU) incorporation assay (Roche Applied Science, Mannheim, Germany).

4.7. SCID Mouse Model of AKI

Animal studies were conducted in accordance with the National Institutes of Health Guide for the Care and Use of Laboratory Animals. All procedures were approved by the Italian Health Ministry (authorization number: 211/2016-PR).

AKI was induced by an intramuscular injection (IM) of glycerol (Sigma) in SCID mice, as described previously [6,20]. Male SCID mice were anesthetized with an IM injection of zolazepam (80 mg/kg) and xilazina (16 mg/kg) and then injected with 8 mL/kg of 50% glycerol in water. Half the dose was injected into each muscle of the inferior hind limbs. Three days after the glycerol injection, the mice were treated intravenously with either 120 µL of the vehicle alone ($n = 7$) or containing 165×10^6 or 82.5×10^6 particles of EVs derived from control MSCs (EV-CTRL, $n = 8$), from MSC-EP

(EV-EP, $n = 8$/doses), or from EP-MSC enriched with specific miRNA mimics (EV-miR127, EV-miR486, EV-miR10a, $n = 6$/group/doses). The mice were sacrificed 5 days after the glycerol injection (2 days after EV treatment).

Blood samples were collected 5 days after glycerol-induced AKI for the measurement of blood urea nitrogen (BUN) and creatinine. BUN was measured by direct quantification of serum urea with a colorimetric assay kit according to the manufacturer's protocol (Arbor Assays, Ann Arbor, MI, USA). Serum creatinine was measured using a colorimetric microplate assay based on the kinetic Jaffe reaction as per the manufacturer's protocol (Quantichrom Creatinine Assay; BioAssay Systems, Hayward, CA, USA).

Renal morphology was evaluated through formalin-fixed paraffin-embedded tissue staining, as previously described [6,20]. Briefly, 5-μm-thick paraffin kidney sections were routinely stained with hematoxylin and eosin (Merck-Millipore) for microscopic evaluation. Luminal hyaline casts and cell necrosis (denudation of the tubular basement membrane) were assessed in non-overlapping fields (10 for each section) using a 40× objective (high-power field [HPF]). The number of casts and tubular profiles showing necrosis were recorded in a single-blind manner.

4.8. Statistical Analyses

Data were analyzed using the GraphPad Prism 6.0 program. Statistical analysis was performed by employing Student's *t*-tests, analysis of variance (ANOVA) with Dunnett's multi-comparison tests or Multiple t test with Helm–Sidak method correction as deemed appropriate. A p-value of <0.05 was considered significant. For the bioinformatic analyses, p values were generated by Mann–Whitney statistical test comparing the median fold change of genes down-regulated in EV treated animals (Log EV treated vs. AKI untreated) that were target of miRNAs with the non-target genes. Nine miRNA families (Table 1) achieved nominal significance ($p < 0.05$).

Author Contributions: S.B. and G.T. performed in vivo studies and tissues analysis; M.T. performed transfection experiments and in vitro assay; F.C. performed in vitro experiments; P.P. performed bioinformatics analyses; S.W. and P.J.Q. data interpretation and revised the manuscript; M.C.D. performed electron microscopy analyses of the vesicle preparations; S.B., M.T., F.C. and G.C. performed study design, data interpretation and manuscript writing. All authors approved the submitted version of the manuscript. M.T. and S.B. equally contributed to this work.

Acknowledgments: The technical assistance of Federica Antico and Massimo Cedrino are gratefully acknowledged.

References

1. Heldring, N.; Mager, I.; Wood, M.J.A.; Le Blanc, K.; Andaloussi, S.E. Therapeutic potential of multipotent mesenchymal stromal cells and their extracellular vesicles. *Hum. Gene Ther.* **2015**, *26*, 506–517. [CrossRef]
2. Lamichhane, T.N.; Sokic, S.; Schardt, J.S.; Raiker, R.S.; Lin, J.W.; Jay, S.M. Emerging roles for extracellular vesicles in tissue engineering and regenerative medicine. *Tissue Eng. Part B Rev.* **2015**, *21*, 45–54. [CrossRef]
3. Robbins, P.D.; Morelli, A.E. Regulation of immune responses by extracellular vesicles. *Nat. Rev. Immunol.* **2014**, *14*, 195–208. [CrossRef]
4. Wang, Y.; He, J.; Pei, X.; Zhao, W. Systematic review and meta-analysis of mesenchymal stem/stromal cells therapy for impaired renal function in small animal models. *Nephrology* **2013**, *8*, 201–218. [CrossRef] [PubMed]
5. Grange, C.; Iampietro, C.; Bussolati, B. Stem cell extracellular vesicles and kidney injury. *Stem Cell Investig.* **2017**, *4*, 90. [CrossRef]
6. Bruno, S.; Tapparo, M.; Collino, F.; Chiabotto, G.; Deregibus, M.C.; Soares Lindoso, R.; Neri, F.; Kholia, S.; Giunti, S.; Wen, S.; et al. Renal Regenerative Potential of Different Extracellular Vesicle Populations Derived from Bone Marrow Mesenchymal Stromal Cells. *Tissue Eng. Part A* **2017**, *23*, 1262–1273. [CrossRef]

7. Tao, S.C.; Yuan, T.; Zhang, Y.L.; Yin, W.J.; Guo, S.C.; Zhang, C.Q. Exosomes derived from miR-140-5p-overexpressing human synovial mesenchymal stem cells enhance cartilage tissue regeneration and prevent osteoarthritis of the knee in a rat model. *Theranostics* **2017**, *7*, 180–195.
8. Lou, G.; Yang, Y.; Liu, F.; Ye, B.; Chen, Z.; Zheng, M.; Liu, Y. MiR-122 modification enhances the therapeutic efficacy of adipose tissue-derived mesenchymal stem cells against liver fibrosis. *J. Cell Mol. Med.* **2017**, *21*, 2963–2973. [CrossRef] [PubMed]
9. Song, J.L.; Zheng, W.; Chen, W.; Qian, Y.; Ouyang, Y.M.; Fan, C.Y. Lentivirus-mediated microRNA-124 gene-modified bone marrow mesenchymal stem cell transplantation promotes the repair of spinal cord injury in rats. *Exp. Mol. Med.* **2017**, *49*, e332. [CrossRef] [PubMed]
10. Li, D.; Zhang, P.; Yao, X.; Li, H.; Shen, H.; Li, X.; Wu, J.; Lu, X. Exosomes Derived From miR-133b-Modified Mesenchymal Stem Cells Promote Recovery After Spinal Cord Injury. *Front. Neurosci.* **2018**, *22*, 845. [CrossRef] [PubMed]
11. Shen, H.; Yao, X.; Li, H.; Li, X.; Zhang, T.; Sun, Q.; Ji, C.; Chen, G. Role of Exosomes Derived from miR-133b Modified MSCs in an Experimental Rat Model of Intracerebral Hemorrhage. *J. Mol. Neurosci.* **2018**, *64*, 421–430. [CrossRef]
12. Collino, F.; Bruno, S.; Incarnato, D.; Dettori, D.; Neri, F.; Provero, P.; Pomatto, M.; Oliviero, S.; Tetta, C.; Quesenberry, P.J.; et al. AKI Recovery Induced by Mesenchymal Stromal Cell-Derived Extracellular Vesicles Carrying MicroRNAs. *J. Am. Soc. Nephrol.* **2015**, *26*, 2349–2360. [CrossRef]
13. Mentkowski, K.I.; Snitzer, J.D.; Rusnak, S.; Lang, J.K. Therapeutic Potential of Engineered Extracellular Vesicles. *AAPS J.* **2018**, *20*, 50. [CrossRef]
14. Janas, T.; Janas, M.M.; Sapoń, K.; Janas, T. Mechanisms of RNA loading into exosomes. *FEBS Lett.* **2015**, *589*, 1391–1398. [CrossRef] [PubMed]
15. Wang, B.; Yao, K.; Huuskes, B.M.; Shen, H.H.; Zhuang, J.; Godson, C.; Brennan, E.P.; Wilkinson-Berka, J.L.; Wise, A.F.; Ricardo, S.D. Mesenchymal Stem Cells Deliver Exogenous MicroRNA-let7c via Exosomes to Attenuate Renal Fibrosis. *Mol. Ther.* **2016**, *24*, 1290–1301. [CrossRef]
16. Sutaria, D.S.; Badawi, M.; Phelps, M.A.; Schmittgen, T.D. Achieving the promise of therapeutic extracellular vesicles: The devil is in details of therapeutic loading. *Pharm. Res.* **2017**, *34*, 1053–1066. [CrossRef] [PubMed]
17. Lou, G.; Song, X.; Yang, F.; Wu, S.; Wang, J.; Chen, Z.; Liu, Y. Exosomes derived from miR-122-modified adipose tissue derived MSCs increase chemosensitivity of hepatocellular carcinoma. *J. Hematol. Oncol.* **2015**, *8*, 122. [CrossRef] [PubMed]
18. Viñas, J.L.; Burger, D.; Zimpelmann, J.; Haneef, R.; Knoll, W.; Campbell, P.; Gutsol, A.; Carter, A.; Allan, D.S.; Burns, K.D. Transfer of microRNA-486-5p from human endothelial colony forming cell-derived exosomes reduces ischemic kidney injury. *Kidney Int.* **2016**, *90*, 1238–1250. [CrossRef] [PubMed]
19. Bruno, S.; Grange, C.; Deregibus, M.C.; Calogero, R.A.; Saviozzi, S.; Collino, F.; Morando, L.; Busca, A.; Falda, M.; Bussolati, B.; et al. Mesenchymal stem cell-derived microvesicles protect against acute tubular injury. *J. Am. Soc. Nephrol.* **2009**, *20*, 1053–1067. [CrossRef]
20. Grange, C.; Tapparo, M.; Bruno, S.; Chatterjee, D.; Quesenberry, P.J.; Tetta, C.; Camussi, G. Biodistribution of mesenchymal stem cell-derived extracellular vesicles in a model of acute kidney injury monitored by optical imaging. *Int. J. Mol. Med.* **2014**, *33*, 1055–1063. [CrossRef]
21. Lindoso, R.S.; Collino, F.; Bruno, S.; Araujo, D.S.; Sant'Anna, J.F.; Tetta, C.; Provero, P.; Quesenberry, P.J.; Vieyra, A.; Einicker-Lamas, M.; et al. Extracellular vesicles released from mesenchymal stromal cells modulate miRNA in renal tubular cells and inhibit ATP depletion injury. *Stem Cells Dev.* **2014**, *23*, 1809–1819. [CrossRef] [PubMed]
22. Deregibus, M.C.; Figliolini, F.; D'Antico, S.; Manzini, P.M.; Pasquino, C.; De Lena, M.; Tetta, C.; Brizzi, M.F.; Camussi, G. Charge-based precipitation of extracellular vesicles. *Int. J. Mol. Med.* **2016**, *38*, 1359–1366. [CrossRef] [PubMed]

6

Molecular Mechanisms of Kidney Injury and Repair in Arterial Hypertension

Laura Katharina Sievers [1,2,3,4,*] and Kai-Uwe Eckardt [1]

1 Department of Nephrology and Medical Intensive Care, Charité-Universitätsmedizin Berlin, 13353 Berlin, Germany; kai-uwe.eckardt@charite.de
2 Max-Delbrück Center for Molecular Medicine in the Helmholtz Association, 13125 Berlin, Germany
3 Experimental and Clinical Research Center, a joint cooperation of Max-Delbrück Center for Molecular Medicine and Charité-Universitätsmedizin Berlin, 13125 Berlin, Germany
4 Berlin Institute of Health (BIH), 10178 Berlin, Germany
* Correspondence: laura-katharina.sievers@charite.de

Abstract: The global burden of chronic kidney disease is rising. The etiologies, heterogeneous, and arterial hypertension, are key factors contributing to the development and progression of chronic kidney disease. Arterial hypertension is induced and maintained by a complex network of systemic signaling pathways, such as the hormonal axis of the renin-angiotensin-aldosterone system, hemodynamic alterations affecting blood flow, oxygen supply, and the immune system. This review summarizes the clinical and histopathological features of hypertensive kidney injury and focusses on the interplay of distinct systemic signaling pathways, which drive hypertensive kidney injury in distinct cell types of the kidney. There are several parallels between hypertension-induced molecular signaling cascades in the renal epithelial, endothelial, interstitial, and immune cells. Angiotensin II signaling via the AT1R, hypoxia induced HIFα activation and mechanotransduction are closely interacting and further triggering the adaptions of metabolism, cytoskeletal rearrangement, and profibrotic TGF signaling. The interplay of these, and other cellular pathways, is crucial to balancing the injury and repair of the kidneys and determines the progression of hypertensive kidney disease.

Keywords: hypertension; kidney; molecular signaling

---

1. Introduction

Arterial hypertension has a large prevalence in the general population and is associated with a wide range of cardiovascular complications and chronic damage to the heart, brain, vasculature, eyes, kidney, and other organs. Hypertensive nephropathy is regarded as the second leading cause of end-stage renal disease (ESRD), outnumbered only by diabetic nephropathy. However, in many cases, it is hard to determine the primary underlying cause of chronic kidney disease (CKD). Arterial hypertension is a typical complication of CKD, irrespective of its etiology, and it is often difficult to differentiate whether increased blood pressure is the cause and/or consequence of impaired kidney function. In any case, coexisting arterial hypertension accelerates the progression of CKD and increases the cardiovascular risk in CKD patients [1]. The clinical course and histopathological characteristics of kidney injury in hypertensive kidney disease may vary, not only on comorbidities, but also in environmental factors and genetic predisposition. For example, patients of black ethnicity are at a much higher risk for rapidly progressing CKD. Given the importance of hypertension for the course of kidney disease, a thorough understanding of the molecular mechanisms of kidney injury and repair, in arterial hypertension, appears fundamental to the development of novel approaches against the progression of CKD worldwide. With the increasing availability of novel therapeutic strategies targeting molecular pathways, a classification of CKD, based on the predominant molecular pathology, rather than clinical correlations/etiologies might become a promising approach in the future.

Arterial hypertension is caused and sustained by a complex network of systemic signaling pathways. The renin-angiotensin-aldosterone-system (RAAS) is one important hormonal axis in hypertension. In addition, several other hormones, such as corticosteroids, catecholamines, thyroid hormones, sex hormones, and others contribute to the regulation of blood pressure. Furthermore, it has been shown that the immune system plays an important role in the development and maintenance of hypertension. For example, the balance between IL17 producing T lymphocytes (Th17) and regulatory T cells (Treg) is dysequilibrated in hypertensive patients, favoring Th17 cells. Other conditions favoring Th17 cells can drive hypertension. In this review we aim to provide a brief overview of clinical and histopathological characteristics of kidney injury in hypertensive kidney disease, and of the systemic signaling pathways and important aspects of the immune system, in arterial hypertension. Moreover, we will describe molecular mechanisms in hypertensive kidney injury and repair, including angiotensin II (Ang II) signaling in different cell types, hypoxia signaling, distinct pro-inflammatory pathways, and TGF-associated profibrotic signaling.

2. Clinical and Histopathological Characteristics of Kidney Injury in Arterial Hypertension

"Hypertensive nephropathy", also known as "hypertensive nephrosclerosis", is traditionally characterized by a combination of pathological changes of the pre- and intra-glomerular microvasculature and the tubulointerstitium. The histopathology can hardly distinguish whether arterial hypertension is the primary cause of kidney dysfunction or whether increased blood pressure occurs as a comorbidity, which drives CKD progression. Thus, the term hypertensive nephropathy summarizes both conditions. The severity of blood pressure elevation often correlates with the degree of renal damage. In many cases, hypertensive nephrosclerosis shows a slow progression, which is historically classified as "benign nephrosclerosis". In contrast, accelerated nephrosclerosis, histopathologically characterized by fibrinoid necrosis and/or myointimal cell proliferation, is classified as "malignant nephrosclerosis" and frequently leads to ESRD [2]. Hypertension-induced kidney damage involves different cell types and anatomical structures in the kidney, including the vasculature, glomeruli, tubulointerstitium, and immune cells. The muscular arteries and arterioles of the kidney parenchyma show progressive intimal thickening during aging, but besides age this process correlates with arterial hypertension [3]. The thickening is caused by collagen deposition and spreading of elastic fibers and myofibroblasts, and ultimately leads to more pulsatile blood flow in kidney arterioles [3]. Another histopathological characteristic of hypertensive nephrosclerosis is arteriosclerosis of the afferent arterioles, also referred to as "afferent arteriolar hyalinosis". These typical hyaline deposits are the consequence of a pathogenetic cascade of atrophy of vascular smooth muscle cells, increased endothelial leakiness and plasma protein extravasation, leading to sub-endothelial protein accumulation [3]. Although this process is associated with hypertension, to some extent, it occurs in all aging kidneys [3]. The glomerular involvement is heterogeneous; there is a side-by-side normal morphology, ischemic, obliterated glomeruli, with collapsed capillaries and focal-segmental-glomerular sclerosis-(FSGS)-like lesions, with partially sclerotic glomerular adhesions.

Another hallmark of hypertensive kidney injury is tubular atrophy, accompanied by interstitial fibrosis. Following a loss of functional nephrons, the surviving nephrons initially maintain total kidney function, but the concomitant hemodynamic adaptations results in an oxygen supply-demand mismatch and ultimately tubulointerstitial hypoxia [4]. Tubulointerstitial hypoxia presumably contributes to the progression of tubular damage and renal functional impairment [5,6]. This relative hypoxia is further aggravated by impaired oxygen delivery to the kidneys during hypertension, due to vasoconstriction hormones, including components of the RAAS, prostaglandins, and endothelin [5].

During the course of CKD, the loss of peritubular capillaries further aggravates tubulointerstitial hypoxia and damage. Hypoxic conditions trigger mitochondrial dysfunction [4] and can activate the transcription factor hypoxia-inducible factor (HIF) [7]. The signaling pathways which promote a maladaptive phenotype at the cellular level will be discussed below. Besides the characteristic vascular adaptations and glomerular pathology, kidney histology of hypertensive nephrosclerosis may also show trans-differentiation and apoptosis of tubular cells, increased peritubular fibrosis, fibroblasts proliferation, and increased interstitial inflammation.

3. Systemic Signaling Pathways and the Immune System in Arterial Hypertension

For decades, the pathophysiology of arterial hypertension has primarily been attributed to vasoconstriction hormones, including RAAS (Figure 1), prostaglandins, and endothelin 1 (ET1). Among these hormonal axes, the RAAS has received particular attention, and was shown to have a crucial influence on blood pressure and target organ damage. This important signaling axis includes several components that are activated stepwise: First, the 452 amino acid peptide pro-hormone angiotensinogen, which is synthesized and excreted by the liver, is cleaved to the ten amino acid peptide Angiotensin I by the protease renin (Figure 1). Angiotensin (Ang) I is then cleaved to the eight amino acid peptide hormone, Ang II, by angiotensin converting enzyme (ACE) (Figure 1). Although, the pro-hormone Ang I and other metabolites of angiontensinogen, such as Ang 1–7, which result from cleavage by other proteases, have effects on the vascular endothelia and other tissues. Here, we will focus on the canonical RAAS signaling and biological effects of Ang II. Ang II binds to the Ang II-receptor 1 (AT1R) in different cell types [8]: In the vasculature, Ang II leads to vasoconstriction and in the adrenal cortex, it increases the secretion of aldosterone (Figure 1). In the kidney, Ang II leads to tubular retention of NaCl and water (Figure 1). Further, Ang II increases the sympathetic activity, which also elevates blood pressure (Figure 1). The systemic vascular tone results from the interplay of many different vasoconstricting and vasodilating stimuli. Within this complex interplay, the pathophysiological relevance of the RAAS for blood pressure regulation is underlined by the clinical significance of RAAS inhibition. State-of-the-art clinical management of arterial hypertension includes, pharmacological targeting of the RAAS with ACE-inhibitors, AT1R blockers, direct renin inhibitors, and aldosterone antagonists [9]. The important pathophysiological contribution and clinical relevance of the RAAS, beyond blood pressure control, is underlined by the fact that treatment with ACE-inhibitors or AT1R blockers shows significant clinical benefits for cardiovascular morbidity and mortality.

ET1 expression may be regulated by inflammatory mediators, shear stress, and glucose. ET1 has an ambiguous role on the vascular tone. Binding of ET1 to the ET1 receptor A (ETA) of vascular smooth muscle cells causes vasoconstriction, while binding to the ET1 receptor B (ETB) has an indirect vasodilating effect via increased release of nitric oxide (NO). ETA antagonists are clinically used in pulmonary arterial hypertension. Further, ETA antagonists may slow the progression of diabetic nephropathy, but until recently, ET1 antagonists are not licensed in arterial hypertension. Sympathetic activity may be induced by central nervous regulation associated with stress, pain, or cold, It is affected by the RAAS and modifies peripheral resistance. In the last years, several non-pharmacological approaches addressing the autonomic nervous system in arterial hypertension have been developed. Renal sympathetic denervation, carotid baroreflex activation therapy, central iliac arteriovenous anastomosis, carotid body ablation, median nerve stimulation, vagal nerve stimulation, and deep brain stimulation continue to be evaluated with respect to their capacity to lower blood pressure and blood pressure associated target organ damage [10].

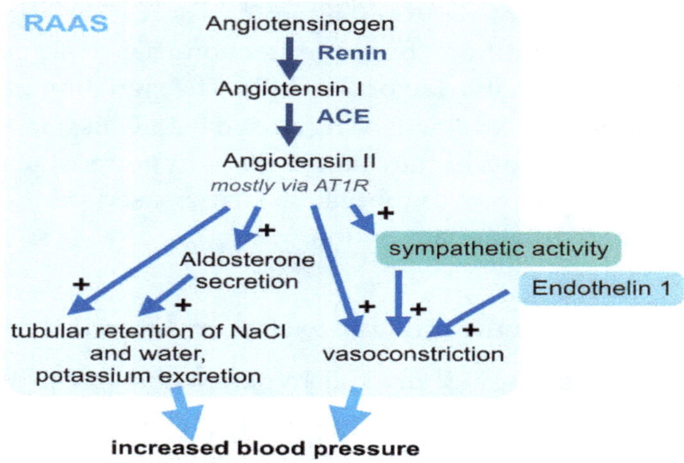

Figure 1. The renin-angiotensin-aldosterone system (RAAS) is a key hormonal axis in the pathogenesis of arterial hypertension. The RAAS combines a regulatory network, including angiotensin II (Ang II) and aldosterone, which increase systemic blood pressure through a concerted mechanism. Angiotensinogen is enzymatically cleaved by renin and angiotensin-converting enzyme (ACE) to generate Angiotensin II, which, mainly via the Ang II receptor 1 (AT1R), stimulates the secretion of aldosterone, acts as a vasoconstrictor and leads to renal tubular retention of NaCl and water. For simplification, the negative feedback loop, which physiologically limits an excess activation of these pathways, is not included in this graph. Besides Ang II, endothelin 1 and increased sympathetic activity, which may be induced by RAAS activation or independent stimuli, also contribute to systemic vasoconstriction and increased peripheral resistance.

Carotid baroreflex activation therapy resulted in a sustained reduction of arterial blood pressure in patients with resistant hypertension in the Rheos Pivotal Trial [11]. Since renal sympathetic over-activity is associated with the pathogenesis and progression of arterial hypertension and CKD, catheter-based renal denervation has been a promising approach in reducing blood pressure and attenuating renal functional decline in hypertensive CKD [12]. Further, meta-analyses have shown beneficial effects in patients with heart failure [12]. After promising animal studies and early trials in patients, subsequent clinical studies could not replicate the positive outcome [12–14]. There are ongoing trials, which aim to resolve the conflicting evidence and to provide data on the long-term safety and efficacy of renal denervation [15–18].

Besides the hormonal and autonomous axes, immune mechanisms play an important role in the pathogenesis of arterial hypertension by contributing to both, the development of hypertension and of hypertensive end-organ damage (Figure 2). $CD4^+$ lymphocytes are key cell types involved in the balance between Treg and Th17 cells, which originate from naive $CD4^+$ cells under specific skewing conditions. Several drivers of hypertension, including Ang II-induced signaling, dietary NaCl, the gut microbiome, at least partly exert their effect via immune mechanisms, and in particular, the regulation of the Treg/Th17 balance (Figure 2). Th17 cells are associated with hypertension and hypertensive end-organ damage, while a protective role is attributed to Treg. For example, it has been shown that Treg deficiency exaggerated Ang II-induced microvascular injury by enhancing immune responses [19]. Ang II was a driver of Treg infiltration in the aortic wall and renal cortex and, in a model of Treg deficient mice, the adoptive transfer of Treg cells prevented Ang II-induced hypertension and vascular injury [20]. Further, it has been demonstrated that Ang II increased the secretion of the pro- inflammatory cytokine IL17 by Th17 cells and that the activation Th17 cells in response to high salt was associated with accelerated fibrosis [21]. Notably, the cytokine IL17 has a differentiated function in diabetic kidney disease: Ablation of intrarenal Th17 cells ameliorated early diabetic nephropathy [22], while the administration of low-dose IL17A had beneficial effects [23]. The ambiguity of IL17 signaling in hypertensive kidney disease remains to be elucidated. Interestingly, the induction of Th17 cells seems to depend on gut microbiota, particularly salt-sensitive lactobacilli.

Increased dietary salt depleted these microbiota, increased Th17 cells, and increased the blood pressure in mice and humans [24]. Besides salt intake, intestinal metabolites, such as the short-chain fatty acid propionate have quantitative effects on the systemic composition of immune cell subsets and blood pressure [25] (Figure 2). Intracellular pathways, that balance the differentiation of Treg and Th17 include. TGFβ, IL6, RORγT, Hippo/TAZ, and HIF-1. All these pathways are directly influenced by Ang II/AT1R signaling. Besides the prominent role of the Treg/Th17 cells in hypertensive end-organ damage, innate immune cells contribute to hypertensive mechanisms. Neutrophils, monocytes/macrophages, dendritic cells, myeloid-derived suppressor cells and innate lymphoid cells may trigger both, blood pressure elevation on the one hand, and profibrotic inflammatory processes in end-organs on the other hand [26]. Innate and adaptive immune mechanisms closely interact in the pathogenesis of hypertension and hypertensive organ damage. For example, monocyte/macrophages and $\gamma\delta$ T cells seem to play a crucial role in the initiation of hypertension by priming adaptive immune cells, thereby triggering vascular inflammation and blood pressure elevation or, if their signaling limits the inflammatory response, protecting against vascular injury [26].

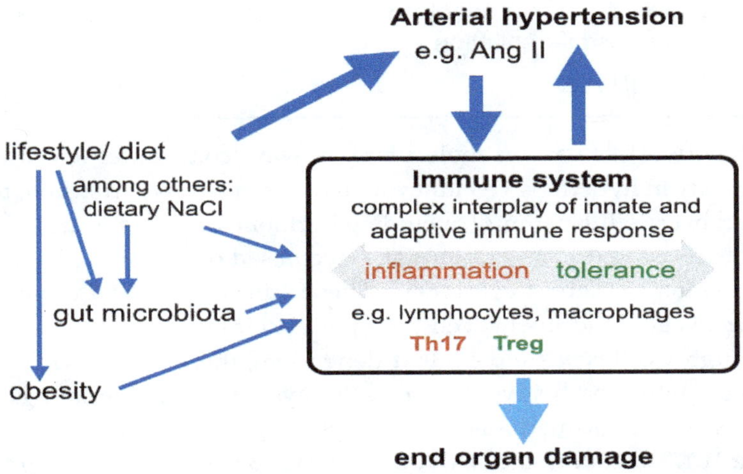

Figure 2. The immune system closely interacts with hormonal and environmental modifiers to control blood pressure. The immune system plays an important role in the pathogenesis of arterial hypertension and hypertensive end-organ damage. Lifestyle factors, such as the dietary nutrient composition and sodium intake directly, and via alterations in the gut microbiome, have influence on the cellular compositions of the immune system. Distinct immune cell subtypes, such as IL17 producing Th17 lymphocytes contribute to increased blood pressure. In parallel, existing arterial hypertension and Ang II favor Th17 polarization of T lymphocytes. Besides the effect of immune cells on blood pressure, the balance of various cells from the adaptive and innate immune system, including lymphocytes and macrophages is critical for end organ damage.

4. Molecular Mechanisms in Hypertensive Kidney Injury

Many different anatomical parts of the kidney, with distinct cell types, are affected by hypertensive kidney injury: Cells forming the nephron, including glomerular podocytes and tubular cells, the vasculature with endothelium and smooth muscle cells, interstital fibroblasts and resident, as well as circulating immune cells of adaptive and innate immune response, are involved (Figure 3). Although novel techniques, such as genome-wide association studies, single cell proteomics or deep sequencing are on the brink of their application in clinical studies, detailed reports scrutinizing cell-type specific molecular mechanisms of hypertensive kidney injury are still missing [27,28]. When subsequently discussing important molecular mechanisms in hypertensive kidney injury and repair, we will focus on the molecular signaling pathways of Ang II signaling, hypoxia, pro- inflammatory signaling, TGF, and profibrotic pathways. Although, the net effect of mechanisms promoting injury and repair is highly cell type- and context-dependent, there are several parallels with regard to the involved molecular signaling pathways across different cell types (Figure 3).

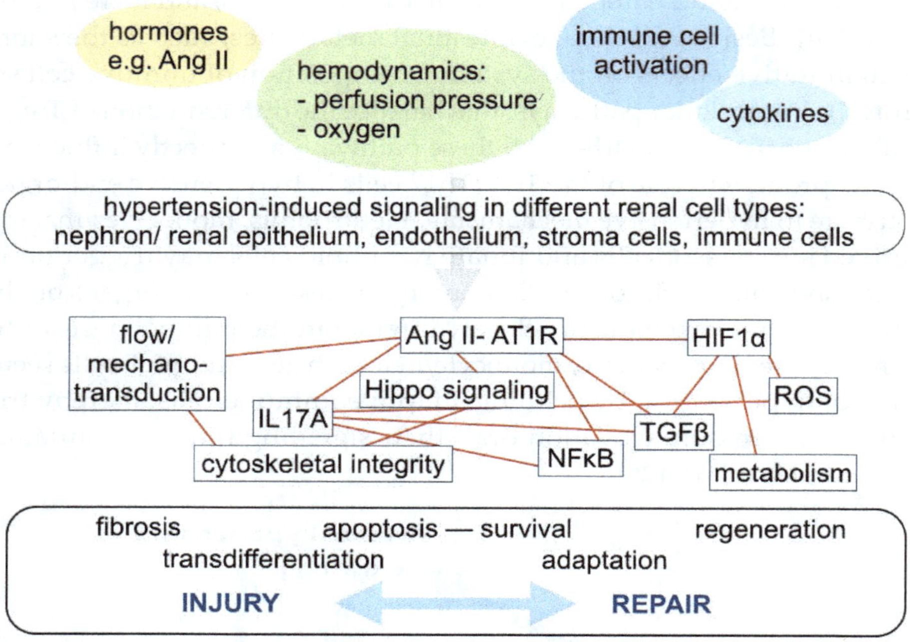

Figure 3. A complex network of various molecular pathways contributes to cellular adaptions, injury, and regenerative capacity in hypertensive kidney injury. In arterial hypertension, the cells in the kidney are exposed to various extracellular stimuli, including hormones, such as Ang II, altered hemodynamics with increased perfusion pressure, and potentially decreased oxygen supply and activated immune cells, which in turn secrete different cytokines. These stimuli affect all renal cell types: Nephron forming renal epithelial cells, endothelial cells, stroma, and immune cells. Although the net effect on injury and repair is highly cell type- and context-dependent, there are several parallels regarding the involved molecular signaling pathways. These pathways, or rather, signaling networks, are highly interrelated. For example, AT1R-mediated Ang II signaling, the Hippo pathway, pro- inflammatory signaling, including IL17 secretion and activation of TGFβ associated profibrotic signaling closely interact. Mechano-transduction and Hippo signaling, among others, influence the cytoskeletal integrity. Hypoxia-inducible factor (HIF) is stabilized by hypoxia, induces metabolic adaptions and may increase TGFβ- associated profibrotic pathways.

The peptide hormone Ang II is an important mediator in the pathophysiology of arterial hypertension, hypertensive end-organ damage, and also hypertensive kidney injury. The AT1R is expressed in various cell types, including podocytes, renal tubular cells, and immune cells. Further, Ang II exerts indirect effects via changes of the glomerular hemodynamics, leading to increased filtration pressure, increased filtration of NaCl and consecutive adaptations of the tubular salt and water handling. Furthermore, Ang II from the systemic circulation increases the tubular expression of angiotensinogen, ACE, renin and AT1R [29]. This feed-forward loop mechanism is at least partly driven by cytokines produced by activated T lymphocytes such as IL6 and IFNγ [30]. Consistent with the prominent glomerular histopathology and the clinical presentation of albuminuria in hypertensive kidney injury, elevated levels of Ang II lead to severe injury of glomerular podocytes with foot process effacement and ultimately podocyte loss. Podocyte depletion is an irreversible hallmark of glomerular injury in CKD, and the beneficial effect of Ang II blockade on the progression of hypertensive CKD correlates with attenuated podocyte loss [31]. Ang II causes podocyte injury via several pathways. Binding of Ang II to the G-protein-coupled AT1R activates an intracellular cascade of kinases, including the activation of phospholipase C, calcium-calmodulin binding, phosphorylation of the protein kinases extracellular-signal regulated kinases (ERK), ribosomal S6 kinase (RSK), protein kinase C (PKC), protein kinase A (PKA), and the activation of adenylate cyclase leading to the generation of cyclic AMP. Already decades ago, it has been demonstrated that a sustained intracellular rise in calcium, as induced by Ang II, has detrimental effects on podocyte viability [32,33]. The calcium influx may be aggravated by simultaneously increased expression of calcium channels, such as TRPC6 [34]. Further, Ang II signaling in podocytes is closely linked to the integrity of the actin cytoskeleton. It has been shown that short term treatment with Ang II regulates the phosphorylation of various actin-associated proteins in podocytes and that e.g., the increased phosphorylation of lymphocyte cytosolic protein 1 (LCP1) leads to alterations in actin bundling, increased filopodia and lamellipodia formation, and membrane ruffling [35]. Besides the regulation of intracellular cytoskeletal components, Ang II has a direct impact on nephrin, a fundamental extracellular adaptor protein crosslinking podocyte at the slit diaphragm. In models of Ang II induced hypertension and kidney injury, nephrin is dephosphorylated in a caveolin-1- [36] and c-Abl [37]-dependent way, ultimately leading to the disintegration of the slit diaphragm. Interestingly, it has been shown that Ang II also regulates the Hippo pathway, a conserved signaling pathway controlling cell proliferation and cell death via a kinase cascade, that regulates the nuclear shuttling of the transcription factors YAP and TAZ. Ang II inactivated the Hippo pathway by decreasing the activity of LATS kinase, consequently increasing the nuclear abundance of the transcription factor YAP in Human Embryonic Kidney cells [38] and TAZ is activated in the tubulointerstitium in mouse models of kidney injury [39]. At the same time, Ang II effects on YAP/TAZ were absent in podocytes, which are postmitotic cells with low baseline Hippo pathway activity [38]. Further, Ang II/AT1R signaling modifies the lipid metabolism and induced lipid droplet accumulation and expression of lipid droplet marker protein in podocytes [40]. The effects of Ang II on renal cells have been extensively studied, but the interrelation of different signaling networks is still not completely understood. Further, Ang II affects the infiltration of immune cells. AT1R signaling drives the differentiation of CD4 lymphocytes to Th17 cells: Silencing of AT1R with siRNA reduced the fraction of Th17 polarized cells and IL17 expression while Ang II treatment increased the secretion of the pro-inflammatory cytokine IL17 by Th17 [21] wheras, in the presence of ACE inhibition with lisinopril, Foxp3 positive Treg were enhanced [41]. Besides the significance of Th17/Treg cells for the development and progression of arterial hypertension and hypertensive end-organ damage, $\gamma\delta$ T-cells contribute to Ang II-induced elevation of blood pressure, endothelial dysfunction, and the activation of innate and adaptive immune response [42]. Further, Ang II increased monocyte chemotactic protein-1 expression in the vasculature, accompanied by higher monocyte/macrophage infiltration and pro-inflammatory macrophage polarization in the renal cortex [19]. Ang II also acts as a pro-fibrogenic cytokine regulating renal cell proliferation, synthesis and degradation of the extracellular matrix by various pathways, e.g., TGFβ [43].

TGFβ is secreted by many different cell types, including monocytes/macrophages, and a key function is the regulation of inflammatory processes and profibrotic signaling. Increased systemic levels of TGFβ are associated with faster CKD progression and TGFβ polymorphisms have been identified as risk factors for ESRD [44,45]. However, the effect of TGFβ is highly context-dependent. Ang II induces the expression of the TGFβ downstream target connective tissue growth factor β (CTGF), which is associated with endothelial mesenchymal transition. The profibrotic action of Ang II may be aggravated by interaction with other pathways such as hypoxia, the activation of plasminogen activator inhibitor-1, or ET1 signaling. Interestingly, the Hippo pathway transcription factor, TAZ, was activated in the renal tubulointerstitium in different models of kidney injury. Nuclear accumulation of TAZ depended on TGFβ1-signaling and went along with fibrosis progression [39]. M2 macrophage polarization, which significantly correlates with kidney fibrosis, is driven by TGFβ1-induced activation of YAP/TAZ, too [46]. The action of bone morphogenetic protein (BMP), which also belongs to the TGF protein family, in the kidney is not completely understood. In healthy renal tubules, BMP is constitutively active and its reactivation, after an injury that suppressed BMP expression, correlates with functional recovery [47].

Ang II, ET1 and catecholamines both exert their function via G-protein coupled receptors (GPCRs), such as the AT1R, ETA, ETA and b-adrenergic receptors. Current pharmacological approaches mainly target these GPCRs. The sensitivity of hormone-induced GPCR activation is modified by G-protein coupled receptor kinases (GRKs), and the regulator of G-Protein Signaling proteins [48]. It has been demonstrated that the dysregulation of the GRK isoforms 2–6 correlates with increased blood pressure, poor response to antihypertensive treatment, and adverse cardiovascular outcomes [49]. Renal fibrosis could be alleviated by the inhibition of the G-protein $\beta\gamma$-subunit in mouse models of cardiorenal syndrome and ischemic acute kidney injury [50]. Further, inhibition of the downstream kinase PKA may reduce profibrotic signaling and profibrogenic epigenetic priming in diabetic kidney disease [51]. Pharmacological modification of GPCR downstream targets may be a promising approach in hypertensive CKD.

Another important mechanism, contributing to hypertensive nephrosclerosis, is hypoxia (Figure 3). Chronic ischemic tubulointerstitial damage, caused by altered hemodynamics, increased oxygen demand, and loss of peritubular capillaries is a hallmark of progressive CKD. Under hypoxic conditions, HIF, and its oxygen-regulated isoforms, HIF1α and HIF2α, are stabilized and promote cellular adaptation to the decreased oxygen supply and influence cell proliferation, survival and metabolism. The increased expression of HIF1α was reported to correlate with glomerular injury and promote hypertensive CKD [52]. HIF1α gene expression in renal endothelia was induced by Ang II in a Nuclear Factor-κB (NFκB)-dependent manner [52]. It has also been shown, that reciprocal positive transcriptional regulation leads to persistent activation of HIF1α and NFκB genes and drives disease progression [52]. The profibrotic action of HIF1α is partly mediated via induction of TGFβ and its proinflammatory downstream target CTGF [53]. Interestingly, HIF2α, which is primarily expressed in non-epithelial cells is associated with ambiguous effects on renal fibrosis: In early stages of CKD, activation of HIF2α worsened renal fibrosis but did not lead to renal functional impairment [54]. In another study, overexpression of HIF2α was sufficient to induce kidney fibrosis [55]. At later stages of CKD, HIF2α activation, in part, activated typical hypoxia-induced target genes of HIF1α such as VEGF, fibronectin, and type 1 collagen but restored the renal vasculature and thereby ameliorated renal dysfunction and fibrosis [54].

Besides the development of hypoxia, the hemodynamic changes associated with a defective renal autoregulation of blood pressure, during hypertensive nephropathy, and other types of chronic kidney disease, are associated with flow- and shear-stress dependent signaling in endothelial cells (Figure 3). In response to increased blood flow, endothelial cells release ATP, which in turn activates endothelial cells or adjacent immune cells, in a paracrine fashion via trinucleotide-receptors, from the ionotropic P2X and metabotropic P2Y receptor family. For example, hypertension correlates with overexpression and activation of the P2 × 7, P2Y12, and P2X1 receptors [56]. The blockade of these receptors inhibits renal vasoconstriction induced by Ang II, restores microvascular dysfunction, and improves the Ang II-associated regional hypoxia [56,57]. In addition to the microvascular implications, the release of inflammatory mediators, such as interleukins in the tubulointerstitium seems to be related to the activation of P2X/P2Y receptors [56]. Secondly, the increased filtration pressure may lead to higher urinary flow and flow-activated signaling pathways in tubular cells, which may lose epithelial characteristics, such as the in the expression of cell junctional proteins [58]. CKD goes along with secretion of pro-inflammatory cytokines by activated immune cells, interstitial cells, and tubular epithelial cells [59]. For example, hypertensive kidney injury correlates with phosphorylation of the cytoskeleton-associated protein cofilin 1, formation of actin stress fibers, nuclear translocation of NFκB and expression of downstream inflammatory factors in renal tubular epithelial cells. [59].

Further, infiltration of IL17 secreting T lymphocytes may lead to vascular dysfunction. IL17 acts on vascular smooth muscle cells and perivascular fibroblasts, in order to increase reactive oxygen species (ROS) production, collagen synthesis, and chemokine production. In parallel, IL 17 reduces the bioavailability of NO and, vasodilatation, enhances vascular stiffness and the recruitment of immune cells [30].

5. Approaches to Foster Regeneration and Repair in Hypertensive Nephropathy

Despite recent advances in the understanding of molecular mechanisms, contributing to hypertensive nephropathy, the interplay between the different signaling networks in each cell type and—even more complex—between distinct cell types, is still incompletely deciphered. However, "omics" approaches such as single-cell proteomics and metabolomics, in conjunction with advanced imaging techniques, comprise excellent opportunities to gain further insight into this complex signaling network. So far, clinical management of hypertensive CKD focusses on the deceleration of CKD progression. A major aim is to stop all comorbidities, which are known to drive the progression of hypertensive CKD: Blood pressure should ideally be normalized, blood glucose control should be excellent, dietary salt may be restricted, and nephrotoxic medications are to be avoided. Further, pharmacological Ang II blockade has beneficial effects on the progression of hypertensive end-organ damage. Therapeutic approaches to other signaling pathways, such as HIF stabilization, ET1 blockade, anti-inflammatory therapy or immunosuppression, have so far either not been tested or not proven safe and efficient. In pre-clinical research, stem cell based approaches are evaluated to improve kidney regeneration in CKD. However, in nephrology in general, and especially with regard to hypertensive nephropathy, regenerative medicine techniques are still in their children's shoes. Studies are carried out with embryonic stem cells, mesenchymal stem cells, adipose stem cells, amniotic fluid stem cells, and renal progenitors, but also pluripotent cells. So far, the results from these studies are conflicting. However, even if stem cells and multipotent cells might not directly differentiate and replace damaged cells, they might produce protective and regenerative factors, and thereby enable functional improvement [60,61].

The bench-to-bedside transition of insight into the molecular mechanisms of CKD in hypertensive patients, and also a profound understanding of the molecular pathogenesis of CKD with other/mixed etiology, may lead to the development novel treatment approaches. Classifying CKD, based on the individual predominant molecular pathology, rather than traditional clinical etiologies would be an important step in developing focused molecular treatments. There is still a long way ahead, but once achieved, personalized medicine holds promise in CKD.

Author Contributions: Conceptualization, L.K.S.; data curation of references, L.K.S. and K.-U.E.; writing—original draft preparation, L.K.S.; writing—review and editing, L.K.S. and K.-U.E.; visualization, L.K.S.; supervision, K.-U.E.

References

1. Scheppach, J.B.; Raff, U.; Toncar, S.; Ritter, C.; Klink, T.; Stork, S.; Wanner, C.; Schlieper, G.; Saritas, T.; Reinartz, S.D.; et al. Blood Pressure Pattern and Target Organ Damage in Patients with Chronic Kidney Disease. *Hypertension* **2018**, *72*, 929–936. [CrossRef] [PubMed]
2. Liang, S.; Le, W.; Liang, D.; Chen, H.; Xu, F.; Chen, H.; Liu, Z.; Zeng, C. Clinico-pathological characteristics and outcomes of patients with biopsy-proven hypertensive nephrosclerosis: A retrospective cohort study. *BMC Nephrol.* **2016**, *17*, 42. [CrossRef]
3. Hill, G.S. Hypertensive nephrosclerosis. *Curr. Opin. Nephrol. Hypertens.* **2008**, *17*, 266–270. [CrossRef]
4. Thomas, J.L.; Pham, H.; Li, Y.; Hall, E.; Perkins, G.A.; Ali, S.S.; Patel, H.H.; Singh, P. Hypoxia-inducible factor-1alpha activation improves renal oxygenation and mitochondrial function in early chronic kidney disease. *Am. J. Physiol. Renal. Physiol.* **2017**, *313*, F282–F290. [CrossRef] [PubMed]
5. Fu, Q.; Colgan, S.P.; Shelley, C.S. Hypoxia: The Force that Drives Chronic Kidney Disease. *Clin. Med. Res.* **2016**, *14*, 15–39. [CrossRef]
6. Venkatachalam, M.A.; Weinberg, J.M.; Kriz, W.; Bidani, A.K. Failed Tubule Recovery, AKI-CKD Transition, and Kidney Disease Progression. *J. Am. Soc. Nephrol.* **2015**, *26*, 1765–1776. [CrossRef]
7. Nangaku, M.; Rosenberger, C.; Heyman, S.N.; Eckardt, K.U. Regulation of hypoxia-inducible factor in kidney disease. *Clin. Exp. Pharmacol. Physiol.* **2013** *40*, 148–157. [CrossRef]
8. Forrester, S.J.; Booz, G.W.; Sigmund, C.D.; Coffman, T.M.; Kawai, T.; Rizzo, V.; Scalia, R.; Eguchi, S. Angiotensin II Signal Transduction: An Update on Mechanisms of Physiology and Pathophysiology. *Physiol. Rev.* **2018**, *98*, 1627–1738. [CrossRef]

9. Reboussin, D.M.; Allen, N.B.; Griswold, M.E.; Guallar, E.; Hong, Y.; Lackland, D.T.; Miller, E.P.R., 3rd.; Polonsky, T.; Thompson-Paul, A.M.; Vupputuri, S. Systematic Review for the 2017 ACC/AHA/AAPA/ABC/ACPM/AGS/APhA/ASH/ASPC/NMA/PCNA Guideline for the Prevention, Detection, Evaluation, and Management of High Blood Pressure in Adults: A Report of the American College of Cardiology/American Heart Association Task Force on Clinical Practice Guidelines. *Circulation* **2018**, *138*, e595–e616.
10. Jordan, J. Device-Based Approaches for the Treatment of Arterial Hypertension. *Curr. Hypertens. Rep.* **2017**, *19*, 59. [CrossRef] [PubMed]
11. Bakris, G.L.; Nadim, M.K.; Haller, H.; Lovett, E.G.; Schafer, J.E.; Bisognano, J.D. Baroreflex activation therapy provides durable benefit in patients with resistant hypertension: Results of long-term follow-up in the Rheos Pivotal Trial. *J. Am. Soc. Hypertens.* **2012**, *6*, 152–158. [CrossRef]
12. Singh, R.R.; Denton, K.M. Renal Denervation. *Hypertension* **2018**, *72*, 528–536. [CrossRef] [PubMed]
13. Persu, A.; Kjeldsen, S.; Staessen, J.A.; Azizi, M. Renal Denervation for Treatment of Hypertension: A Second Start and New Challenges. *Curr. Hypertens. Rep.* **2016**, *18*, 6. [CrossRef]
14. Symplicity HTN-2 Investigators; Esler, M.D.; Krum, H.; Sobotka, P.A.; Schlaich, M.P.; Schmieder, R.E.; Bohm, M. Renal sympathetic denervation in patients with treatment-resistant hypertension (The Symplicity HTN-2 Trial): A randomised controlled trial. *Lancet* **2010**, *376*, 1903–1909.
15. Mahfoud, F.; Bohm, M.; Schmieder, R.; Narkiewicz, K.; Ewen, S.; Ruilope, L.; Schlaich, M.; Williams, B.; Fahy, M.; Mancia, G. Effects of renal denervation on kidney function and long-term outcomes: 3-year follow-up from the Global SYMPLICITY Registry. *Eur. Heart J.* **2019**. [CrossRef]
16. Townsend, R.R.; Mahfoud, F.; Kandzari, D.E.; Kario, K.; Pocock, S.; Weber, M.A.; Ewen, S.; Tsioufis, K.; Tousoulis, D.; Sharp, A.S.P.; et al. Catheter-based renal denervation in patients with uncontrolled hypertension in the absence of antihypertensive medications (SPYRAL HTN-OFF MED): A randomised, sham-controlled, proof-of-concept trial. *Lancet* **2017**, *390*, 2160–2170. [CrossRef]
17. Azizi, M.; Schmieder, R.E.; Mahfoud, F.; Weber, M.A.; Daemen, J.; Davies, J.; Basile, J.; Kirtane, A.J.; Wang, Y.; Lobo, M.D.; et al. Endovascular ultrasound renal denervation to treat hypertension (RADIANCE-HTN SOLO): A multicentre, international, single-blind, randomised, sham-controlled trial. *Lancet* **2018**, *391*, 2335–2345. [CrossRef]
18. Kandzari, D.E.; Bohm, M.; Mahfoud, F.; Townsend, R.R.; Weber, M.A.; Pocock, S.; Tsioufis, K.; Tousoulis, D.; Choi, J.W.; East, C.; et al. Effect of renal denervation on blood pressure in the presence of antihypertensive drugs: 6-month efficacy and safety results from the SPYRAL HTN-ON MED proof-of-concept randomised trial. *Lancet* **2018**, *391*, 2346–2355. [CrossRef]
19. Mian, M.O.; Barhoumi, T.; Briet, M.; Paradis, P.; Schiffrin, E.L. Deficiency of T-regulatory cells exaggerates angiotensin II-induced microvascular injury by enhancing immune responses. *J. Hypertens.* **2016**, *34*, 97–108. [CrossRef]
20. Barhoumi, T.; Kasal, D.A.; Li, M.W.; Shbat, L.; Laurant, P.; Neves, M.F.; Paradis, P.; Schiffrin, E.L. T regulatory lymphocytes prevent angiotensin II-induced hypertension and vascular injury. *Hypertension* **2011**, *57*, 469–476. [CrossRef]
21. Mehrotra, P.; Patel, J.B.; Ivancic, C.M.; Collett, J.A.; Basile, D.P. Th-17 cell activation in response to high salt following acute kidney injury is associated with progressive fibrosis and attenuated by AT-1R antagonism. *Kidney Int.* **2015**, *88*, 776–784. [CrossRef]
22. Kim, S.M.; Lee, S.H.; Lee, A.; Kim, D.J.; Kim, Y.G.; Kim, S.Y.; Jeong, K.H.; Lee, T.W.; Ihm, C.G.; Lim, S.J.; et al. Targeting T helper 17 by mycophenolate mofetil attenuates diabetic nephropathy progression. *Transl. Res.* **2015**, *166*, 375–383. [CrossRef]
23. Mohamed, R.; Jayakumar, C.; Chen, F.; Fulton, D.; Stepp, D.; Gansevoort, R.T.; Ramesh, G. Low-Dose IL-17 Therapy Prevents and Reverses Diabetic Nephropathy, Metabolic Syndrome, and Associated Organ Fibrosis. *J. Am. Soc. Nephrol.* **2016**, *27*, 745–765. [CrossRef]
24. Wilck, N.; Matus, M.G.; Kearney, S.M.; Olesen, S.W.; Forslund, K.; Bartolomaeus, H.; Haase, S.; Mahler, A.; Balogh, A.; Marko, L.; et al. Salt-responsive gut commensal modulates TH17 axis and disease. *Nature* **2017**, *551*, 585–589. [CrossRef] [PubMed]
25. Bartolomaeus, H.; Balogh, A.; Yakoub, M.; Homann, S.; Marko, L.; Hoges, S.; Tsvetkov, D.; Krannich, A.; Wundersitz, S.; Avery, E.G.; et al. The Short-Chain Fatty Acid Propionate Protects from Hypertensive Cardiovascular Damage. *Circulation* **2018**. [CrossRef] [PubMed]

26. Higaki, A.; Caillon, A.; Paradis, P.; Schiffrin, E.L. Innate and Innate-Like Immune System in Hypertension and Vascular Injury. *Curr. Hypertens. Rep.* **2019**, *21*, 4. [CrossRef]
27. Warren, H.R.; Evangelou, E.; Cabrera, C.P.; Gao, H.; Ren, M.; Mifsud, B.; Ntalla, I.; Surendran, P.; Liu, C.; Cook, J.P.; et al. Corrigendum: Genome-wide association analysis identifies novel blood pressure loci and offers biological insights into cardiovascular risk. *Nat. Genet.* **2017**, *49*, 1558. [CrossRef] [PubMed]
28. Delles, C.; Carrick, E.; Graham, D.; Nicklin, S.A. Utilizing proteomics to understand and define hypertension: Where are we and where do we go? *Expert Rev. Proteomics* **2018**, *15*, 581–592. [CrossRef]
29. Giani, J.F.; Janjulia, T.; Taylor, B.; Bernstein, E.A.; Shah, K.; Shen, X.Z.; McDonough, A.A.; Bernstein, K.E.; Gonzalez-Villalobos, R.A. Renal generation of angiotensin II and the pathogenesis of hypertension. *Curr. Hypertens. Rep.* **2014**, *16*, 477. [CrossRef] [PubMed]
30. McMaster, W.G.; Kirabo, A.; Madhur, M.S.; Harrison, D.G. Inflammation, immunity, and hypertensive end-organ damage. *Circ. Res.* **2015**, *116*, 1022–1033. [CrossRef]
31. Fukuda, A.; Wickman, L.T.; Venkatareddy, M.P.; Sato, Y.; Chowdhury, M.A.; Wang, S.Q.; Shedden, K.A.; Dysko, R.C.; Wiggins, J.E.; Wiggins, R.C. Angiotensin II-dependent persistent podocyte loss from destabilized glomeruli causes progression of end stage kidney disease. *Kidney Int.* **2012**, *81*, 40–55. [CrossRef]
32. Gloy, J.; Henger, A.; Fischer, K.G.; Nitschke, R.; Mundel, P.; Bleich, M.; Schollmeyer, P.; Greger, R.; Pavenstadt, H. Angiotensin II depolarizes podocytes in the intact glomerulus of the Rat. *J. Clin. Invest.* **1997**, *99*, 2772–2781. [CrossRef]
33. Henger, A.; Huber, T.; Fischer, K.G.; Nitschke, R.; Mundel, P.; Schollmeyer, P.; Greger, R.; Pavenstadt, H. Angiotensin II increases the cytosolic calcium activity in rat podocytes in culture. *Kidney Int.* **1997**, *52*, 687–693. [CrossRef] [PubMed]
34. Nijenhuis, T.; Sloan, A.J.; Hoenderop, J.G.; Flesche, J.; van Goor, H.; Kistler, A.D.; Bakker, M.; Bindels, R.J.; de Boer, R.A.; Moller, C.C.; et al. Angiotensin II contributes to podocyte injury by increasing TRPC6 expression via an NFAT-mediated positive feedback signaling pathway. *Am. J. Pathol.* **2011**, *179*, 1719–1732. [CrossRef]
35. Schenk, L.K.; Moller-Kerutt, A.; Klosowski, R.; Wolters, D.; Schaffner-Reckinger, E.; Weide, T.; Pavenstadt, H.; Vollenbroker, B. Angiotensin II regulates phosphorylation of actin-associated proteins in human podocytes. *FASEB J.* **2017**, *31*, 5019–5035. [CrossRef] [PubMed]
36. Ren, Z.; Liang, W.; Chen, C.; Yang, H.; Singhal, P.C.; Ding, G. Angiotensin II induces nephrin dephosphorylation and podocyte injury: Role of caveolin-1. *Cell Signal.* **2012**, *24*, 443–450. [CrossRef]
37. Yang, Q.; Ma, Y.; Liu, Y.; Liang, W.; Chen, X.; Ren, Z.; Wang, H.; Singhal, P.C.; Ding, G. Angiotensin II down-regulates nephrin-Akt signaling and induces podocyte injury: Roleof c-Abl. *Mol. Biol. Cell* **2016**, *27*, 197–208. [CrossRef] [PubMed]
38. Wennmann, D.O.; Vollenbroker, B.; Eckart, A.K.; Bonse, J.; Erdmann, F.; Wolters, D.A.; Schenk, L.K.; Schulze, U.; Kremerskothen, J.; Weide, T.; et al. The Hippo pathway is controlled by Angiotensin II signaling and its reactivation induces apoptosis in podocytes. *Cell Death Dis.* **2014**, *5*, e1519. [CrossRef]
39. Anorga, S.; Overstreet, J.M.; Falke, L.L.; Tang, J.; Goldschmeding, R.G.; Higgins, P.J.; Samarakoon, R. Deregulation of Hippo-TAZ pathway during renal injury confers a fibrotic maladaptive phenotype. *FASEB J.* **2018**, *32*, 2644–2657. [CrossRef]
40. Yang, Y.; Yang, Q.; Yang, J.; Ma, Y.; Ding, G. Angiotensin II induces cholesterol accumulation and injury in podocytes. *Sci. Rep.* **2017**, *7*, 10672. [CrossRef]
41. Platten, M.; Youssef, S.; Hur, E.M.; Ho, P.P.; Han, M.H.; Lanz, T.V.; Phillips, L.K.; Goldstein, M.J.; Bhat, R.; Raine, C.S.; et al. Blocking angiotensin-converting enzyme induces potent regulatory T cells and modulates TH1- and TH17-mediated autoimmunity. *Proc. Natl. Acad. Sci. USA* **2009**, *106*, 14948–14953. [CrossRef]
42. Caillon, A.; Mian, M.O.R.; Fraulob-Aquino, J.C.; Huo, K.G.; Barhoumi, T.; Ouerd, S.; Sinnaeve, P.R.; Paradis, P.; Schiffrin, E.L. gammadelta T Cells Mediate Angiotensin II-Induced Hypertension and Vascular Injury. *Circulation* **2017**, *135*, 2155–2162. [CrossRef]
43. Ruster, C.; Wolf, G. Angiotensin II as a morphogenic cytokine stimulating renal fibrogenesis. *J. Am. Soc. Nephrol.* **2011**, *22*, 1189–1199. [CrossRef]
44. Suthanthiran, M.; Li, B.; Song, J.O.; Ding, R.; Sharma, V.K.; Schwartz, J.E.; August, P. Transforming growth factor-beta 1 hyperexpression in African-American hypertensives: A novel mediator of hypertension and/or target organ damage. *Proc. Natl. Acad. Sci. USA* **2000**, *97*, 3479–3484. [CrossRef]
45. Suthanthiran, M.; Gerber, L.M.; Schwartz, J.E.; Sharma, V.K.; Medeiros, M.; Marion, R.; Pickering, T.G.; August, P. Circulating transforming growth factor-beta1 levels and the risk for kidney disease in African Americans. *Kidney Int.* **2009**, *76*, 72–80. [CrossRef]

46. Feng, Y.; Liang, Y.; Zhu, X.; Wang, M.; Gui, Y.; Lu, Q.; Gu, M.; Xue, X.; Sun, X.; He, W.; et al. The signaling protein Wnt5a promotes TGFbeta1-mediated macrophage polarization and kidney fibrosis by inducing the transcriptional regulators Yap/Taz. *J. Biol. Chem.* **2018**, *293*, 19290–19302. [CrossRef]
47. Vigolo, E.; Marko, L.; Hinze, C.; Muller, D.N.; Schmidt-Ullrich, R.; Schmidt-Ott, K.M. Canonical BMP signaling in tubular cells mediates recovery after acute kidney injury. *Kidney Int.* **2019**, *95*, 108–122. [CrossRef] [PubMed]
48. Brinks, H.L.; Eckhart, A.D. Regulation of GPCR signaling in hypertension. *Biochim. Biophys. Acta* **2010**, *1802*, 1268–1275. [CrossRef]
49. Yang, J.; Villar, V.A.; Armando, I.; Jose, P.A.; Zeng, C. G Protein-Coupled Receptor Kinases: Crucial Regulators of Blood Pressure. *J. Am. Heart Assoc.* **2016**, *5*, e003519. [CrossRef] [PubMed]
50. Kamal, F.A.; Travers, J.G.; Schafer, A.E.; Ma, Q.; Devarajan, P.; Blaxall, B.C. G Protein-Coupled Receptor-G-Protein betagamma-Subunit Signaling Mediates Renal Dysfunction and Fibrosis in Heart Failure. *J. Am. Soc. Nephrol.* **2017**, *28*, 197–208. [CrossRef]
51. Deb, D.K.; Bao, R.; Li, Y.C. Critical role of the cAMP-PKA pathway in hyperglycemia-induced epigenetic activation of fibrogenic program in the kidney. *FASEB J.* **2017**, *31*, 2065–2075. [CrossRef]
52. Luo, R.; Zhang, W.; Zhao, C.; Zhang, Y.; Wu, H.; Jin, J.; Zhang, W.; Grenz, A.; Eltzschig, H.K.; Tao, L.; et al. Elevated Endothelial Hypoxia-Inducible Factor-1alpha Contributes to Glomerular Injury and Promotes Hypertensive Chronic Kidney Disease. *Hypertension* **2015**, *66*, 75–84. [CrossRef]
53. Eckardt, K.U.; Bernhardt, W.M.; Weidemann, A.; Warnecke, C.; Rosenberger, C.; Wiesener, M.S.; Willam, C. Role of hypoxia in the pathogenesis of renal disease. *Kidney Int. Suppl.* **2005**, *99*, S46–S51. [CrossRef]
54. Kong, K.H.; Oh, H.J.; Lim, B.J.; Kim, M.; Han, K.H.; Choi, Y.H.; Kwon, K.; Nam, B.Y.; Park, K.S.; Park, J.T.; et al. Selective tubular activation of hypoxia-inducible factor-2alpha has dual effects on renal fibrosis. *Sci. Rep.* **2017**, *7*, 11351. [CrossRef]
55. Schietke, R.E.; Hackenbeck, T.; Tran, M.; Gunther, R.; Klanke, B.; Warnecke, C.L.; Knaup, K.X.; Shukla, D.; Rosenberger, C.; Koesters, R.; et al. Renal tubular HIF-2alpha expression requires VHL inactivation and causes fibrosis and cysts. *PLoS ONE* **2012**, *7*, e31034. [CrossRef]
56. Franco, M.; Bautista-Perez, R.; Perez-Mendez, O. Purinergic receptors in tubulointerstitial inflammatory cells: A pathophysiological mechanism of salt-sensitive hypertension. *Acta Physiol. (Oxf)* **2015**, *214*, 75–87. [CrossRef]
57. Menzies, R.I.; Howarth, A.R.; Unwin, R.J.; Tam, F.W.; Mullins, J.J.; Bailey, M.A. Inhibition of the purinergic P2X7 receptor improves renal perfusion in angiotensin-II-infused rats. *Kidney Int.* **2015**, *88*, 1079–1087. [CrossRef]
58. Maggiorani, D.; Dissard, R.; Belloy, M.; Saulnier-Blache, J.S.; Casemayou, A.; Ducasse, L.; Gres, S.; Belliere, J.; Caubet, C.; Bascands, J.L.; et al. Shear Stress-Induced Alteration of Epithelial Organization in Human Renal Tubular Cells. *PLoS ONE* **2015**, *10*, e0131416. [CrossRef] [PubMed]
59. Wang, Q.Z.; Gao, H.Q.; Liang, Y.; Zhang, J.; Wang, J.; Qiu, J. Cofilin1 is involved in hypertension-induced renal damage via the regulation of NF-kappaB in renal tubular epithelial cells. *J. Transl. Med.* **2015**, *13*, 323. [CrossRef]
60. Hickson, L.J.; Eirin, A.; Lerman, L.O. Challenges and opportunities for stem cell therapy in patients with chronic kidney disease. *Kidney Int.* **2016**, *89*, 767–778. [CrossRef] [PubMed]
61. Peired, A.J.; Sisti, A.; Romagnani, P. Mesenchymal Stem Cell-Based Therapy for Kidney Disease: A Review of Clinical Evidence. *Stem Cells Int.* **2016**, *2016*, 4798639. [CrossRef] [PubMed]

7

Mesenchymal Stem Cells—Potential Applications in Kidney Diseases

Benjamin Bochon [1,†], Magdalena Kozubska [2,†], Grzegorz Surygała [3,†], Agnieszka Witkowska [4], Roman Kuźniewicz [5], Władysław Grzeszczak [5] and Grzegorz Wystrychowski [5,*]

1 Psychiatric Services of Thurgovia, Academic Teaching Hospital of the Medical University of Salzburg, 8596 Münsterlingen, Switzerland; benjaminbochon@yahoo.com
2 General Practice, 43-426 Dębowiec, Poland; magdalena.kozubska@interia.eu
3 Regional Blood Donation and Blood Treatment Centre, 40-074 Katowice, Poland; gregorian08@wp.pl
4 DaVita Dialysis, 42-700 Lubliniec, Poland; witkowskaaga@op.pl
5 Department of Internal Medicine, Diabetology and Nephrology, School of Medicine with the Division of Dentistry in Zabrze, Medical University of Silesia in Katowice, 41-800 Zabrze, Poland; rkuzniewicz@sum.edu.pl (R.K.); wgrzeszczak@sum.edu.pl (W.G.)
* Correspondence: gwystrychowski@sum.edu.pl
† These authors contributed equally to this paper.

Abstract: Mesenchymal stem cells constitute a pool of cells present throughout the lifetime in numerous niches, characteristic of unlimited replication potential and the ability to differentiate into mature cells of mesodermal tissues in vitro. The therapeutic potential of these cells is, however, primarily associated with their capabilities of inhibiting inflammation and initiating tissue regeneration. Owing to these properties, mesenchymal stem cells (derived from the bone marrow, subcutaneous adipose tissue, and increasingly urine) are the subject of research in the settings of kidney diseases in which inflammation plays the key role. The most advanced studies, with the first clinical trials, apply to ischemic acute kidney injury, renal transplantation, lupus and diabetic nephropathies, in which beneficial clinical effects of cells themselves, as well as their culture medium, were observed. The study findings imply that mesenchymal stem cells act predominantly through secreted factors, including, above all, microRNAs contained within extracellular vesicles. Research over the coming years will focus on this secretome as a possible therapeutic agent void of the potential carcinogenicity of the cells.

Keywords: mesenchymal stem cell; mesodermal stem cell; renal ischemia-reperfusion; inflammation; kidney transplantation; microRNA; extracellular vesicles; exosomes

1. Introduction

Chronic kidney disease (CKD) affects ~10% of the general population, leading to the deterioration of the quality of life and premature death due to cardiovascular complications. On one hand, chronic renal insufficiency arises as a consequence of continuous insidious kidney damage and scarring in such common diseases as high blood pressure, diabetes, or nephrolithiasis, and, fortunately not as frequent, various forms of chronic glomerulonephritis. On the other, CKD gets instigated or aggravated with incidents of acute kidney injury (AKI), due to such insults as ischemia, infection, autoimmune reaction or toxins like radiological contrast or drugs. The possibilities of pharmacological prevention or attenuation of chronic renal failure are limited to controlling cardiovascular risk factors (usually not optimal), avoidance of potential renal toxins (often unfeasible), or causal treatment of AKI whenever possible (with variable efficiency and frequent complications). In the light of medical advances in other areas, this shortage of therapeutic options raises understandable frustration among patients and their physicians. Stem cell-based therapies may lead to the expected breakthrough in the treatment of kidney diseases.

2. Mesenchymal Stem Cells

2.1. Types of Stem Cells

Stem cells, owing to their unique ability to replicate and differentiate into specialized organ cells, provide the tissues with the ability to regenerate and survive most injuries [1]. Four types of these cells are defined according to their differentiation potential. In the embryonic period, the early stages of ontogenesis occur owing to the unlimited abilities of totipotent zygotic cells, replaced over time by pluripotent embryonic cells that differentiate into cells of all three germ layers, but no longer have the ability to differentiate into placental cells [2]. Beyond this phase, pluripotent cells that resemble the embryonic stem cells can be obtained by dedifferentiation of fibroblasts or epithelial cells in vitro (induced pluripotent stem cells) [3]. Throughout the lifetime, somatic stem cells are preserved within numerous niches—multipotent ones, which transform into all cells of a given tissue (e.g., bone marrow progenitor cells) or unipotent ones that can only differentiate into one type of mature cell (e.g., cells of the basal layer of the epidermis) [4].

At present, the cells under the most extensive investigations in experimental biology and medicine are mesenchymal (mesodermal) stem cells (MSC) that occur in the human body in mesodermal tissues, including placenta, amniotic fluid, umbilical cord tissues, bone marrow, adipose tissue, testis or lungs [5].

2.2. Regenerative Properties of MSC

MSC exhibit multipotent properties in vitro—when treated with appropriate chemical compounds they have the ability to differentiate into all mesodermal lineage cells, such as fibroblasts, osteocytes, chondrocytes, adipocytes or myocytes [6]. Few studies indicate that they can also transform into cells of endodermal or ectodermal origin [7]. Whereas this vast differentiation potential is of interest and conceivable use in the ex vivo generation of injured tissue replacements, there is only scarce evidence that MSC takes advantage of it in vivo [8]. Most data show that they rather promote tissue repair processes by the means of cell-to-cell interactions or secreted biomaterial, including antioxidant, antiapoptotic and growth factors (GF), such as Epithelial GF, Vascular Endothelial GF (VEGF), Transforming GF (TGF) α and β, Fibroblast GF, Insulin-like GF type 1, and others [9] that stimulate divisions of local progenitor cells. Studies show that these compounds are released from MSC in the free state or contained within spherical vesicles of a 30–100 nm diameter—exosomes of an endosomal origin or microvesicles budding from the cellular membrane. These extracellular vesicles allow signal transmission between the cells not only through the transported proteins, but also mRNAs and microRNAs [10]. Multiple microRNA particles have been identified within MSC extracellular vesicles and their patterns differ considerably between experimental models of different ischemic/inflammatory diseases [11]. Of great importance is homing of MSC to the ischemic, necrotic or inflamed sites, as a result of their membrane expression of chemokine receptors and integrins [5], responsiveness to damage associated molecular patterns [12] or mitochondria released from dead cells with their engulfment [13]. This tropism reduces the distance of secreted products to their target locations and allows an additional way of restoring local homeostasis by MSC—intercellular transfer of mitochondria [14]. Substituting defective native mitochondria with MSC-derived fully operational ones provides ATP for most needed anabolic reactions [15] and has been shown to revive damaged alveolar or corneal epithelia [16,17]. According to most reports mitochondria are moved to the damaged cells by means of nanotube tunneling [18], microvesicles [19] or cellular fusion, as recently comprehensively reviewed [20].

MSC are increasingly used in reconstructive surgery. In countries with less stringent legal restrictions (such as Japan and South Korea), they are used as a replicative matrix for renewal of joint surfaces and regeneration of facial defects (which requires collagen scaffolding) or as a source of cytokines and GFs stimulating natural healing in periodontal disease and skin wounds [21]. Their usefulness is examined in experimental models of corneal damage, lung, spinal cord and brain injuries [22].

2.3. *Immunomodulatory Properties of MSC*

Beside their regenerative potential, MSC are characterized by the ability to modulate immune responses. Of note, they are characterized by low expression of MHC class I antigens and no expression of MHC class II antigens or B7-1, B7-2 and CD40 costimulatory molecules. This implies that the infusion of allogeneic stem cells does not induce a clinically significant immune response [23]. Most importantly, exposure to MSC in vitro or their systemic administration in large amounts (~10^6–10^8 cells) inhibits Th17 lymphocytes, augments the pool and activity of regulatory T-cells, and increases expression of anti-inflammatory cytokines like IL-10, subsequently blunting inflammatory reaction [24]. Their use in the treatment of autoimmune diseases, such as inflammatory diseases of the joints [25] or intestines [26] has been tested with good results. Contrary to initial assumptions, studies with infusions of exogenous MSC showed that their anti-inflammatory effect is not primarily the result of the direct interaction with immune cells in the target inflamed tissue, but they can act from distance by the means of their secretome, at least partially contained within exosomes or microvesicles [27]. Meticulously isolated extracellular vesicles of umbilical cord MSC (by means of size-exclusion chromatography) have been shown to exert a potent immunosuppressant effect in vitro, in contrast to other fractions of the MSC conditioned medium [28].

A British group has recently found that immunosuppressive activity of human bone marrow MSC in the experimental model of an established severe inflammatory reaction (MSC intravenous infusion on the third day of graft-versus-host disease in mice) relies on their apoptosis. The reductions of the lung and spleen pools of graft-versus-host disease effector T-cells were detectable either when MSC were lysed and engulfed by recipient's NK or CD8+ T cells in an antigen-independent way or when apoptosis was induced in MSC prior to their infusion. Based on the results with the additional use of an inhibitor of indoleamine 2,3-dioxygenase, the authors concluded that increased expression and release of this anti-inflammatory cytokine by recipient's phagocytes upon MSC apoptosis is the mediator of the immunosuppressive effect [29]. However, it can be reasoned that this very mechanism does not exclude the role of extracellular vesicles and microRNAs which can be extensively released from the apoptotic cells. Somewhat in line with the latter study, the key role of apoptosis of MSC with the self-activation of IL-1/IL-1R/NFκB pathway induced by caspases, has been implicated in the increased secretion of Prostaglandin E2 by MSC and consequential proinflammatory M1→ anti-inflammatory M2 macrophage transition [30].

2.4. *Source of MSC for Research Purposes*

Mesenchymal stem cells can be obtained from fetal tissues, umbilical cord blood or Wharton's Jelly, which for obvious reasons limits this route of acquisition to the perinatal period. In males, they may be acquired throughout a lifetime from testis [31], but due to greater accessibility, MSC for research purposes are derived mostly from bone marrow or subcutaneous adipose tissue. Fat may become preferential as a source of MSC not only owing to less invasive procurement, but also due to higher MSC concentration than in bone marrow, lesser expression of MHC class I antigens, and greater replicative and secretory potential of MSC [32,33] (Table 1). MSC can also be obtained from induced pluripotent stem cells by their differentiation in vitro [34], which constitutes another life-long, yet technically much more challenging way of acquisition.

Table 1. Differences in the properties of bone marrow and fat mesenchymal stem cells.

Differentiating Characteristic	Bone Marrow MSC	Adipose MSC
Stability in culture	Lower	Higher
Aging	More advanced	Less advanced
Replicative potential	Lower	Higher
Immunomodulatory properties	Lower	Higher

2.5. *Kidney as a Source of MSC*

A promising method of a non-invasive collection of MSC is their isolation from urine. In 2008, for the first time, Zhang et al. from North Carolina identified cells present in the urine in the amount of 2–7/100 mL that adhere to plastic and form colonies of differentiated daughter cells expressing membrane markers characteristic of urothelial, endothelial, and interstitial cells, or myocytes [35]. In further studies, the differentiation of these cells in appropriate culture media to the endo, ecto- and mesodermal lineage was achieved [36]. In contrast to MSC, urine-derived cells (up to 75% of them) show telomerase activity, which is associated with their higher replicative potential, apparently not associated with an increased risk of tumorigenesis [37]. The origin of these cells is most likely glomerular—MSC-like cells with a vast differentiation potential were isolated from the renal cortical decapsulated glomeruli [38] and shown nephroprotective in the renal ischemia-reperfusion injury (IRI) [39]. These cells seem distinct from the renal perivascular MSC-like cells that possess lesser differentiating capabilities (no adipogenesis), but also compelling kidney reparative properties confirmed in the tubular epithelial cell line injury in vitro or non-ischemic AKI in mice [40].

3. Research on the Use of Mesenchymal Stem Cells in Kidney Diseases

Potential applications of MSC in kidney diseases primarily take advantage of their secretory capabilities and aim to enhance the natural regenerative processes in the settings of AKI, and in the bolder perspective, even induce such processes in CKD. On the other hand, MSC can be used to grow renal cells in vitro to replace damaged native cells. In this context, cultures of kidney fragments (organoids) with subsequent implantations are to be considered, despite all technical complexity. Thirdly, the use of immunomodulatory properties of MSC can play an important role in the treatment of inflammatory kidney disease, such as primary and secondary glomerulonephritis, or in the prevention of rejection of the transplanted kidney. Finally, urinary isolation of cells that are functionally similar to MSC can significantly increase the availability of the material for all these therapeutic options.

3.1. *Attempts to Replace Damaged Kidney Tissue*

Kidney organogenesis includes mutually stimulating processes of the growth and differentiation of the intermediate mesoderm cells—to the ureteric bud (mesonephric duct protrusion) and to the metanephric blastema. They further transform respectively into the urinary tract system (up to connecting tubules), or nephrons, renal interstitium and endothelium [41]. Development of a new kidney by recapitulating organogenesis in whole or in part in vitro is an intensively studied area of tissue engineering. As research from the 1990s showed, appropriate sets of GFs can induce early stages of the development of an isolated ureteric bud, as well as metanephric blastema [42,43]. However, it remains problematic to derive cells with fetal characteristics from an adult, as well as to provide vascularization of the developing tissue. The first issue is currently being investigated with the use of induced pluripotent cells obtained from fibroblasts. In several cases, these cells (as well as embryonic MSC) were successfully cultured over <4 weeks into three-dimensional organoids with structural and functional characteristics of nephron complexes. The applied protocols included the use of such stimulants as Fibroblast GF-9, WNT-signaling pathway agonist, and activin [44,45]. Recent works by van den Berg et al. showed that renal organoids generated from human embryonic or induced pluripotent stem cells, became efficiently vascularized upon kidney subcapsular implantation in mice. Compared to organoids cultured continuously in vitro, those that were placed in vivo on the 18th day of the three-dimensional growth featured a more advanced structural maturation regarding glomerular endothelium, filtration barrier (slit diaphragm formation), tubular epithelium polarization and differentiation, as well as peritubular vascularization, when assessed on the 28th day since implantation [46].

A different way of generating a kidney replacement is through colonization of an acellular connective tissue scaffold with cells of a high replicative and differentiating potential or mature renal cells. The use of mature renal cells would eliminate the possible risk of cancer associated with stem cell divisions, but is much more technically difficult. A more feasible approach is through intra-arterial and intra-ureteral infusions of multipotent cells, which in response to the scaffold environment and native or exogenous GFs would differentiate into glomerular endothelial and epithelial or tubular cells, respectively. In order to obtain an intact acellular, sterile connective tissue scaffold of the kidney, an organ retrieved from another organism is infused with detergents like sodium lauryl sulfate or nonionic surfactants [47]. A successful repopulation of digested rat kidneys with rat fetal cells has been reported by the authors from Boston in 2013. The umbilical vein endothelial cells infused into renal artery produced endothelial layer in the entire renal circulation, whereas neonatal kidney cell suspension administered into the ureter resulted in the settlement of cells in their physiological niches of the urinary tract, beginning from podocytes down to connecting tubules. Such regenerated kidneys perfused in vitro with a solution containing crystalloids, glucose, albumin, amino acids, creatinine and urea showed partial functionality in the production of "urine", creatinine filtration (10–25% of the physiological level) and albumin retention (47% of the physiological level). In contrast, after orthotopic implantation, despite adequate blood flow and absence of bleeding or clotting and urine production of ~1/3 of physiological volume, they featured only a negligible excretion of urea and creatinine [48]. Similar results were obtained by another team of researchers from China [49]. On the other hand, Italian researchers did not manage to obtain sealed layers of cells in the distal parts of the renal circulation and proximal sections of the nephrons despite various protocols of embryonic MSC administration [50]. This area of research is awaiting verification of the usefulness of bone marrow or adipose MSC.

In the context of kidney regeneration, it is of note, that Iranian authors intend to assess effects of intravenous infusion of autologous bone marrow MSC on the course of autosomal dominant polycystic kidney disease [51].

3.2. *Induction of Repair Processes after Acute Kidney Injury*

One of the major study areas of MSC has been their influence on the course of renal IRI, being the most frequent cause of AKI and occurring in the clinical settings of shock, cardiac arrest, extracorporeal circulation and peritransplantation period. In addition to apoptosis caused by an energy deficiency and acidosis during ischemia, reperfusion results in further tissue damage, due to oxidative stress and inflammatory reaction. Studies conducted so far have shown that MSC infusion alleviates IRI of the kidney. Regardless of the mode of MSC administration (to the renal artery or intravenously, at various times in relation to IRI), the animal models showed a milder course of acute kidney failure [52], with reductions of oxidative damage and local expression of inflammatory cytokines [53], increased renal pool of regulatory T lymphocytes [54], faster regeneration of renal tubular epithelium [55], and reduction of subsequent fibrosis of the renal interstitium [56].

Intravenous infusion of MSC (derived from induced pluripotent stem cells) was equally nephroprotective in the model of toxin-induced AKI. In mice 2×10^5 MSC, injected 2 h after administration of Adriamycin, mitigated proteinuria and renal failure present on day 7 in controls. This could be attributed to the observed inhibition of oxidative stress and apoptosis in the tubular cells [57].

As already mentioned, these beneficial effects of MSC result from their secretory properties, not replicative-differentiating potential. In an experiment conducted by a German-American team, rats subjected to 40-min ischemia of both kidneys were administered labelled allogenic bone marrow-derived

MSC (10^6 cells) to the aorta immediately after or 24 h after renal reperfusion. In both cases, two hours after the end of the infusion, MSC were found in the renal tissue (within the glomerular and peritubular capillaries), but were not detected, neither did differentiate to other cells, during the subsequent 22 and 70 h of observation. Nevertheless, faster normalization of renal excretory function, reduced renal expression of proinflammatory cytokines (Interleukin-1β, Tumor Necrosis Factor α, Interferon γ) and higher renal expression of anti-inflammatory and antiapoptotic factors, such as Interleukin-10, basic Fibroblast GF, TGF α and Bcl-2 were observed at the conclusion of observation [58].

The fraction of MSC secretome responsible for this nephroprotective effect may be largely RNA, as shown by Italian researchers. Microvesicles isolated from human bone marrow MSC medium (30 μg), administered intravenously to rats after a 45-min ischemia of the sole kidney, attenuated acute renal failure and atrophy of tubular cells, whereas subjecting these microvesicles to RNase abolished their beneficial effects in this experimental model [59]. Further studies in rodents and cell lines by this largely Torino-based group revealed that the nephroprotective effect of microvesicles derived from bone marrow MSC in AKI may be owing to high contents of a few microRNA families (miR-483–5p, -191, -28–3p, -423–5p, -744, -129–3p, -24, and miR-148a) that get transferred to tubular epithelial cells. This results in altered expression of at least 165 genes involved in cellular adhesion and extracellular matrix remodeling, including downregulation of the transcription of fibrinogen-α subunit [60]. Furthermore, extracellular vesicles secreted by the bone marrow MSC were shown by this group to be heterogeneous in size and contents, with the exosomal fraction to diminish apoptosis and enhance proliferation of tubular cells undergoing hypoxia/reperfusion in vitro. This fraction was rich in the microRNA families involved in kidney regeneration (miR-100, -21, -24, -214, -34a, -127, -30c, -29a, -125b, -10b, -let-7c, -99a, -17 and miR-20a) [61]. Another study showed that also the above mentioned glomerular MSC-like cells (obtained from human renal cortex) and their extracellular vesicles alleviate AKI in mice by promoting tubular cell proliferation when infused intravenously at reperfusion following a 35-min sole kidney ischemia (10^5 cells or 400×10^6 vesicles, respectively). Interestingly, the injected vesicles were homing to the injured tubular cells (and not glomeruli) where they were visible for up to 6 h after infusion, contrary to the administered vesicles obtained from dermal fibroblasts, which did not accumulate in the kidney and consequently showed no effects whatsoever. In line with earlier studies, the nephroprotective properties of the vesicles derived from the glomerular MSC-like cells were eliminated in case they had been pretreated with high-concentration RNase and 62 microRNAs were found to be specifically abundant in these extracellular vesicles [39].

Similar to MSC, the MSC-derived extracellular vesicles were found to protect kidneys also from a toxic injury. The above quoted Italian group of Camussi showed that human bone marrow MSC (75×10^3) or their microvesicles (15 μg) alleviated AKI to the same extent when administered intravenously on the third day after glycerol injection in mice. Moreover MSC microvesicles were homing and getting incorporated into tubular cells in vivo only in glycerol-exposed animals, and not in controls, and their antiapoptotic effects were RNA-dependent [62]. Correspondingly positive renal outcomes were obtained by these authors in the mouse model of cisplatin-induced lethal AKI, in which MSC-secreted microvesicles (100 μg) were infused 8 h after cisplatin injection. Importantly, nearly half of the animals were alive after three weeks, and when injections of the microvesicles were repeated every four days, 80% of mice survived [63].

The very same model of toxic AKI was used by German investigators to show that the renoprotective properties of MSC secretome can be enhanced by hypoxic preconditioning of the MSC culture. Such treatment of mouse adipose MSC (0.5% oxygen for 48 h) increased their expression of VEGF and by >2-fold its secretion, as well as that of other 63 proteins. This corresponded with a moderately alleviated course of AKI following infusion of the hypoxia-preconditioned MSC medium (at 24 h after cisplatin injection), as compared to the non-manipulated MSC medium [64]. Significantly positive renal outcomes were obtained by another group in the rat model of renal IRI with the administration of hypoxia-preconditioned (1% oxygen for 24 h) human adipose MSC at reperfusion.

Like in the former study, these cells showed higher expression of VEGF than naïve MSC. Furthermore, in vivo they featured greater antioxidant and antiapoptotic properties [65].

More light on the possible cellular mechanisms of the regenerative properties of the MSC extracellular vesicles was shed by Chinese groups. In studies conducted in the rat models of renal IRI, urologists from Shanghai have shown that 100 μg microvesicles derived from the human umbilical cord mesenchyme alleviated kidney macrophage infiltration, tubular apoptosis and AKI when intravenously infused at reperfusion. This may be due to the revealed attenuation of the renal expression of fractalkine (itself a potent chemoattractant), likely mediated by a transfer of certain microRNAs to renal cells [66]. RNA transfer from MSC extracellular vesicles to tubular cells was also shown by these authors to underlie the increase of tubular VEGF synthesis and attenuation of AKI, as well as renal fibrosis, in rats that were administered the vesicles at reperfusion of the solitary kidney [67]. Other experiments showed that additional effectors of the MSC vesicles in the tubular cell nuclei of the kidneys subjected to IRI may be Nrf2/antioxidant response element with subsequent overexpression of antioxidant enzymes [68] or the Sox9 transcription factor enhancing tubular cell proliferation and diminishing kidney fibrosis [69] (one of the few studies with the use of human adipose-derived MSC and their vesicles).

On the other hand, another group from the same university have convincingly shown that a transfer of protein may also take part in the nephroprotective effects of MSC and their vesicles. It was found by these researchers that extracellular vesicles derived from human induced pluripotent stem cell-derived MSC exert a potent nephroprotective effect in the renal IRI by a transfer of protein that inhibits programmed inflammatory cell death (necroptosis) [70]. 10^{12} extracellular vesicles delivered intravenously 1 h before bilateral 30-min kidney ischemia decreased the kidney histological damage and the degree of renal failure in rats at 48 h after ischemia. Analyses in vitro showed that this phenomenon relied on a transfer of the transcription factor Specificity protein-1 to the renal proximal tubule cells with subsequent activation of nuclear expression of sphingosine kinase-1. This enzyme phosphorylates dihydrosphingosine into sphinganine-1-phosphate, a compound shown to alleviate the extent of IRI [71].

The use of MSC in the clinical setting of renal ischemia (not related to kidney transplantation) was the subject of a study conducted by researchers from Minnesota. Fourteen patients with unilateral renal artery stenosis were administered autologous adipose-derived MSC (10^5 or 2.5×10^5 cells/kg body weight) to the stenotic renal artery. After the subsequent three months blood flows increased in both the stenotic and the contralateral kidney, and glomerular filtration was higher by 21% compared to the control group [72]. Somewhat contrary to these results, MSC were ineffective in the setting of postoperative AKI that occurred within 24 h from cardiac surgery. Intraaortic infusion of allogenic bone marrow-derived MSC (2×10^6 cells / kg body weight within 48 h from the operation) in 67 patients did not improve kidney function nor 30-day mortality. In fact, patients who received the MSC suspension showed a tendency to a worse prognosis in the postoperative period [73]. As noted by the authors, such results indicate that MSC may not be as effective in the environment of an established inflammatory reaction as in its prevention, like with the pretreatment of anticipated ischemic AKI. Nevertheless, a clinical trial is planned by a team from Massachusetts in patients with AKI treated with continuous renal replacement therapy, in which patient's blood will be exposed to MSC across a semipermeable membrane of a hollow fiber extracorporeal device inserted into the hemodiafiltration circuit [74]. This would prevent any MSC-induced immunization, eliminate the risk of uncontrolled MSC replication, but expectantly provide a constant influx of the cells' beneficial products into the patient.

3.3. *Immunomodulation of Kidney Transplantation*

IRI is an inherent element of kidney transplantation and is manifested in the peritransplant period as the delayed graft function. The therapeutic potential of MSC in this setting is additionally related to a possible immunosuppressive effect, which may increase the effectiveness of pharmacological prophylaxis of the transplant rejection. The animal studies and scarce observations in humans, despite varying protocols of application, encourage the use of MSC-based therapies in kidney transplant patients, with no clear preference of any of the cell sources (autologous, donor-derived, third-party).

In rats in which allogeneic or syngeneic kidney transplantation was performed, infusion of allogeneic bone marrow MSC into the graft artery during reperfusion reduced the organ infiltration with CD8+ lymphocytes and monocytes, and alleviated failure of the rejected graft [75]. MSC were likewise effective with intravenous administrations. Syngeneic MSC infused in this way during kidney transplantation reduced the expression of inflammatory cytokines in the graft in rats [76]. In mice MSC administered intravenously 24 h before kidney transplantation increased the pool of regulatory T-cells in the spleen and prolonged survival of the transplanted kidney (which was not observed with the infusion performed at 24 h post-transplantation) [77]. In addition, Spanish researchers reported that MSCs can also be effective in the treatment of chronic graft nephropathy—intravenous infusion at 11 weeks after renal transplantation in rats resulted in reduced proteinuria, diminished inflammatory infiltration of the interstitium, and lesser interstitial fibrosis/tubular atrophy at 24 weeks after organ transplantation [78].

In one of the pioneer studies of human MSC use in renal transplantation, adipose MSC derived from the perirenal fat of the living kidney donor or the third-party MSC, inhibited similarly both pre- and post-transplant anti-donor and anti-third party alloreactivity of recipient's T lymphocytes [79]. This finding was followed by the first clinical studies of the MSC use in the living-donor kidney transplant recipients conducted in Italy. In total, two patients underwent intravenous administration of autologous bone marrow MSC at one week after transplantation (1.7×10^6 and 2.0×10^6 cells per kg body weight, respectively), while the other two were given autologous MSC 24 h prior to kidney graft implantation (2.0×10^6 cells per kg body weight intravenously). Over the five- to seven-year follow-up the mean renal function yearly decline rate was lower by ~70% than in non-MSC treated transplanted patients [80]. However, the MSC recipients showed considerable variability in the clinical course with one patient developing calcineurin inhibitor-free graft tolerance, whilst the other one experiencing acute graft rejection at two weeks after transplantation—both patients being ones that were given MSC before kidney implantation. Nevertheless, there was no elevation in the frequency of infections or neoplasms in the MSC-treated subjects. With the exception of one patient, a ~50% reduction in the blood percentage of memory CD8+ T cells was observed at 12 months post-transplantation compared with the pre-transplant levels, a phenomenon not seen in any of the controls [80].

In another pilot study, authors from China infused donor-derived bone marrow MSC into the graft renal artery during reperfusion and intravenously at one month after kidney transplantation in six recipients. This allowed the reduction of tacrolimus dosing by ~50% (with C0 ~4 vs. ~7 μg/L in controls) without episodes of rejection within 12 months of observation [81]. The immunosuppressive efficacy of MSC in the late post-transplant period was studied by Dutch researchers, who applied autologous bone marrow MSC in six kidney transplant recipients with subclinical rejection or histological progression of graft nephropathy at six months after transplantation. Two intravenous infusions of 10^6 cells/kg body weight each, in a week interval, eliminated peri-tubular cellular infiltrates at 12 months after transplantation, and patients' blood monocytes were characterized by diminished replication in vitro. It is notable, however, that CMV or BKV infection occurred in three of these patients [82].

In the largest clinical trial conducted so far 105 Chinese renal transplant recipients were administered autologous MSC at graft reperfusion and again after two weeks in place of anti-IL-2 receptor antibodies. Such induction of immunosuppression was associated with faster organ regeneration in the first month after transplantation, as well as a lower rate of cellular rejection (7.6% vs. 21.6% in the control group) and its milder course in the six-month follow-up [83].

On the other hand, studies appeared that denied effects of intravenous infusions of MSC on the kidney transplant outcome—improvement of renal allograft function and rat survival was found only when allogeneic fat MSC were injected into the graft artery, and not when they were administered intravenously at implantation [84]. Even more discouraging are the recent findings of another Chinese team of researchers, who injected allogeneic umbilical cord blood MSC to 21 recipients intravenously immediately prior to transplantation (2×10^6/kg body weight) and, additionally, to graft artery at reperfusion (5×10^6), on top of the standard immunosuppression. In the period of one-year follow-up, no statistically significant differences were found against the controls in terms of postoperative and infectious complications, renal function, frequency of rejection nor survival time of the kidney transplant [85]. Of note, one experimental study from Germany also found unfavorable effects of MSC infusion in the peritransplant period—rats given syngeneic or donor-derived bone marrow MSC intravenously four days before kidney transplantation showed symptoms of more severe cellular and humoral rejection and worse graft function on the 10th day after graft implantation [86].

3.4. Immunomodulation of Primary Glomerulonephritis

Inflammatory glomerulopathies constitute another area of potential clinical applications of the MSC. The few conducted experimental studies have shown their beneficial effect on the course of these diseases. For example, in an animal model of membranoproliferative glomerulonephritis, intravenous infusion of allogeneic fetal MSC reduced glomerular expression of proinflammatory cytokines, decreased monocyte infiltrates, mesangial hyperplasia, synthesis of connective tissue matrix and proteinuria. Interestingly, in this study the MSC culture medium inhibited mesangial expression of TNFα and monocyte chemoattractant protein 1 (MCP-1) in vitro [87]. Likewise, in the rat model of focal segmental glomerulosclerosis (doxorubicin-induced nephropathy), several intravenous infusions of bone marrow MSC increased glomerular VEGF synthesis, which was accompanied by attenuations of: Glomerular monocyte infiltration, apoptosis of the podocytes, and the extent of podocyte-parietal epithelial bridging [88].

A key role of MSC secretome in their actions was revealed in a rat model of experimental anti-glomerular basement membrane disease, in which intraperitoneal administration of human MSC medium over the 10 days since induction of disease reduced renal proinflammatory cytokine expression, increased plasma MCP-1 concentration and shifted the glomerular macrophage infiltration into the dominance of the anti-inflammatory M2 cells. This was associated with the lesser formation of crescents, reduction of proteinuria and improvement of glomerular filtration [89]. Similar favorable results were obtained in rats that received human MSC intravenously on the fourth day of the same type of rapidly progressive glomerulonephritis. Beside a smaller degree of histological and functional renal disorders, increased expression of anti-inflammatory cytokines, as well as reduced TGF β, collagen I and III mRNA concentrations in the kidney cortex were found in these rats on day 13 of the disease [90].

The use of MSC in primary glomerulonephritis in human patients has been described in two case reports from Italy. In the first one, a 13-year-old boy experienced a relapse of focal segmental glomerulosclerosis in the kidney graft on the second day after the transplantation. Intensification of immunosuppressive therapy with rituximab did not bring remission and the patient underwent weekly plasmapheresis, which only temporarily reduced the amount of proteinuria. Therefore, at month 7 after the transplantation, the patient was given two intravenous infusions of allogeneic bone marrow MSC (1×10^6 cells/kg body weight each), which was repeated after further three and seven months. In the 22-month follow-up from the first infusion, proteinuria remained stable without the need to perform plasmapheresis, the plasma concentration of Epidermal GF and TGF α decreased, and serum creatinine oscillated around 0.9 mg/dL [91]. In the second case, autologous bone marrow MSC (1.5×10^6 cells/kg body weight) were given intravenously to a 73-year-old patient with pANCA-positive rapidly progressive glomerulonephritis, whose treatment with steroid and cyclophosphamide was ineffective, and rituximab was discontinued due to severe oral candidiasis. Seven days after administration of MSC, serum creatinine decreased from 7.8 to 2.2 mg/dL, which was accompanied by normalization of urinary sediment, a significant reduction in the pANCA titer, and decrease in serum cytokine concentrations, as well as an increase in the regulatory T-cell pool in the blood. The MSC infusion was repeated after eight months, due to the recurrence of the disease with similar efficiency (serum creatinine 1.9 mg/dL), and over the next 11 months of observation, the patient's condition was good and did not require any treatment [92].

3.5. Immunomodulation of Lupus Nephritis

Systemic lupus erythematosus is a multisystem condition that involves kidneys in approximately 60% of cases. Since the standard immunosuppressive treatment is mostly insufficient in patients with severe proliferative lupus nephritis [93], the cell-based therapies are a promising alternative owing to their immunomodulatory properties. To date, many pre-clinical studies regarding the use of MSC transplantation in the context of lupus nephritis therapy have been performed giving mostly positive outcomes in terms of proteinuria and renal histopathology, as reviewed lately [94]. In one of the most recent experimental studies, Tani et al. applied systemic treatment with low-dose allogenic bone marrow MSC (10^6 cells/kg body weight intravenously) in a mouse model of spontaneously developing lupus with co-occurring glomerulonephritis. The therapeutic strategy was the early MSC administration (18–22 weeks of age) in order to investigate its potential interference with the developing disease, as well as to compare the outcomes of a single and multiple cell infusions. MSC treatment resulted in a significant delay of proteinuria appearance with the most beneficial results in mice that received multiple cell administrations. Nevertheless, histopathological nephritis scores did not differ from the controls and some harmful effects of MSC were observed, such as significantly higher B-cell deposition in kidneys of mice that received multiple MSC doses and decreased levels of regulatory T-cells after both single and multiple MSC injections [95].

The MSC-based therapies are used increasingly in Chinese patients with lupus nephritis, and often with good outcomes in terms of clinical remission [96] or blood Treg/Th17 balance [97]. However, there is still a shortage of randomized, double-blind, placebo-controlled trials. In 2017 Deng et al. presented a randomized clinical study comparing the efficacy of a standard immunosuppressive treatment (methylprednisolone and cyclophosphamide applied intravenously, followed by maintenance oral prednisolone and mycophenolate mofetil) with ($n = 12$) or without ($n = 6$) a co-administration of human umbilical cord MSC (two intravenous injections of 2×10^8 cells in total) [98]. The primary endpoint was remission of nephritis (combined partial and complete remission) defined with specified values of serum creatinine, urinary red blood cells and proteinuria in the 12-month follow-up. Remission was noted in 75% of patients in the MSC-treated group and in 83% of patients in the placebo group. The reduction of proteinuria was comparable and no significant difference in serum creatinine levels between the two groups was noted. When it comes to secondary endpoints (clinical symptom scores, complement concentration, anti-dsDNA antibody and ANA titers, death and commencement of permanent dialysis or renal transplantation), no significant differences were observed, either, and the trial was terminated ahead of schedule. The newest report regarding the application of MSC in the lupus nephritis came from Spain and suggests the efficacy of the cells in the most severe cases. Three patients who demonstrated class IV active proliferative lupus nephritis, were treated with allogenic bone marrow MCS (9×10^7 of cells infused intravenously) at the exacerbation of the disease [99]. One week after MSC infusion a considerable decrease of proteinuria was observed in all patients and maintained throughout the course of a nine-month follow-up. The complete clinical symptom remission in two patients and partial remission to the mild activity of the disease in the third patient were noted and call for a randomized and controlled trial in such patients.

Of note, so far no animal or clinical studies have been reported with the application of MSC extracellular vesicles in the lupus nephropathy, although the rationale for such investigations have been formulated [100,101].

3.6. Therapeutic Potential in Diabetic Kidney Disease

Glomerular microinflammation takes part in the pathogenesis of diabetic nephropathy, albeit is not the target of standard immunosuppressive treatment, due to its small intensity and possible metabolic complications of such therapies. Not surprisingly, the interest of researchers has recently focused on MSC and the studies of their use in diabetic nephropathy are consequently, and somewhat paradoxically, more advanced than in gross inflammatory glomerulopathies.

On one hand, MSC can indirectly prevent kidney damage or inhibit its progression by improving glycemic control of diabetes, as shown in experimental and clinical studies. In the mouse model of established streptozotocin-induced type 1 diabetes, intravenous administrations of human bone marrow MSC or their medium induced regeneration of pancreatic islets and subsequently reduced blood glucose levels by 30–35% [102,103]. MSC may also hinder type 2 diabetes: Myoblasts pre-exposed to the MSC medium featured lower expression of proinflammatory cytokines, increased synthesis and expression of the GLUT4 glucose transporter, and consequently less compromised insulin sensitivity upon 24-h exposure to a palmitate solution. MSC medium was as effective in this regard as a metformin solution [104]. The influence of MSC on the course of type 2 diabetes in humans has been evaluated so far in several studies conducted in small groups of patients, and with considerable methodological differences—in terms of the origin of administered cells, dose and route of administration (intravenous, pancreatic artery), or the use of controls. In the majority of these works, increases in the blood C-peptide concentrations and reductions of hemoglobin A1c levels were observed for several months after the MSC infusions, with no effects on the peripheral insulin resistance [105,106].

The nephroprotective properties of MSC in diabetic nephropathy have been revealed in experimental models of type 1 diabetes. Intravenous infusion of allogeneic bone marrow MSC in the late phase of streptozotocin-induced diabetes resulted in the reduction of albuminuria and the degree of glomerular filtration impairment in rodents. In the renal tissue of these animals, reduced oxidative stress, as well as diminished expressions of proinflammatory cytokines, apoptotic proteins and TGF β were observed, whereas expressions of nephrin, podocin, bone morphogenetic protein 7 and VEGF were augmented [107,108].

The immunomodulatory effects of MSC-secreted factors, rather than the cells themselves, have been implicated by a study in mice with streptozotocin-induced or high-fat diet-induced diabetes. In both models, intravenous infusions of both rat bone marrow MSC or their medium reduced alike renal proinflammatory cytokine expression and macrophage infiltration. This was accompanied by attenuated albuminuria and diminished interstitial fibrosis [109]. The key role of the MSC-secreted extracellular vesicles could be deduced from only scarce renal localization of the administered MSC and the fact of obtaining comparable beneficial histological effects in the kidney after subcapsular administration of exosomes previously isolated from MSC [109]. The nephroprotective effects of factors secreted by the MSC were also indicated by the results of a study in rats with streptozotocin-induced diabetes that were injected intravenously with exosomes derived from the aforementioned pluripotent MSC-like cells isolated from human urine. In these animals, no mesangial expansion, reduced renal expression of apoptotic proteins, as well as diminished albuminuria were found in comparison to the control group [110]. Recently, Ebrahim et al. succeeded in clarifying the mechanisms of the beneficial effects of bone marrow MSC exosomes in type 1 diabetic nephropathy in rats, showing their capability of improving tubular cell autophagy, as seen with the electron microscopy and reflected in the reduced renal expression of the mechanistic target of rapamycin. This was accompanied by significantly reduced expression of fibronectin and TGF β with diminished fibrosis and improved function of the kidneys [111].

In the years 2015–2016, the first reports emerged on the use of allogeneic multipotent mesenchymal precursor cells in patients with type 2 diabetes. The cellular suspension was obtained from the bone marrow by a selection of cells with membrane expression of alkaline phosphatase STRO-3 (rexlemestrocel-L, currently in the second phases of clinical verification in groups of patients with various medical conditions). In the first of these works, these cells were given in the amount of $0.3–2 \times 10^6$/kg body weight to 45 patients with inadequately controlled type 2 diabetes. In the second one the same preparation was given to patients with diabetic renal insufficiency (eGFR 20–50 mL/min/1.73 m^2) at a dose of 150×10^6 or 300×10^6 cells (both groups numbering 10 patients). During the 12 weeks following infusions, no significant side effects or immunization of patients with donor antigens were noted. In this relatively short period of observation, there was however no significant effect of the tested preparation on the clinical parameters related to diabetes and renal failure [112,113].

4. Conclusions

The presented review of published works on the use of mesenchymal stem cells in kidney diseases shows the greatest advancement of experimental research in the fields of AKI, kidney transplantation, and diabetic or lupus nephropathies (Table 2). The majority of results indicate the reparative, immunosuppressive and antifibrotic effects of factors released from MSC in the environment of low-grade inflammation (as in the case of diabetic glomerulopathy) or in prevention/alleviation of a developing inflammatory injury (as with pretreatment of the anticipated ischemic AKI, early treatment of ischemic or toxic tubular injury or administration preceding/concurrent with kidney graft implantation). The efficacy of MSC secretome in the milieu of an established renal inflammation or injury (as with post-IRI administration) seems less uniform.

Table 2. Intensity and outcomes of the studies of MSC or MSC secretome in the major renal settings.

Kidney Disease Setting		Animal Studies		Human Studies	
		MSC	MSC Medium or EVs	MSC	MSC Medium or EVs
Acute kidney injury	ischemic	↑↑↑	↑↑↑	↑↓	○
	non-ischemic	↑↑	↑↑	○	○
Kidney transplantation	pre-/intra-implantation	↑↑	○	↑↑	○
	post-implantation	↓	○	↑	○
Chronic allograft nephropathy		↑	○	↑	○
Glomerulo-nephritis	primary	↑↑	↑	↑	○
	lupus	↑↑↑	○	↑↓	○
Diabetic kidney disease		↑↑	↑↑	○	○

MSC—mesenchymal stem cells; EVs—extracellular vesicles; ○ no conducted studies; ↑ single conducted study or a few case reports, positive outcomes; ↑↑ several conducted studies, mostly positive outcomes; ↑↑↑ numerous conducted studies, mostly positive outcomes; ↑↓ several conducted studies, conflicting outcomes; ↓ single conducted study, negative outcomes.

The most promising MSC product in the context of renal regeneration/immunosuppression appears to be microRNAs contained within extracellular vesicles (Figure 1). Membranous protection enables their homing to the injured tissue and subsequent epigenetic modulation of the local expression of reparative cytokines and transcription/growth factors. Studies show that also MSC-secreted proteins or mitochondria take part in tissue regeneration. However, the role of freely released transcription/growth factors or cell-to-cell mitochondrial transfer may be limited to MSC infused to the aorta or renal artery, for the assured proximity to the injured cells. On the other hand, the intravenously administered MSC, which largely get trapped and apoptotic in the lungs, may dispatch both proteins and mitochondria within extracellular vesicles that shall be able to reach the injured or inflamed kidneys. Of importance for the future clinical applications, the secretory reparative potential of MSC can be enhanced in culture, as with hypoxic preconditioning.

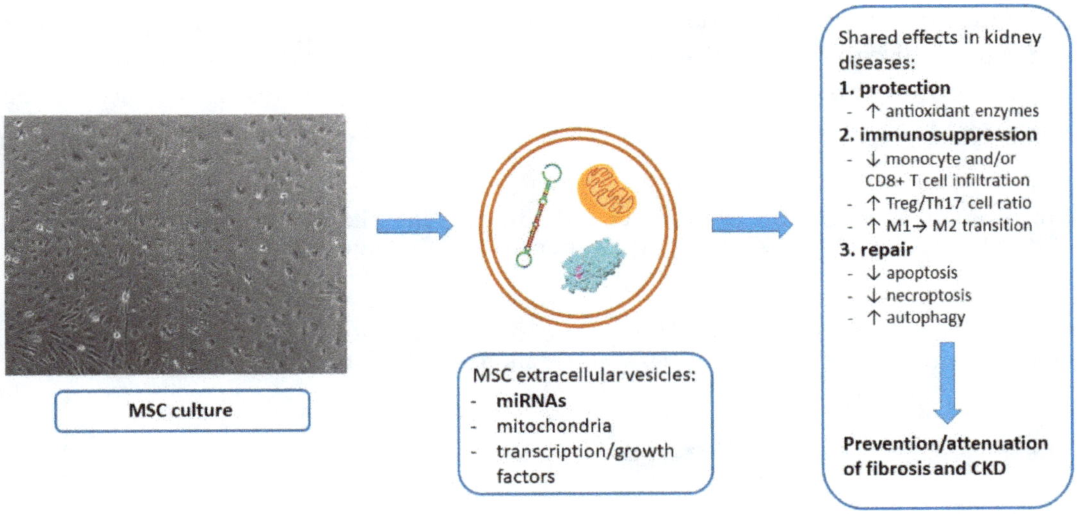

Figure 1. Shared major mechanisms of nephroprotection with exogenous MSC/MSC-derived products in renal diseases.

It is striking that the number of clinical trials with the use of MSC in kidney diseases so far has remained disproportionately low considering their therapeutic potential emerging from experimental studies (placebo-controlled trials are particularly in demand). For example, in the last three years there has been only one reported use of MSC in renal transplant recipients [85]. This may be related to the fact that the outcomes of the pioneer uses of MSC in patients have not been uniformly favorable. Also, and likely more importantly, shortage of trials can be attributed to reservations that both scientists and bioethical boards may have towards applications of allogenic cells with high mitotic potential, as such associated with the risk of immunization or cancer.

Thus far, there have been findings of MSC enhancing divisions in cancer cell lines [114] and augmenting the metastatic potential of co-administered cancerous cells in animals [115]. Nevertheless, there has been no report of de novo carcinogenesis in vivo following MSC infusion, neither in animals nor in humans. One reported case of angiomyeloproliferative renal lesions was related to percutaneous renal injections of not MSC, but peripheral blood-derived autologous hematopoietic cells [116]. Moreover, it has been shown that MSC can actually inhibit the progression of cancerous tumors. In hamsters with induced premalignant stages of squamous cell carcinoma of the mouth cavity, they decreased the progression of lesions (except for the largest doses) [117]. Less optimistic are the latest discoveries in the field of MSC immunogenicity. Contrary to the assumptions of its negligibility due to lack of expression of HLA class II antigens, equine bone marrow stromal cells treated with a proinflammatory cytokine (Interferon γ) expressed MHC class II antigens on their cellular membrane and stimulated the proliferation of T lymphocytes in vitro [118]. It is not certain whether this process also takes place in vivo—current applications in humans do not indicate significant immunogenicity of allogeneic MSC, although it is necessary to bear in mind the relatively short periods of observation in the conducted studies [119].

All these objections direct the researchers' interest into microvesicles or exosomes secreted by MSC. In particular, microRNAs contained within are considered equally efficient, but potentially not tumorigenic and less immunogenic therapeutic objects. Although increasingly used in animal models, their applicability in clinical trials is dulled by the lack of sufficient knowledge of the consequences of administering exogenous molecules with such high stability as microRNAs [120]. On the other hand, it has to be noted that this very characteristic may constitute the observed effectiveness of systemically administered MSC-derived vesicles in kidney disease models.

Regardless of all question marks, the secretory products of mesenchymal stem cells deserve further research in experimental and subsequently clinical studies, providing a chance for the most awaited breakthrough in the treatment of the inflammatory and, especially, ever more frequent autoimmune diseases with renal involvement. Finally, commenting on the concerns of possible side effects of MSC-based therapies, it can be questioned whether the widely used classical immunosuppressive drugs—source of common infectious, metabolic and cancerous complications—would ever be approved for the clinical use at the present-day level of safety expectations.

Author Contributions: Concept, writing—review and editing, G.W.; literature search, writing—original draft preparation, B.B., M.K., G.S., A.W., R.K., and G.W.; supervision, W.G. and G.W.

Acknowledgments: We acknowledge Wojciech Wystrychowski for providing an image of human adipose MSC culture in a subconfluent state, as well as Krzysztof Gajdzik for his assistance in editing the paper.

Abbreviations

ANA	Anti-Nuclear Antibody
AKI	Acute Kidney Injury
CKD	Chronic Kidney Disease
dsDNA	double stranded Deoxyribonucleic Acid
eGFR	estimated Glomerular Filtration Rate
HLA	Human Leukocyte Antigen
IRI	Ischemia-Reperfusion Injury
MCP	Monocyte Chemoattractant Protein
MHC	Major Histocompatibility Complex
MSC	Mesenchymal (mesodermal) stem cells
pANCA	perinuclear Anti-Neutrophil Cytoplasmic Antibody
RNA	Ribonucleic Acid
TGF	Transforming Growth Factor
VEGF	Vascular Endothelial Growth Factor

References

1. Bonaventura, G.; Chamayou, S.; Liprino, A.; Guglielmino, A.; Fichera, M.; Caruso, M.; Barcellona, M.L. Different Tissue-Derived Stem Cells: A Comparison of Neural Differentiation Capability. *PLoS ONE* **2015**, *10*, e0140790. [CrossRef] [PubMed]
2. Mitalipov, S.; Wolf, D. Totipotency, pluripotency and nuclear reprogramming. *Adv. Biochem. Eng. Biotechnol.* **2009**, *114*, 185–199.
3. Yu, J.; Vodyanik, M.A.; Smuga-Otto, K.; Antosiewicz-Bourget, J.; Frane, J.L.; Tian, S.; Nie, J.; Jonsdottir, G.A.; Ruotti, V.; Stewart, R.; et al. Induced pluripotent stem cell lines derived from human somatic cells. *Science* **2007**, *318*, 1917–1920. [CrossRef]
4. Biehl, J.K.; Russell, B. Introduction to stem cell therapy. *J. Cardiovasc Nurs* **2009**, *24*, 98–103; quiz 104–105. [CrossRef] [PubMed]
5. Kim, N.; Cho, S.-G. Clinical applications of mesenchymal stem cells. *Korean J. Intern. Med.* **2013**, *28*, 387–402. [CrossRef]
6. Kariminekoo, S.; Movassaghpour, A.; Rahimzadeh, A.; Talebi, M.; Shamsasenjan, K.; Akbarzadeh, A. Implications of mesenchymal stem cells in regenerative medicine. *Artif. Cells Nanomed. Biotechnol.* **2016**, *44*, 749–757. [CrossRef]
7. Jeon, B.-G.; Jang, S.-J.; Park, J.-S.; Subbarao, R.B.; Jeong, G.-J.; Park, B.-W.; Rho, G.-J. Differentiation potential of mesenchymal stem cells isolated from human dental tissues into non-mesodermal lineage. *Animal Cells and Systems* **2015**, *19*, 321–331. [CrossRef]
8. Seo, M.J.; Suh, S.Y.; Bae, Y.C.; Jung, J.S. Differentiation of human adipose stromal cells into hepatic lineage in vitro and in vivo. *Biochem. Biophys. Res. Commun.* **2005**, *328*, 258–264. [CrossRef]
9. Murphy, M.B.; Moncivais, K.; Caplan, A.I. Mesenchymal stem cells: environmentally responsive therapeutics for regenerative medicine. *Exp. Mol. Med.* **2013**, *45*, e54. [CrossRef]

10. Belting, M.; Wittrup, A. Nanotubes, exosomes, and nucleic acid-binding peptides provide novel mechanisms of intercellular communication in eukaryotic cells: implications in health and disease. *J. Cell Biol.* **2008**, *183*, 1187–1191. [CrossRef]
11. Qiu, G.; Zheng, G.; Ge, M.; Wang, J.; Huang, R.; Shu, Q.; Xu, J. Mesenchymal stem cell-derived extracellular vesicles affect disease outcomes via transfer of microRNAs. *Stem Cell Res. Ther.* **2018**, *9*, 320. [CrossRef] [PubMed]
12. Lotfi, R.; Eisenbacher, J.; Solgi, G.; Fuchs, K.; Yildiz, T.; Nienhaus, C.; Rojewski, M.T.; Schrezenmeier, H. Human mesenchymal stem cells respond to native but not oxidized damage associated molecular pattern molecules from necrotic (tumor) material. *Eur. J. Immunol.* **2011**, *41*, 2021–2028. [CrossRef]
13. Mahrouf-Yorgov, M.; Augeul, L.; Da Silva, C.C.; Jourdan, M.; Rigolet, M.; Manin, S.; Ferrera, R.; Ovize, M.; Henry, A.; Guguin, A.; et al. Mesenchymal stem cells sense mitochondria released from damaged cells as danger signals to activate their rescue properties. *Cell Death Differ.* **2017**, *24*, 1224–1238. [CrossRef]
14. Spees, J.L.; Olson, S.D.; Whitney, M.J.; Prockop, D.J. Mitochondrial transfer between cells can rescue aerobic respiration. *Proc. Natl. Acad. Sci. USA* **2006**, *103*, 1283–1288. [CrossRef] [PubMed]
15. Wang, X.; Gerdes, H.-H. Transfer of mitochondria via tunneling nanotubes rescues apoptotic PC12 cells. *Cell Death Differ.* **2015**, *22*, 1181–1191. [CrossRef] [PubMed]
16. Jiang, D.; Gao, F.; Zhang, Y.; Wong, D.S.H.; Li, Q.; Tse, H.-F.; Xu, G.; Yu, Z.; Lian, Q. Mitochondrial transfer of mesenchymal stem cells effectively protects corneal epithelial cells from mitochondrial damage. *Cell Death Dis.* **2016**, *7*, e2467. [CrossRef] [PubMed]
17. Islam, M.N.; Das, S.R.; Emin, M.T.; Wei, M.; Sun, L.; Westphalen, K.; Rowlands, D.J.; Quadri, S.K.; Bhattacharya, S.; Bhattacharya, J. Mitochondrial transfer from bone-marrow-derived stromal cells to pulmonary alveoli protects against acute lung injury. *Nat. Med.* **2012**, *18*, 759–765. [CrossRef] [PubMed]
18. Liu, K.; Ji, K.; Guo, L.; Wu, W.; Lu, H.; Shan, P.; Yan, C. Mesenchymal stem cells rescue injured endothelial cells in an in vitro ischemia-reperfusion model via tunneling nanotube like structure-mediated mitochondrial transfer. *Microvasc. Res.* **2014**, *92*, 10–18. [CrossRef] [PubMed]
19. Phinney, D.G.; Di Giuseppe, M.; Njah, J.; Sala, E.; Shiva, S.; St Croix, C.M.; Stolz, D.B.; Watkins, S.C.; Di, Y.P.; Leikauf, G.D.; et al. Mesenchymal stem cells use extracellular vesicles to outsource mitophagy and shuttle microRNAs. *Nat. Commun.* **2015**, *6*, 8472. [CrossRef]
20. Torralba, D.; Baixauli, F.; Sánchez-Madrid, F. Mitochondria Know No Boundaries: Mechanisms and Functions of Intercellular Mitochondrial Transfer. *Front. Cell Dev. Biol.* **2016**, *4*, 107. [CrossRef]
21. Kim, Y.-J.; Jeong, J.-H. Clinical application of adipose stem cells in plastic surgery. *J. Korean Med. Sci.* **2014**, *29*, 462–467. [CrossRef]
22. Wei, X.; Yang, X.; Han, Z.; Qu, F.; Shao, L.; Shi, Y. Mesenchymal stem cells: A new trend for cell therapy. *Acta Pharmacol. Sin.* **2013**, *34*, 747–754. [CrossRef]
23. Le Blanc, K. Immunomodulatory effects of fetal and adult mesenchymal stem cells. *Cytotherapy* **2003**, *5*, 485–489. [CrossRef] [PubMed]
24. Luz-Crawford, P.; Kurte, M.; Bravo-Alegría, J.; Contreras, R.; Nova-Lamperti, E.; Tejedor, G.; Noël, D.; Jorgensen, C.; Figueroa, F.; Djouad, F.; et al. Mesenchymal stem cells generate a CD4+CD25+Foxp3+ regulatory T cell population during the differentiation process of Th1 and Th17 cells. *Stem Cell Res. Ther.* **2013**, *4*, 65. [CrossRef]
25. Maumus, M.; Guérit, D.; Toupet, K.; Jorgensen, C.; Noël, D. Mesenchymal stem cell-based therapies in regenerative medicine: applications in rheumatology. *Stem Cell Res. Ther.* **2011**, *2*, 14. [CrossRef]
26. Duran, N.E.; Hommes, D.W. Stem cell-based therapies in inflammatory bowel disease: Promises and pitfalls. *Therap Adv. Gastroenterol.* **2016**, *9*, 533–547. [CrossRef]
27. Zhang, B.; Yin, Y.; Lai, R.C.; Tan, S.S.; Choo, A.B.H.; Lim, S.K. Mesenchymal stem cells secrete immunologically active exosomes. *Stem Cells Dev.* **2014**, *23*, 1233–1244. [CrossRef] [PubMed]
28. Monguió-Tortajada, M.; Roura, S.; Gálvez-Montón, C.; Pujal, J.M.; Aran, G.; Sanjurjo, L.; la Franquesa, M.; Sarrias, M.-R.; Bayes-Genis, A.; Borràs, F.E. Nanosized UCMSC-derived extracellular vesicles but not conditioned medium exclusively inhibit the inflammatory response of stimulated T cells: implications for nanomedicine. *Theranostics* **2017**, *7*, 270–284. [CrossRef] [PubMed]
29. Galleu, A.; Riffo-Vasquez, Y.; Trento, C.; Lomas, C.; Dolcetti, L.; Cheung, T.S.; von Bonin, M.; Barbieri, L.; Halai, K.; Ward, S.; et al. Apoptosis in mesenchymal stromal cells induces in vivo recipient-mediated immunomodulation. *Sci. Transl. Med.* **2017**, *9*. [CrossRef]

30. Bartosh, T.J.; Ylöstalo, J.H.; Bazhanov, N.; Kuhlman, J.; Prockop, D.J. Dynamic compaction of human mesenchymal stem/precursor cells into spheres self-activates caspase-dependent IL1 signaling to enhance secretion of modulators of inflammation and immunity (PGE2, TSG6, and STC1). *Stem Cells* **2013**, *31*, 2443–2456. [CrossRef] [PubMed]
31. De Chiara, L.; Famulari, E.S.; Fagoonee, S.; van Daalen, S.K.M.; Buttiglieri, S.; Revelli, A.; Tolosano, E.; Silengo, L.; van Pelt, A.M.M.; Altruda, F. Characterization of Human Mesenchymal Stem Cells Isolated from the Testis. *Stem Cells Int.* **2018**, *2018*, 4910304. [CrossRef] [PubMed]
32. Strioga, M.; Viswanathan, S.; Darinskas, A.; Slaby, O.; Michalek, J. Same or not the same? Comparison of adipose tissue-derived versus bone marrow-derived mesenchymal stem and stromal cells. *Stem Cells Dev.* **2012**, *21*, 2724–2752. [CrossRef]
33. Melief, S.M.; Zwaginga, J.J.; Fibbe, W.E.; Roelofs, H. Adipose tissue-derived multipotent stromal cells have a higher immunomodulatory capacity than their bone marrow-derived counterparts. *Stem Cells Transl. Med.* **2013**, *2*, 455–463. [CrossRef]
34. Lian, Q.; Zhang, Y.; Zhang, J.; Zhang, H.K.; Wu, X.; Zhang, Y.; Lam, F.F.-Y.; Kang, S.; Xia, J.C.; Lai, W.-H.; et al. Functional mesenchymal stem cells derived from human induced pluripotent stem cells attenuate limb ischemia in mice. *Circulation* **2010**, *121*, 1113–1123. [CrossRef]
35. Zhang, Y.; McNeill, E.; Tian, H.; Soker, S.; Andersson, K.-E.; Yoo, J.J.; Atala, A. Urine derived cells are a potential source for urological tissue reconstruction. *J. Urol.* **2008**, *180*, 2226–2233. [CrossRef]
36. Bharadwaj, S.; Liu, G.; Shi, Y.; Wu, R.; Yang, B.; He, T.; Fan, Y.; Lu, X.; Zhou, X.; Liu, H.; et al. Multipotential differentiation of human urine-derived stem cells: potential for therapeutic applications in urology. *Stem Cells* **2013**, *31*, 1840–1856. [CrossRef]
37. Zhang, D.; Wei, G.; Li, P.; Zhou, X.; Zhang, Y. Urine-derived stem cells: A novel and versatile progenitor source for cell-based therapy and regenerative medicine. *Genes Dis.* **2014**, *1*, 8–17. [CrossRef] [PubMed]
38. Bruno, S.; Bussolati, B.; Grange, C.; Collino, F.; di Cantogno, L.V.; Herrera, M.B.; Biancone, L.; Tetta, C.; Segoloni, G.; Camussi, G. Isolation and characterization of resident mesenchymal stem cells in human glomeruli. *Stem Cells Dev.* **2009**, *18*, 867–880. [CrossRef]
39. Ranghino, A.; Bruno, S.; Bussolati, B.; Moggio, A.; Dimuccio, V.; Tapparo, M.; Biancone, L.; Gontero, P.; Frea, B.; Camussi, G. The effects of glomerular and tubular renal progenitors and derived extracellular vesicles on recovery from acute kidney injury. *Stem Cell Res. Ther.* **2017**, *8*, 24. [CrossRef]
40. Leuning, D.G.; Reinders, M.E.J.; Li, J.; Peired, A.J.; Lievers, E.; de Boer, H.C.; Fibbe, W.E.; Romagnani, P.; van Kooten, C.; Little, M.H.; et al. Clinical-Grade Isolated Human Kidney Perivascular Stromal Cells as an Organotypic Cell Source for Kidney Regenerative Medicine. *Stem Cells Transl. Med.* **2017**, *6*, 405–418. [CrossRef] [PubMed]
41. Grobstein, C. Inductive epitheliomesenchymal interaction in cultured organ rudiments of the mouse. *Science* **1953**, *118*, 52–55. [CrossRef]
42. Barasch, J.; Yang, J.; Ware, C.B.; Taga, T.; Yoshida, K.; Erdjument-Bromage, H.; Tempst, P.; Parravicini, E.; Malach, S.; Aranoff, T.; et al. Mesenchymal to epithelial conversion in rat metanephros is induced by LIF. *Cell* **1999**, *99*, 377–386. [CrossRef]
43. Sakurai, H.; Bush, K.T.; Nigam, S.K. Identification of pleiotrophin as a mesenchymal factor involved in ureteric bud branching morphogenesis. *Development* **2001**, *128*, 3283–3293.
44. Takasato, M.; Er, P.X.; Chiu, H.S.; Little, M.H. Generation of kidney organoids from human pluripotent stem cells. *Nat. Protoc.* **2016**, *11*, 1681–1692. [CrossRef]
45. Morizane, R.; Lam, A.Q.; Freedman, B.S.; Kishi, S.; Valerius, M.T.; Bonventre, J.V. Nephron organoids derived from human pluripotent stem cells model kidney development and injury. *Nat. Biotechnol.* **2015**, *33*, 1193–1200. [CrossRef] [PubMed]
46. van den Berg, C.W.; Ritsma, L.; Avramut, M.C.; Wiersma, L.E.; van den Berg, B.M.; Leuning, D.G.; Lievers, E.; Koning, M.; Vanslambrouck, J.M.; Koster, A.J.; et al. Renal Subcapsular Transplantation of PSC-Derived Kidney Organoids Induces Neo-vasculogenesis and Significant Glomerular and Tubular Maturation In Vivo. *Stem Cell Reports* **2018**, *10*, 751–765. [CrossRef]
47. Caralt, M.; Uzarski, J.S.; Iacob, S.; Obergfell, K.P.; Berg, N.; Bijonowski, B.M.; Kiefer, K.M.; Ward, H.H.; Wandinger-Ness, A.; Miller, W.M.; et al. Optimization and critical evaluation of decellularization strategies to develop renal extracellular matrix scaffolds as biological templates for organ engineering and transplantation. *Am. J. Transplant.* **2015**, *15*, 64–75. [CrossRef]

48. Song, J.J.; Guyette, J.P.; Gilpin, S.E.; Gonzalez, G.; Vacanti, J.P.; Ott, H.C. Regeneration and experimental orthotopic transplantation of a bioengineered kidney. *Nat. Med.* **2013**, *19*, 646–651. [CrossRef] [PubMed]
49. Guan, Y.; Liu, S.; Sun, C.; Cheng, G.; Kong, F.; Luan, Y.; Xie, X.; Zhao, S.; Zhang, D.; Wang, J.; et al. The effective bioengineering method of implantation decellularized renal extracellular matrix scaffolds. *Oncotarget* **2015**, *6*, 36126–36138. [CrossRef]
50. Remuzzi, A.; Figliuzzi, M.; Bonandrini, B.; Silvani, S.; Azzollini, N.; Nossa, R.; Benigni, A.; Remuzzi, G. Experimental Evaluation of Kidney Regeneration by Organ Scaffold Recellularization. *Sci Rep.* **2017**, *7*, 43502. [CrossRef] [PubMed]
51. Makhlough, A.; Shekarchian, S.; Moghadasali, R.; Einollahi, B.; Hosseini, S.E.; Jaroughi, N.; Bolurieh, T.; Baharvand, H.; Aghdami, N. Safety and tolerability of autologous bone marrow mesenchymal stromal cells in ADPKD patients. *Stem Cell Res. Ther.* **2017**, *8*, 116. [CrossRef]
52. Sheashaa, H.; Lotfy, A.; Elhusseini, F.; Aziz, A.A.; Baiomy, A.; Awad, S.; Alsayed, A.; El-Gilany, A.-H.; Saad, M.-A.A.A.; Mahmoud, K.; et al. Protective effect of adipose-derived mesenchymal stem cells against acute kidney injury induced by ischemia-reperfusion in Sprague-Dawley rats. *Exp. Ther. Med.* **2016**, *11*, 1573–1580. [CrossRef]
53. Chen, Y.-T.; Sun, C.-K.; Lin, Y.-C.; Chang, L.-T.; Chen, Y.-L.; Tsai, T.-H.; Chung, S.-Y.; Chua, S.; Kao, Y.-H.; Yen, C.-H.; et al. Adipose-derived mesenchymal stem cell protects kidneys against ischemia-reperfusion injury through suppressing oxidative stress and inflammatory reaction. *J. Transl. Med.* **2011**, *9*, 51. [CrossRef] [PubMed]
54. Hu, J.; Zhang, L.; Wang, N.; Ding, R.; Cui, S.; Zhu, F.; Xie, Y.; Sun, X.; Wu, D.; Hong, Q.; et al. Mesenchymal stem cells attenuate ischemic acute kidney injury by inducing regulatory T cells through splenocyte interactions. *Kidney Int.* **2013**, *84*, 521–531. [CrossRef] [PubMed]
55. Cao, H.; Qian, H.; Xu, W.; Zhu, W.; Zhang, X.; Chen, Y.; Wang, M.; Yan, Y.; Xie, Y. Mesenchymal stem cells derived from human umbilical cord ameliorate ischemia/reperfusion-induced acute renal failure in rats. *Biotechnol. Lett.* **2010**, *32*, 725–732. [CrossRef]
56. Donizetti-Oliveira, C.; Semedo, P.; Burgos-Silva, M.; Cenedeze, M.A.; Malheiros, D.M.A.C.; Reis, M.A.; Pacheco-Silva, A.; Câmara, N.O.S. Adipose tissue-derived stem cell treatment prevents renal disease progression. *Cell Transplant.* **2012**, *21*, 1727–1741. [CrossRef]
57. Wu, H.J.; Yiu, W.H.; Wong, D.W.L.; Li, R.X.; Chan, L.Y.Y.; Leung, J.C.K.; Zhang, Y.; Lian, Q.; Lai, K.N.; Tse, H.F.; et al. Human induced pluripotent stem cell-derived mesenchymal stem cells prevent adriamycin nephropathy in mice. *Oncotarget* **2017**, *8*, 103640–103656. [CrossRef]
58. Tögel, F.; Hu, Z.; Weiss, K.; Isaac, J.; Lange, C.; Westenfelder, C. Administered mesenchymal stem cells protect against ischemic acute renal failure through differentiation-independent mechanisms. *Am. J. Physiol. Renal Physiol.* **2005**, *289*, F31–F42. [CrossRef] [PubMed]
59. Gatti, S.; Bruno, S.; Deregibus, M.C.; Sordi, A.; Cantaluppi, V.; Tetta, C.; Camussi, G. Microvesicles derived from human adult mesenchymal stem cells protect against ischaemia-reperfusion-induced acute and chronic kidney injury. *Nephrol. Dial. Transplant.* **2011**, *26*, 1474–1483. [CrossRef]
60. Collino, F.; Bruno, S.; Incarnato, D.; Dettori, D.; Neri, F.; Provero, P.; Pomatto, M.; Oliviero, S.; Tetta, C.; Quesenberry, P.J.; et al. AKI Recovery Induced by Mesenchymal Stromal Cell-Derived Extracellular Vesicles Carrying MicroRNAs. *J. Am. Soc. Nephrol.* **2015**, *26*, 2349–2360. [CrossRef]
61. Collino, F.; Pomatto, M.; Bruno, S.; Lindoso, R.S.; Tapparo, M.; Sicheng, W.; Quesenberry, P.; Camussi, G. Exosome and Microvesicle-Enriched Fractions Isolated from Mesenchymal Stem Cells by Gradient Separation Showed Different Molecular Signatures and Functions on Renal Tubular Epithelial Cells. *Stem Cell Rev.* **2017**, *13*, 226–243. [CrossRef]
62. Bruno, S.; Grange, C.; Deregibus, M.C.; Calogero, R.A.; Saviozzi, S.; Collino, F.; Morando, L.; Busca, A.; Falda, M.; Bussolati, B.; et al. Mesenchymal stem cell-derived microvesicles protect against acute tubular injury. *J. Am. Soc. Nephrol.* **2009**, *20*, 1053–1067. [CrossRef] [PubMed]
63. Bruno, S.; Grange, C.; Collino, F.; Deregibus, M.C.; Cantaluppi, V.; Biancone, L.; Tetta, C.; Camussi, G. Microvesicles derived from mesenchymal stem cells enhance survival in a lethal model of acute kidney injury. *PLoS ONE* **2012**, *7*, e33115. [CrossRef]
64. Overath, J.M.; Gauer, S.; Obermüller, N.; Schubert, R.; Schäfer, R.; Geiger, H.; Baer, P.C. Short-term preconditioning enhances the therapeutic potential of adipose-derived stromal/stem cell-conditioned medium in cisplatin-induced acute kidney injury. *Exp. Cell Res.* **2016**, *342*, 175–183. [CrossRef]

65. Zhang, W.; Liu, L.; Huo, Y.; Yang, Y.; Wang, Y. Hypoxia-pretreated human MSCs attenuate acute kidney injury through enhanced angiogenic and antioxidative capacities. *BioMed Res. Int.* **2014**, *2014*, 462472. [CrossRef]
66. Zou, X.; Zhang, G.; Cheng, Z.; Yin, D.; Du, T.; Ju, G.; Miao, S.; Liu, G.; Lu, M.; Zhu, Y. Microvesicles derived from human Wharton's Jelly mesenchymal stromal cells ameliorate renal ischemia-reperfusion injury in rats by suppressing CX3CL1. *Stem Cell Res. Ther.* **2014**, *5*, 40. [CrossRef] [PubMed]
67. Zou, X.; Gu, D.; Xing, X.; Cheng, Z.; Gong, D.; Zhang, G.; Zhu, Y. Human mesenchymal stromal cell-derived extracellular vesicles alleviate renal ischemic reperfusion injury and enhance angiogenesis in rats. *Am. J. Transl. Res.* **2016**, *8*, 4289–4299.
68. Zhang, G.; Zou, X.; Huang, Y.; Wang, F.; Miao, S.; Liu, G.; Chen, M.; Zhu, Y. Mesenchymal Stromal Cell-Derived Extracellular Vesicles Protect Against Acute Kidney Injury Through Anti-Oxidation by Enhancing Nrf2/ARE Activation in Rats. *Kidney Blood Press. Res.* **2016**, *41*, 119–128. [CrossRef] [PubMed]
69. Zhu, F.; Chong Lee Shin, O.L.S.; Pei, G.; Hu, Z.; Yang, J.; Zhu, H.; Wang, M.; Mou, J.; Sun, J.; Wang, Y.; et al. Adipose-derived mesenchymal stem cells employed exosomes to attenuate AKI-CKD transition through tubular epithelial cell dependent Sox9 activation. *Oncotarget* **2017**, *8*, 70707–70726. [CrossRef]
70. Yuan, X.; Li, D.; Chen, X.; Han, C.; Xu, L.; Huang, T.; Dong, Z.; Zhang, M. Extracellular vesicles from human-induced pluripotent stem cell-derived mesenchymal stromal cells (hiPSC-MSCs) protect against renal ischemia/reperfusion injury via delivering specificity protein (SP1) and transcriptional activating of sphingosine kinase 1 and inhibiting necroptosis. *Cell Death Dis.* **2017**, *8*, 3200.
71. Awad, A.S.; Ye, H.; Huang, L.; Li, L.; Foss, F.W.; Macdonald, T.L.; Lynch, K.R.; Okusa, M.D. Selective sphingosine 1-phosphate 1 receptor activation reduces ischemia-reperfusion injury in mouse kidney. *Am. J. Physiol. Renal Physiol.* **2006**, *290*, F1516–F1524. [CrossRef]
72. Saad, A.; Dietz, A.B.; Herrmann, S.M.S.; Hickson, L.J.; Glockner, J.F.; McKusick, M.A.; Misra, S.; Bjarnason, H.; Armstrong, A.S.; Gastineau, D.A.; et al. Autologous Mesenchymal Stem Cells Increase Cortical Perfusion in Renovascular Disease. *J. Am. Soc. Nephrol.* **2017**, *28*, 2777–2785. [CrossRef] [PubMed]
73. Swaminathan, M.; Stafford-Smith, M.; Chertow, G.M.; Warnock, D.G.; Paragamian, V.; Brenner, R.M.; Lellouche, F.; Fox-Robichaud, A.; Atta, M.G.; Melby, S.; et al. Allogeneic Mesenchymal Stem Cells for Treatment of AKI after Cardiac Surgery. *J. Am. Soc. Nephrol.* **2018**, *29*, 260–267. [CrossRef]
74. Miller, B.L.K.; Garg, P.; Bronstein, B.; LaPointe, E.; Lin, H.; Charytan, D.M.; Tilles, A.W.; Parekkadan, B. Extracorporeal Stromal Cell Therapy for Subjects With Dialysis-Dependent Acute Kidney Injury. *Kidney Int Rep.* **2018**, *3*, 1119–1127. [CrossRef]
75. De Martino, M.; Zonta, S.; Rampino, T.; Gregorini, M.; Frassoni, F.; Piotti, G.; Bedino, G.; Cobianchi, L.; Dal Canton, A.; Dionigi, P.; et al. Mesenchymal stem cells infusion prevents acute cellular rejection in rat kidney transplantation. *Transplant. Proc.* **2010**, *42*, 1331–1335. [CrossRef]
76. Hara, Y.; Stolk, M.; Ringe, J.; Dehne, T.; Ladhoff, J.; Kotsch, K.; Reutzel-Selke, A.; Reinke, P.; Volk, H.-D.; Seifert, M. In vivo effect of bone marrow-derived mesenchymal stem cells in a rat kidney transplantation model with prolonged cold ischemia. *Transpl. Int.* **2011**, *24*, 1112–1123. [CrossRef]
77. Casiraghi, F.; Azzollini, N.; Todeschini, M.; Cavinato, R.A.; Cassis, P.; Solini, S.; Rota, C.; Morigi, M.; Introna, M.; Maranta, R.; et al. Localization of mesenchymal stromal cells dictates their immune or proinflammatory effects in kidney transplantation. *Am. J. Transplant.* **2012**, *12*, 2373–2383. [CrossRef] [PubMed]
78. Franquesa, M.; Herrero, E.; Torras, J.; Ripoll, E.; Flaquer, M.; Gomà, M.; Lloberas, N.; Anegon, I.; Cruzado, J.M.; Grinyó, J.M.; et al. Mesenchymal stem cell therapy prevents interstitial fibrosis and tubular atrophy in a rat kidney allograft model. *Stem Cells Dev.* **2012**, *21*, 3125–3135. [CrossRef] [PubMed]
79. Crop, M.J.; Baan, C.C.; Korevaar, S.S.; Ijzermans, J.N.M.; Alwayn, I.P.J.; Weimar, W.; Hoogduijn, M.J. Donor-derived mesenchymal stem cells suppress alloreactivity of kidney transplant patients. *Transplantation* **2009**, *87*, 896–906. [CrossRef]
80. Perico, N.; Casiraghi, F.; Todeschini, M.; Cortinovis, M.; Gotti, E.; Portalupi, V.; Mister, M.; Gaspari, F.; Villa, A.; Fiori, S.; et al. Long-Term Clinical and Immunological Profile of Kidney Transplant Patients Given Mesenchymal Stromal Cell Immunotherapy. *Front. Immunol.* **2018**, *9*, 1359. [CrossRef] [PubMed]
81. Peng, Y.; Ke, M.; Xu, L.; Liu, L.; Chen, X.; Xia, W.; Li, X.; Chen, Z.; Ma, J.; Liao, D.; et al. Donor-derived mesenchymal stem cells combined with low-dose tacrolimus prevent acute rejection after renal transplantation: A clinical pilot study. *Transplantation* **2013**, *95*, 161–168. [CrossRef] [PubMed]

82. Reinders, M.E.J.; de Fijter, J.W.; Roelofs, H.; Bajema, I.M.; de Vries, D.K.; Schaapherder, A.F.; Claas, F.H.J.; van Miert, P.P.M.C.; Roelen, D.L.; van Kooten, C.; et al. Autologous bone marrow-derived mesenchymal stromal cells for the treatment of allograft rejection after renal transplantation: Results of a phase I study. *Stem Cells Transl. Med.* **2013**, *2*, 107–111. [CrossRef] [PubMed]
83. Tan, J.; Wu, W.; Xu, X.; Liao, L.; Zheng, F.; Messinger, S.; Sun, X.; Chen, J.; Yang, S.; Cai, J.; et al. Induction therapy with autologous mesenchymal stem cells in living-related kidney transplants: A randomized controlled trial. *JAMA* **2012**, *307*, 1169–1177. [CrossRef] [PubMed]
84. Iwai, S.; Sakonju, I.; Okano, S.; Teratani, T.; Kasahara, N.; Yokote, S.; Yokoo, T.; Kobayash, E. Impact of ex vivo administration of mesenchymal stem cells on the function of kidney grafts from cardiac death donors in rat. *Transplant. Proc.* **2014**, *46*, 1578–1584. [CrossRef]
85. Sun, Q.; Huang, Z.; Han, F.; Zhao, M.; Cao, R.; Zhao, D.; Hong, L.; Na, N.; Li, H.; Miao, B.; et al. Allogeneic mesenchymal stem cells as induction therapy are safe and feasible in renal allografts: Pilot results of a multicenter randomized controlled trial. *J. Transl Med.* **2018**, *16*, 52. [CrossRef]
86. Seifert, M.; Stolk, M.; Polenz, D.; Volk, H.-D. Detrimental effects of rat mesenchymal stromal cell pre-treatment in a model of acute kidney rejection. *Front. Immunol* **2012**, *3*, 202. [CrossRef]
87. Tsuda, H.; Yamahara, K.; Ishikane, S.; Otani, K.; Nakamura, A.; Sawai, K.; Ichimaru, N.; Sada, M.; Taguchi, A.; Hosoda, H.; et al. Allogenic fetal membrane-derived mesenchymal stem cells contribute to renal repair in experimental glomerulonephritis. *Am. J. Physiol. Renal Physiol.* **2010**, *299*, F1004–F1013. [CrossRef]
88. Zoja, C.; Garcia, P.B.; Rota, C.; Conti, S.; Gagliardini, E.; Corna, D.; Zanchi, C.; Bigini, P.; Benigni, A.; Remuzzi, G.; et al. Mesenchymal stem cell therapy promotes renal repair by limiting glomerular podocyte and progenitor cell dysfunction in adriamycin-induced nephropathy. *Am. J. Physiol. Renal Physiol.* **2012**, *303*, F1370–F1381. [CrossRef] [PubMed]
89. Iseri, K.; Iyoda, M.; Ohtaki, H.; Matsumoto, K.; Wada, Y.; Suzuki, T.; Yamamoto, Y.; Saito, T.; Hihara, K.; Tachibana, S.; et al. Therapeutic effects and mechanism of conditioned media from human mesenchymal stem cells on anti-GBM glomerulonephritis in WKY rats. *Am. J. Physiol. Renal Physiol.* **2016**, *310*, F1182–F1191. [CrossRef] [PubMed]
90. Suzuki, T.; Iyoda, M.; Shibata, T.; Ohtaki, H.; Matsumoto, K.; Shindo-Hirai, Y.; Kuno, Y.; Wada, Y.; Yamamoto, Y.; Kawaguchi, M.; et al. Therapeutic effects of human mesenchymal stem cells in Wistar-Kyoto rats with anti-glomerular basement membrane glomerulonephritis. *PLoS ONE* **2013**, *8*, e67475. [CrossRef]
91. Belingheri, M.; Lazzari, L.; Parazzi, V.; Groppali, E.; Biagi, E.; Gaipa, G.; Giordano, R.; Rastaldi, M.P.; Croci, D.; Biondi, A.; et al. Allogeneic mesenchymal stem cell infusion for the stabilization of focal segmental glomerulosclerosis. *Biologicals* **2013**, *41*, 439–445. [CrossRef]
92. Gregorini, M.; Maccario, R.; Avanzini, M.A.; Corradetti, V.; Moretta, A.; Libetta, C.; Esposito, P.; Bosio, F.; Dal Canton, A.; Rampino, T. Antineutrophil cytoplasmic antibody-associated renal vasculitis treated with autologous mesenchymal stromal cells: Evaluation of the contribution of immune-mediated mechanisms. *Mayo Clin. Proc.* **2013**, *88*, 1174–1179. [CrossRef]
93. Jiménez, S.; Cervera, R.; Font, J.; Ingelmo, M. The epidemiology of systemic lupus erythematosus. *Clin. Rev. Allergy Immunol.* **2003**, *25*, 3–12. [CrossRef]
94. Sattwika, P.D.; Mustafa, R.; Paramaiswari, A.; Herningtyas, E.H. Stem cells for lupus nephritis: A concise review of current knowledge. *Lupus* **2018**, *27*, 1881–1897. [CrossRef]
95. Tani, C.; Vagnani, S.; Carli, L.; Querci, F.; Kühl, A.A.; Spieckermann, S.; Cieluch, C.P.; Pacini, S.; Fazzi, R.; Mosca, M. Treatment with Allogenic Mesenchymal Stromal Cells in a Murine Model of Systemic Lupus Erythematosus. *Int J. Stem Cells* **2017**, *10*, 160–168. [CrossRef] [PubMed]
96. Gu, F.; Wang, D.; Zhang, H.; Feng, X.; Gilkeson, G.S.; Shi, S.; Sun, L. Allogeneic mesenchymal stem cell transplantation for lupus nephritis patients refractory to conventional therapy. *Clin. Rheumatol.* **2014**, *33*, 1611–1619. [CrossRef] [PubMed]
97. Wang, D.; Huang, S.; Yuan, X.; Liang, J.; Xu, R.; Yao, G.; Feng, X.; Sun, L. The regulation of the Treg/Th17 balance by mesenchymal stem cells in human systemic lupus erythematosus. *Cell. Mol. Immunol.* **2017**, *14*, 423–431. [CrossRef]
98. Deng, D.; Zhang, P.; Guo, Y.; Lim, T.O. A randomised double-blind, placebo-controlled trial of allogeneic umbilical cord-derived mesenchymal stem cell for lupus nephritis. *Ann. Rheum. Dis.* **2017**, *76*, 1436–1439. [CrossRef]

99. Barbado, J.; Tabera, S.; Sánchez, A.; García-Sancho, J. Therapeutic potential of allogeneic mesenchymal stromal cells transplantation for lupus nephritis. *Lupus* **2018**, *27*, 2161–2165. [CrossRef]
100. Sharma, J.; Hampton, J.M.; Valiente, G.R.; Wada, T.; Steigelman, H.; Young, M.C.; Spurbeck, R.R.; Blazek, A.D.; Bösh, S.; Jarjour, W.N.; et al. Therapeutic Development of Mesenchymal Stem Cells or Their Extracellular Vesicles to Inhibit Autoimmune-Mediated Inflammatory Processes in Systemic Lupus Erythematosus. *Front. Immunol.* **2017**, *8*, 526. [CrossRef]
101. Perez-Hernandez, J.; Redon, J.; Cortes, R. Extracellular Vesicles as Therapeutic Agents in Systemic Lupus Erythematosus. *Int. J. Mol. Sci* **2017**, *18*, 717. [CrossRef]
102. Gao, X.; Song, L.; Shen, K.; Wang, H.; Qian, M.; Niu, W.; Qin, X. Bone marrow mesenchymal stem cells promote the repair of islets from diabetic mice through paracrine actions. *Mol. Cell. Endocrinol.* **2014**, *388*, 41–50. [CrossRef]
103. Lee, R.H.; Seo, M.J.; Reger, R.L.; Spees, J.L.; Pulin, A.A.; Olson, S.D.; Prockop, D.J. Multipotent stromal cells from human marrow home to and promote repair of pancreatic islets and renal glomeruli in diabetic NOD/scid mice. *Proc. Natl. Acad. Sci. USA* **2006**, *103*, 17438–17443. [CrossRef]
104. Shree, N.; Bhonde, R.R. Conditioned Media From Adipose Tissue Derived Mesenchymal Stem Cells Reverse Insulin Resistance in Cellular Models. *J. Cell. Biochem.* **2017**, *118*, 2037–2043. [CrossRef]
105. Liu, X.; Zheng, P.; Wang, X.; Dai, G.; Cheng, H.; Zhang, Z.; Hua, R.; Niu, X.; Shi, J.; An, Y. A preliminary evaluation of efficacy and safety of Wharton's jelly mesenchymal stem cell transplantation in patients with type 2 diabetes mellitus. *Stem Cell Res. Ther.* **2014**, *5*, 57. [CrossRef]
106. Hu, J.; Li, C.; Wang, L.; Zhang, X.; Zhang, M.; Gao, H.; Yu, X.; Wang, F.; Zhao, W.; Yan, S.; et al. Long term effects of the implantation of autologous bone marrow mononuclear cells for type 2 diabetes mellitus. *Endocr. J.* **2012**, *59*, 1031–1039. [CrossRef]
107. Ezquer, F.; Giraud-Billoud, M.; Carpio, D.; Cabezas, F.; Conget, P.; Ezquer, M. Proregenerative Microenvironment Triggered by Donor Mesenchymal Stem Cells Preserves Renal Function and Structure in Mice with Severe Diabetes Mellitus. *BioMed Res. Int.* **2015**, *2015*, 164703. [CrossRef]
108. Abdel Aziz, M.T.; Wassef, M.A.A.; Ahmed, H.H.; Rashed, L.; Mahfouz, S.; Aly, M.I.; Hussein, R.E.; Abdelaziz, M. The role of bone marrow derived-mesenchymal stem cells in attenuation of kidney function in rats with diabetic nephropathy. *Diabetol. Metab. Syndr.* **2014**, *6*, 34. [CrossRef] [PubMed]
109. Nagaishi, K.; Mizue, Y.; Chikenji, T.; Otani, M.; Nakano, M.; Konari, N.; Fujimiya, M. Mesenchymal stem cell therapy ameliorates diabetic nephropathy via the paracrine effect of renal trophic factors including exosomes. *Sci. Rep.* **2016**, *6*, 34842. [CrossRef]
110. Jiang, Z.; Liu, Y.; Niu, X.; Yin, J.; Hu, B.; Guo, S.; Fan, Y.; Wang, Y.; Wang, N. Exosomes secreted by human urine-derived stem cells could prevent kidney complications from type I diabetes in rats. *Stem Cell Res. Ther.* **2016**, *7*, 24. [CrossRef] [PubMed]
111. Ebrahim, N.; Ahmed, I.A.; Hussien, N.I.; Dessouky, A.A.; Farid, A.S.; Elshazly, A.M.; Mostafa, O.; Gazzar, W.B.E.; Sorour, S.M.; Seleem, Y.; et al. Mesenchymal Stem Cell-Derived Exosomes Ameliorated Diabetic Nephropathy by Autophagy Induction through the mTOR Signaling Pathway. *Cells* **2018**, *7*, 226. [CrossRef]
112. Packham, D.K.; Fraser, I.R.; Kerr, P.G.; Segal, K.R. Allogeneic Mesenchymal Precursor Cells (MPC) in Diabetic Nephropathy: A Randomized, Placebo-controlled, Dose Escalation Study. *EBioMedicine* **2016**, *12*, 263–269. [CrossRef]
113. Skyler, J.S.; Fonseca, V.A.; Segal, K.R.; Rosenstock, J. MSB-DM003 Investigators Allogeneic Mesenchymal Precursor Cells in Type 2 Diabetes: A Randomized, Placebo-Controlled, Dose-Escalation Safety and Tolerability Pilot Study. *Diabetes Care* **2015**, *38*, 1742–1749. [CrossRef]
114. Sasser, A.K.; Mundy, B.L.; Smith, K.M.; Studebaker, A.W.; Axel, A.E.; Haidet, A.M.; Fernandez, S.A.; Hall, B.M. Human bone marrow stromal cells enhance breast cancer cell growth rates in a cell line-dependent manner when evaluated in 3D tumor environments. *Cancer Lett.* **2007**, *254*, 255–264. [CrossRef]
115. Zhu, W.; Xu, W.; Jiang, R.; Qian, H.; Chen, M.; Hu, J.; Cao, W.; Han, C.; Chen, Y. Mesenchymal stem cells derived from bone marrow favor tumor cell growth in vivo. *Exp. Mol. Pathol.* **2006**, *80*, 267–274. [CrossRef]
116. Thirabanjasak, D.; Tantiwongse, K.; Thorner, P.S. Angiomyeloproliferative lesions following autologous stem cell therapy. *J. Am. Soc. Nephrol.* **2010**, *21*, 1218–1222. [CrossRef]
117. Bruna, F.; Plaza, A.; Arango, M.; Espinoza, I.; Conget, P. Systemically administered allogeneic mesenchymal

stem cells do not aggravate the progression of precancerous lesions: A new biosafety insight. *Stem Cell Res. Ther.* **2018**, *9*, 137. [CrossRef]

118. Schnabel, L.V.; Pezzanite, L.M.; Antczak, D.F.; Felippe, M.J.B.; Fortier, L.A. Equine bone marrow-derived mesenchymal stromal cells are heterogeneous in MHC class II expression and capable of inciting an immune response in vitro. *Stem Cell Res. Ther.* **2014**, *5*, 13. [CrossRef]
119. Lohan, P.; Treacy, O.; Griffin, M.D.; Ritter, T.; Ryan, A.E. Anti-Donor Immune Responses Elicited by Allogeneic Mesenchymal Stem Cells and Their Extracellular Vesicles: Are We Still Learning? *Front. Immunol.* **2017**, *8*, 1626. [CrossRef]
120. Sohel, M.H. Extracellular/Circulating MicroRNAs: Release Mechanisms, Functions and Challenges. *Achiev. Life Sci.* **2016**, *10*, 175–186. [CrossRef]

8

Potential and Therapeutic Efficacy of Cell-based Therapy using Mesenchymal Stem Cells for Acute/Chronic Kidney Disease

Chul Won Yun [1] **and Sang Hun Lee** [1,2,*]

1 Medical Science Research Institute, Soonchunhyang University Seoul Hospital, Seoul 04401, Korea; skydbs113@naver.com
2 Department of Biochemistry, Soonchunhyang University College of Medicine, Cheonan 34538, Korea
* Correspondence: ykckss1114@nate.com

Abstract: Kidney disease can be either acute kidney injury (AKI) or chronic kidney disease (CKD) and it can lead to the development of functional organ failure. Mesenchymal stem cells (MSCs) are derived from a diverse range of human tissues. They are multipotent and have immunomodulatory effects to assist in the recovery from tissue injury and the inhibition of inflammation. Numerous studies have investigated the feasibility, safety, and efficacy of MSC-based therapies for kidney disease. Although the exact mechanism of MSC-based therapy remains uncertain, their therapeutic value in the treatment of a diverse range of kidney diseases has been studied in clinical trials. The use of MSCs is a promising therapeutic strategy for both acute and chronic kidney disease. The mechanism underlying the effects of MSCs on survival rate after transplantation and functional repair of damaged tissue is still ambiguous. The paracrine effects of MSCs on renal recovery, optimization of the microenvironment for cell survival, and control of inflammatory responses are thought to be related to their interaction with the damaged kidney environment. This review discusses recent experimental and clinical findings related to kidney disease, with a focus on the role of MSCs in kidney disease recovery, differentiation, and microenvironment. The therapeutic efficacy and current applications of MSC-based kidney disease therapies are also discussed.

Keywords: mesenchymal stem cells; acute and chronic kidney disease; exosome; natural products

---

1. Introduction

Kidney disease, including acute kidney injury (AKI) and chronic kidney disease (CKD), is a significant global public health problem, with incidence and mortality rates increasing in recent decades [1,2]. AKI is experienced by one fifth of all adults and one third of all children worldwide. It is characterized by sudden kidney failure or a rapid loss of kidney function [3]. AKI has many potential causes, including renal ischemia from low blood pressure, crush injury, inflammation, and urinary tract obstruction or infection [4,5]. It is diagnosed based on elevated blood urea nitrogen (BUN) and creatinine concentrations, or decreased urine output [5]. Chronic kidney disease (CKD) is characterized by a progressive loss of kidney function, leading to end-stage renal disease (ESRD) and the accumulation of collagen, caused by inflammation, resulting in fibrosis [6,7]. At the end stage of CKD, an irreversible loss of renal function is treated with dialysis or kidney transplantation. AKI can also result in ESRD, leading to an increased risk of CKD or worsening of CKD symptoms [8]. Additionally, CKD is a progressive disease, causing significant morbidity and mortality. Although pharmaceutical or surgical therapies may improve overall kidney function, they cannot enhance the regeneration and functional recovery of the surrounding tissues affected by kidney damage. Therefore, there is a need to develop more effective strategies for treating kidney injury.

Human mesenchymal stem cells (MSCs) are isolated from diverse tissues, including bone marrow and adipose tissue. They have the characteristics of multipotent cells, with multi-lineage differentiation, self-renewal, and proliferative potential [9–11]. There is some evidence indicating that MSCs originate from renal pericytes, which form a network around the microvasculature [12]. In addition, MSCs can secrete many different cytokines and growth factors, which regulate immune activity and enhance the potential of expansion and differentiation of host cells, thus promoting the recovery of damaged tissues [13]. They also play critical roles in the modulation of renal blood flow, capillary permeability, endothelial cell survival, and immunological responses [14]. Therefore, MSCs with potential angiogenic and immunomodulatory properties, are also a promising source of cells for the recovery of damaged sites and the treatment of various pathological conditions, such as renal injury and renal failure, making them an ideal therapeutic strategy for regenerative kidney therapy [15,16]. For effective MSC-based treatment of kidney disease, it is important to study the therapeutic mechanisms of MSCs and explore ways of enhancing the efficiency of MSC-based therapy.

In this review, we first summarize the various types of kidney disease and then explore the application of MSC-based therapies. The potential therapeutic effects of MSCs, their mechanisms of action, and techniques for enhancing MSC functionality are then discussed.

2. The Mechanisms of MSC-based Therapy for Kidney Disease

MSCs may have several origins, such as bone-morrow [17], adipose [18], and umbilical cord [19], and can be used to treat various renal diseases. The therapeutic effects of MSC-based therapy are associated with characteristics including multipotency, self-renewal, secretion of factors related to proliferation and survival, immunomodulation, and homing [20–22]. MSCs differentiate into various organ lineages, such as bone, cartilage, and adipose [23]. The differentiation potential of MSCs has increasing interest due to the potential to treat diverse diseases and improve novel clinical perspectives on MSC function. Recent evidence indicates that MSCs differentiate into epithelial-like cells. One study has demonstrated that MSCs generate keratinocytes and multiple skin cell types, which can then be processed for use in wound repair procedures [24]. In a mouse model of ischemia/kidney reperfusion injury, administered MSCs differentiated into renal tubular epithelium, which induced tissue structural integrity and tissue recovery [25]. In addition, recent studies have indicated that the benefits of MSC injection are related to the ability of MSCs to secrete several cytokines, chemokines, and growth factors. Several observations have revealed that the major role of MSCs include secretion of multiple biologically active factors that exert effects on local cellular environments. Other studies have demonstrated that these factors protected against apoptosis of adjacent cells and induced cell proliferation, as well as promoting the regeneration of damaged renal tissue [26]. There is also much evidence that has demonstrated that MSCs injected into damaged tissue sites for repair interacted closely with local microenvironments, including inflammatory responses and hypoxic tissues, and stimulated cells to secrete several growth factors related to tissue regeneration factors [5,27].

In addition, modulation of the immune system is another characteristic of MSCs and these cells were effective in treating several immune disorders in humans and animal models [28,29]. Although the mechanism of immunomodulatory function is not fully clear, cell-to-cell contact, and/or the secretion of soluble immunosuppressive factors is thought to contribute. Several studies have revealed that MSCs interact with multiple immune cells and display an ability to suppress excessive inflammatory responses [30,31]. Furthermore, inflammation induced tissue damage is a critical process triggered in response to injury and disease, MSCs could be used for the treatment of tissue or organ injury associated with intense inflammatory activity, such as kidney failure, heart injury. Finally, the homing mechanism of MSCs is related to their ability to reach damaged sites via interaction with signal molecules secreted by injured tissue and MSC receptors [32]. Some studies have revealed that MSCs migrate to areas of inflammation [33,34], and then further promote homing into damaged tissues by enhancing paracrine effects. Furthermore some studies have suggested that overexpression by MSCs of CXCR4, or serine protease kallikrein, which are homing receptors, improved renal function and enhanced anti-inflammatory effects in renal injury [35,36]. Another study confirmed that IGF1-pretreated MSCs displayed increased expression of IGF1 and CXCR4 in bmMSCs, and enhanced cell migration and renal protective effects [37]. Therefore, several mechanisms and complex signaling contribute to the therapeutic effects of MSC-based therapy, and further studies are necessary to enhance the efficacy of MSC-based therapy to treat kidney disease.

3. MSC-based Therapy for Kidney Disease

The promising properties of MSCs, such as regeneration and differentiation, has generated considerable interest and spurred numerous studies in various diseases. Preclinical results have demonstrated the therapeutic efficacy of MSCs in reducing acute and chronic kidney injuries in animal models. Therefore, early-phase clinical trials have been performed to investigate the safety and efficacy of allogenic MSC infusion [38] (Figure 1).

A symptom of AKI is acute renal failure, which is the sudden loss of kidney function. Mesenchymal stem cells (MSCs) are one option for the treatment of AKI [39], due to their physiological activities related to inflammation, apoptosis, angiogenesis, and immunomodulation [40]. The administration of MSCs has been shown to improve renal function and protect against tubular injury in a mouse model of AKI [41]. This was accompanied by an increase in M2 macrophage infiltration and the conversion of activated macrophages to an anti-inflammatory phenotype. These findings suggest that MSCs can protect against AKI through the anti-inflammatory activation of macrophages, which assists in the recovery from tubular injury. MSCs have also been shown to contribute to improved renal function in an in vivo canine acute kidney injury model, by decreasing BUN and creatinine levels and recovering renal lesions [42]. Another study has suggested that MSCs treatment improves glomerular filtration, renal function, and alleviates oxidative stress-induced cell senescence and inflammation and increases the proliferation of kidney cells in an ischemia/reperfusion injury (IRI)-induced acute kidney injury model [43].

In addition, numerous studies in a range of different mouse models have suggested that novel therapeutic strategies using MSCs can be developed to treat AKI. One such study showed AKI-protective effects when using MSC-based therapy, but failed to confirm that the injected MSCs were incorporated into tubules, vessels, or other specific compartments of the kidney [44]. Further studies demonstrated that the subcellular mechanisms of MSC-mediated protection did not act directly at the sites of damage. One study indicated that the protective effects of MSCs are due to the secretion of factors that have paracrine effects [22]. Another study suggested that MSCs produce and secrete extracellular vesicles, which then lead to renal-protective effects [45]. The mortality rate in AKI patients is approximately 50%. Most surviving patients recover full renal function, but some develop CKD, requiring further treatment, such as dialysis and renal transplantation [46]. Clinical trials using MSC-based therapies are currently underway to investigate the safety and efficacy of allogenic MSC administration. One such trial (NCT00733876), performed in 2013, was a phase I exploratory study of 16 patients [5,26] aimed at estimating the safety and efficacy of bone marrow-derived MSC injection in patients at high risk of developing AKI after on-pump cardiac surgery [47]. No specific or serious adverse effects were observed during a six-month follow-up period during this trial. These observations indicate that the administration of MSCs is safe at the doses used and has protective effects on renal function. Another clinical trial (NCT01275612) performed in oncology patients with cisplatin-mediated AKI, has completed phase II. This study aims to test the feasibility and safety of ex vivo proliferative MSCs as a treatment to recover kidney function.

CKD is diagnosed based on increased serum creatinine levels, low estimated glomerular filtration rate (eGFR), or urinary abnormalities for at least three months [48]. CKD is associated with a significant increase in the risk of atherosclerosis and type 2 diabetes [49]. Moreover, CKD is closely related to cardiovascular disease, which is the cause of mortality in almost 50% of CKD patients [50]. Some patients with CKD develop ESRD and show increased risk factors for cardiovascular disease.

Considering the high cost of renal replacement therapy, effective treatment of progressive CKD is required, [49]. Therefore, there is a need to develop novel therapeutic strategies to treat CKD.

CKD is a global public health problem, due to the high cost of treatment and its major impact on the health of affected patients [51]. CKD is associated with a high risk of diabetics, hypertension, and cardiovascular disease and results in the loss of kidney function [52]. The kidneys play an important role in eliminating toxic metabolites, such as uremic toxins. When the function of kidney is weakened, these toxic substances accumulate in the blood and result in biochemically toxic effects in numerous tissues and organs, which results in additional complications, including cardiovascular disease, anemia, and neurological disorders [53,54]. The administration of MSCs induces anti-inflammatory and anti-fibrotic effects in CKD models [17,55] and is a promising cell-based therapy for chronic kidney disease. Uremic toxins, such as p-cresol (PC) and indoxyl sulfate (IS), reduce the functionality of MSCs in CKD patients [18]. A recent study has suggested that the toxic product, p-cresol, leads to mitochondrial dysfunction in adipose-derived (ad) MSCs from CKD patients and inhibits the therapeutic effects of cell-based therapy. Pioglitazone, which is used to treat CKD, protects against PC-induced apoptosis and improves mitochondrial function via upregulation of PINK1 [19]. In addition, the transplantation of MSCs enhances renal function and increases the expression and activity of ATPase in a rat model of CKD with renovascular hypertension. Moreover, MSCs improve renal morphology and reduce fibrosis in the kidney [20]. MSC treatment alleviates renal fibrosis and chronic inflammation by reducing collagen deposition and modulating chemokine and cytokine expression in a CKD model [56]. These results demonstrate that MSC treatment has protective effects by regulating inflammation and proliferation and, thus, reducing renal damage and improving kidney function.

A major symptom of CKD is the reduced regenerative capacity of the kidney. Several studies have indicated that MSCs induce regenerative effects in animal CKD models [21]. Some studies have suggested that the administration of MSCs provides significant renal protection by decreasing inflammatory infiltrates, fibrosis, and glomerulosclerosis [22]. In addition, four clinical trials are currently assessing the safety and efficacy of MSC-based therapies to treat CKD. One clinical trial using autologous bone-marrow (bm) was performed in 2014 and phase I exploratory study of six patients (NCT02166489). This study is aimed to evaluate the safety and tolerability of bmMSC administration in CKD patients. No cell-related adverse effects was observed during 12 months after bmMSC administration. This study is limited the therapeutic effects of MSCs due to small sample size, the lack of a control group, and a short follow-up; further study is necessary to confirm the efficacy of bmMSC to treat CKD [57]. Another clinical trial using adMSC was performed in 2013 and phase I exploratory study of six patients (NCT01840540). This study is aimed to test the safety and toxicity of adMSC administration in CKD paitents. adMSC is confirmed the potential of clinical usage and characteristics of MSC marker [58]. Other clinical trials are using autologous bmMSCs (NCT02195323) and using AD-MSCs (NCT02266394 and NCT01840540). These clinical studies are either ongoing or are completed, but the results are not yet published.

Diabetes mellitus usually progresses to CKD, despite recent developments in its clinical management [59]. In addition, diabetic kidney disease (DKD), also known as diabetic nephropathy (DN), can cause kidney damage [60]. DKD is caused by a complex mechanism involving the kidney and other organs and tissues. The five-year mortality rate for DKD patients is approximately 39%, which is similar to the mortality rates of many cancers. However, there have been no successful, specific therapies developed to treat DKD. The current treatment involves early detection, glycemic control, and regulation of blood pressure. Several studies have indicated that MSC administration improves DKD symptoms, including elevated serum creatinine and BUN levels and glomerular hypertrophy [24,25,61]. These results indicate that the systemic administration of MSCs induces beneficial effects via their anti-inflammatory properties in animal models of DKD. MSCs have been shown to reduce the levels of inflammatory factors, such as TNFa, IL-6, and IL-1b and the infiltration of macrophages [25,61]. A clinical trial, aimed at developing novel treatments for DKD using MSC-based therapies, is ongoing (NCT02585622). This clinical study is investigating the safety, feasibility, tolerability, and efficacy of bmMSC therapy in a diabetic mouse model [62] (Table 1).

Table 1. The effects of mesenchymal stem cells (MSCs) in the treatment of kidney disease.

Pathological Condition	Type of Source	Findings	Reference
Acute Kidney Injury (AKI)	BM-derived MSC	Protection against kidney tubular injury, M2 macrophage infiltration and reduction of inflammatory responses, improvement of renal function	[41]
AKI	UC-derived MSC	Decrease in BUN and creatinine levels, recovery of renal lesions and cell senescence, improvement of glomerular filtration, induction of proliferation	[42,43]
Clinical trial (AKI)	BM-derived MSC	Phase I, exploratory study of 16 patients, estimating safety and efficacy of MSC administration	NCT00733876 [5,26,47]
Clinical trial (AKI)	BM-derived MSC	Phase II, oncology patients with cisplatin-mediated AKI, testing of the feasibility and safety of MSC therapy, treatment to recover kidney function	NCT01275612
Chronic kidney disease (CKD)	AD-derived MSC	Recovery of MSC functionality, such as mitochondrial dysfunction via treatment of pioglitazone, reduction of p-cresol mediated apoptosis	[19]
CKD with renovascular hypertension	BM-derived MSC	Enhancement of renal function, increase of ATPase activity, improvement of renal morphology, decrease of renal fibrosis	[20]
CKD	BM-derived MSC	Alleviation of renal fibrosis and chronic inflammation, reduction of collagen deposition, modulation of chemokine and cytokine expression	[56]
Clinical trial (CKD)	BM-derived MSC	Phase I, evaluation of safety and tolerability of MSC administration, improvement of renal function	NCT02166489 [57]
Clinical trial (CKD)	BM-derived MSC	Phase I, test of safety of MSC administration	NCT02195323
Clinical trial (CKD)	AD-derived MSC	Phase I, investigation of safety and toxicity of MSC administration, confirmation of the characteristics of MSC markers, classical and non-classical markers.	NCT01840540 [58]
Clinical trial (CKD)	AD-derived MSC	Phase I, ongoing clinical trial, measurement of blood and urinary markers for kidney function	NCT02266394
Diabetic kidney disease (DKD)	BM-derived MSC	Reduction of creatinine and BUN levels, improvement of glomerular hypertrophy, anti-inflammatory effects	[61]
Clinical trial (DKD)	BM-derived MSC	Phase I, Phase II, ongoing clinical trial, investigation of the safety, feasibility, tolerability, and efficacy of MSC therapy	NCT02585622 [62]

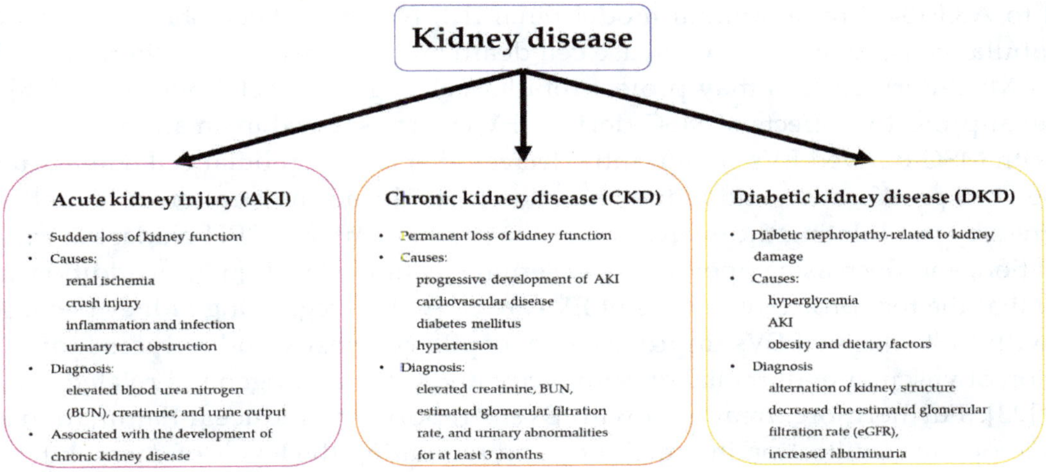

Figure 1. A schema illustrating an overview of kidney disease, with its diverse symptoms.

4. The Therapeutic Strategy of Exosomes Derived MSCs in the Treatment of Kidney Disease

Extracellular vesicles (EVs) are small vesicles secreted by MSCs and endocytic compartments. Exosomes are a type of EV, 30–100 nm in diameter, that are derived from the plasma membrane and micro-vesicles (100–1000 nm), and are released into the extracellular environment. Some studies have suggested that exosomes contain cytokines, proteins, mRNAs, miRNAs, and rRNAs [27–30]. In addition, a recent study demonstrated that miRNAs, mRNAs, and proteins from EVs are able to regulate cellular signaling pathways in recipient cells [31]. Indeed, there is a considerable amount of data indicating that the administration of MSC-derived EVs is safe and can enhance kidney function in numerous animal models of AKI and CKD. Therefore, MSC-derived EVs may be a potential therapeutic agent for renal disease (Figure 2).

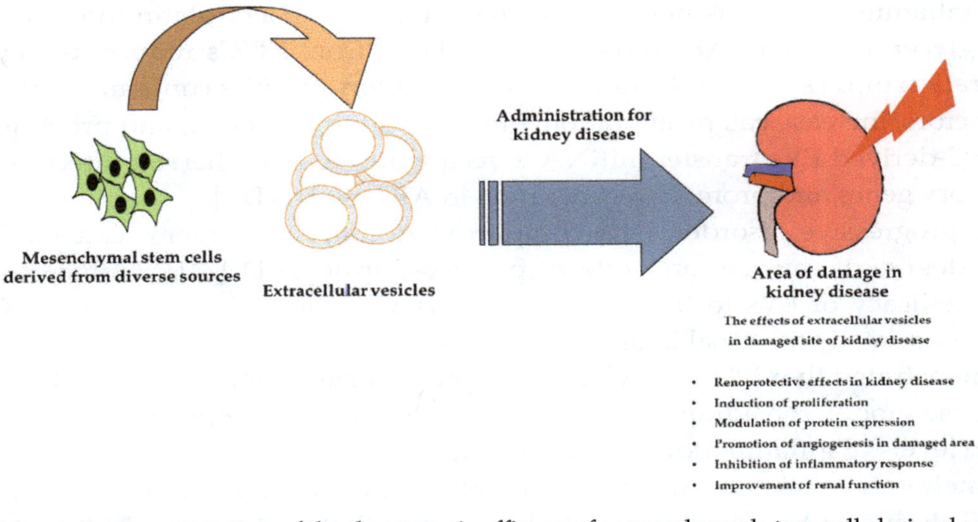

Figure 2. Schematic representation of the therapeutic efficacy of mesenchymal stem cell-derived extracellular vesicles for the treatment of kidney disease.

Renal ischemia/reperfusion injury (IRI) is one of the causes of acute kidney injury. It occurs as a result of a sudden blockage of blood flow to the kidney, with a subsequent restoration of flow and re-oxygenation. It is significantly associated with morbidity and mortality in AKI patients [63]. In addition, AKI is a potential risk factor for progressive CKD [32], but there is currently no effective therapy for AKI. One study has suggested that human adMSC-derived exosomes inhibit the AKI-CKD transition via modulation of SOX9, which is a transcription factor related to the development of kidney disease in mouse model of AKI [33]. The pathogenesis of renal IRI is unclear, but ischemic conditions and the generation of reactive oxygen species can induce inflammation and cell death, which lead to AKI [34]. In an animal model renal IRI, EVs have been shown to incorporate into damaged tubular cells, where they decrease cell death and increase cell proliferation. These results suggest that MSC-derived EVs may protect tubular cells against metabolic stress [36]. In another study, the renal-protective effects of MSC-derived EVs were assessed in an animal model of renal IRI. Treatment with MSC-derived EVs significantly decreased epithelial tubular cell damage and apoptosis and increased cell proliferation and kidney function [35]. The administration of EVs attenuates renal oxidative stress by modulating the expression of the pro-oxidant, NADPH oxidase 2, enhancing renal cell proliferation, and decreasing apoptosis and serum creatinine levels [37]. In addition, some studies have shown that the renoprotective effects of EVs are caused by regulating kidney neovascularization. Treatment with MSC-derived EVs improves renal capillary density and reduces kidney fibrosis via the expression of vascular endothelial growth factor and other angiogenesis-related mRNAs in a rat AKI model [23]. Furthermore, treatment with EVs is reported to reduce inflammation after AKI by reducing macrophage infiltration in the kidney and regulating the levels of chemokines and related immune responses via the actions of miRNAs carried by the EVs [64].

Drug-induced nephrotoxicity is a one of the common causes of AKI, with an incidence as high as 60% [65,66]. Several clinical treatments, such as anti-inflammatory drugs, antibiotics, and contrast agents, are toxic to renal cells and compromise renal function by changing intraglomerular hemodynamics, inducing inflammation, and increasing uric acid deposition [67]. Recent studies have shown that MSC-derived EVs have beneficial effects in the treatment of drug-induced nephropathy. The anticancer drug, cisplatin, can induce nephropathy and lead to an increase in BUN and creatinine levels, oxidative stress, and apoptosis [68,69]. The administration of human umbilical cord (huc) MSC-derived exosomes improves cisplatin-mediated renal damage in AKI rat models and NRK-52E cells [70]. The therapeutic effects of exosomes on cisplatin-induced kidney damage occur via a decrease in oxidative stress and apoptosis and enhanced cell proliferation. In addition, cisplatin-induced nephrotoxicity results in mitochondrial apoptosis and the induction of an inflammatory response in the kidney [71]. The administration of hucMSC-derived exosomes inhibits mitochondrial apoptosis and the release of inflammatory cytokines by inducing autophagy in a cisplatin-induced nephrotoxicity model. In a glycerol-induced AKI model, EVs isolated from MSCs reduce kidney damage [72]. The administration of EVs induces tubular cell proliferation and EVs containing mRNAs, miRNAs, and growth factors, increase cell proliferation, improve kidney function, and promote AKI recovery. Moreover, MSC-derived EVs transfer miRNA to recipient cells and, thereby, affect the expression of pro-inflammatory genes and promote regeneration in AKI models [73].

CKD is a progressive disorder, with complex symptoms and diverse causes. Several factors influence the degree of severity and rate of progression of CKD [74]. Numerous studies have confirmed the efficacy of EVs to treat CKD. Renovascular disease (RVD) is one of the causes of CKD [75]. It is associated with renal injury, poor renal function, and metabolic syndrome [76]. A recent study has demonstrated that MSC-derived EVs improve renal function and structural recovery [77]. In a renal disease model, the administration of MSC-derived EVs improves renal inflammation by decreasing the levels of inflammatory cytokines, such as TNF-α, IL-6, and IL-1-β. Moreover, in this model, EVs ameliorate renal fibrosis and enhance renal function, thus demonstrating renoprotective effects of MSC-derived EVs. Another study has shown that MSC-derived EVs contain a diverse array of pro-angiogenic genes and proteins, which promote angiogenesis and vascular recovery [78]. Moreover, the administration of EVs increases microcirculation and decreases tissue damage in the kidney and improves renal function. The unilateral ureteral obstruction (UUO) model, which induces renal inflammation, apoptosis, and fibrosis, is a popular experimental model to study mechanisms associated with kidney diseases, such as AKI and CKD [79]. Recent studies have tested the efficacy of MSC-derived EVs in the treatment of kidney disease in UUO animal models. EV administration restores epithelial-mesenchymal transition (EMT) morphological changes induced by renal fibrosis, by modulating TGF-β, E-cadherin, and αSMA expression in HK2 cells and improves renal function in animal models [80]. In addition, EVs isolated from kidney-derived MSCs have been shown to ameliorate EMT morphological changes and enhance the proliferation of TGF-β1-treated human umbilical vein epithelial cells and suppress inflammatory cell infiltration and renal fibrosis in UUO mouse models [81]. One clinical trial has investigated the renoprotective efficacy of MSC-derived EVs in patients with CKD. Treatment with MSC-derived EVs resulted in significant recovery of eGFR, creatinine, and BUN levels. EV treatment not only decreased TNF-α levels, but also increased IL-10 levels in CKD patients and this ameliorated the inflammatory immune reaction. Moreover, kidney biopsies revealed that EV administration increased the levels of renal regeneration and differentiation markers [82]. These results suggest that MSC-derived EV therapy decreases inflammation and improves renal function in patients with CKD.

DN is a severe complication of diabetes mellitus and is a major cause of CKD [83]. Treatment with MSC-derived exosomes results in improved renal function and repair of damaged renal tissues by modulating autophagy and fibrotic markers in a diabetic mouse model [84]. MSC-derived EV therapy has been shown to prevent the effects of DN progression and reduce urine volume and albumin excretion. Moreover, EV therapy protects podocytes and tubular epithelial cells from apoptosis and promotes vascular regeneration and cell survival [85] (Table 2).

Table 2. The effects of MSC-derived extracellular vesicles in the treatment of kidney disease.

Pathological Condition	Type of Source	Findings	Reference
Renal ischemic/Reperfusion injury (IRI)	BM-MSC derived exosomes	Inhibition of AKI-CKD transition, modulation of SOX9	[33]
Renal IRI	BM-MSC derived exosomes	Recovery of damaged tubular cells, decrease in cell death, enhancement of cell proliferation, protection for metabolic stress	[36]
Renal IRI	BM-MSC derived exosomes	Decrease in epithelial tubular cell damage and apoptosis, improvement of cell proliferation and kidney function	[35]
AKI	UC-MSC derived exosomes	Enhancement of renal capillary density, reduction of kidney fibrosis, modulation of vascular endothelial growth factor and angiogenesis-related mRNAs	[23]
AKI	UC-MSC derived exosomes	Reduction of inflammation and macrophage infiltration, modulation of chemokine levels and immune response	[64]
Drug-induced nephrotoxicity (DN-AKI)	UC-MSC derived exosomes	Decrease in oxidative stress and apoptosis, improvement in cell proliferation, inhibition of inflammation, induction of autophagy	[70,71]
AKI	BM-MSC derived exosomes	Induction of tubular cell proliferation, improvement of kidney function, promotion of kidney regeneration	[72]
CKD	BM-derived MSC	Reduction of inflammation, amelioration of renal fibrosis, enhancement of renal function	[77]
CKD in unilateral ureteral obstruction (UUO)	BM-MSC derived exosomes	Reduced renal fibrosis and improved renal function	[80]
CKD in UUO	kidney-MSC derived exosomes	Reduction in EMT morphological change, enhancement of cell proliferation, suppression of inflammatory cell infiltration and renal fibrosis	[81]
Clinical trial (CKD)	UC-MSC derived exosomes	Reno-protective efficacy of MSC derived EVs, recovery of eGFR, creatinine, and BUN, reduction of inflammatory immune reaction, renal regeneration	[82]
DN-CKD	BM-MSC derived exosomes	Improvement in renal function, repair of damaged renal tissue, modulation of autophagy	[84]
DN-CKD	Urine-MSC derived exosomes	Prevention of DN progression, reduction of urine volume and albumin excretion, protection of podocytes and tubular epithelial cells, promotion of vascular regeneration and cell survival	[85]

5. Enhancement of MSC Functionality to Improve their Therapeutic Effects in Kidney Disease

MSC-based therapy has been widely studied for the treatment of kidney disease and has been shown to result in improved renal function and the recovery of damaged renal tissues in animal studies and clinical trials [6]. However, MSC-based therapy is limited by the low survival rate of MSCs when used to treat severe kidney disease [86]. Several factors, such as anoikis, ischemia, inflammation, and ROS production reduce the efficacy of MSC-based therapies [87,88]. Some studies have suggested that the preconditioning of MSCs protects them from the harmful environment at site of damage and improves their function. These pretreatment methods include incubation with cytokines or natural or chemical compounds and the application of supporting materials (Figure 3).

Many cytokines and natural/chemical compounds have been shown to have protective effects by enhancing cell survival and proliferation and modulating downstream pathways [89]. Docosahexaenoic acid (DHA) is a necessary omega-3 fatty acid found in blood and in the kidney. 14S,21R-dihydroxy-doxosa 4Z,7Z19Z,12E,16Z,19Z-hexaenoic acid (14S,21R-dHDHA) has been identified as a new DHA-derived lipid mediator and treatment with this compound has been shown to enhance the function of MSCs. In vitro and in IRI mouse models, the usage of this compound is revealed that MSCs treated with 14S,21R-dHDHA show reduced apoptosis and inflammatory responses, and improved renal function [90]. Other studies have shown that the pharmacological agent, S-nitroso N-acetyl penicillamine (SNP), a nitric oxide donor associated with cyto-protective and tissue-protective effects, promotes MSC functionality by increasing cell proliferation and survival in a renal ischemia model [91]. Moreover, the administration of SNP-treated MSCs results in a significant improvement in renal function and increases the expression of pro-survival and pro-angiogenic factors in ischemic renal tissue. Darbepoetin-α (DPO) is an erythropoietic agent that shows similar protective and hematopoietic effects and reduces kidney damage in an animal model of renal IRI [92]. DPO-treated MSCs also improve renal function and kidney structure in an ischemic renal disease model.

Atorvastatin (Ator) has diverse biological activities, including anti-apoptosis, antioxidant, and anti-inflammatory effects [93]. Ator-treated MSCs induced renoprotective effects, including improved renal function and enhanced survival of engrafted MSCs in impaired kidneys in an IRI model. Melatonin, a pineal gland secretory hormone associated with the regulation of circadian rhythms and homeostasis, also enhances the function of MSCs via several biological activities [94–96]. Pretreatment with melatonin significantly increases the survival of MSCs injected into damaged sites and the surviving MSCs improved angiogenesis, increased renal cell proliferation, and enhanced renal function in a renal ischemia model [88]. In addition, in a model of ischemic disease associated with CKD, melatonin pretreatment ameliorated oxidative stress and senescence by enhancing PrP^{C}-mediated mitochondrial function [97]. In an in vivo model of ischemia, the administration of melatonin-pretreated MSCs increased the secretion of angiogenic cytokines and the survival of engrafted MSCs in CKD-associated ischemic sites. Fucoidan is a sulfated polysaccharide extracted from brown algae and seaweed. It shows diverse biological activities, such as anti-inflammation and antioxidant effects [98]. In a p-cresol-induced CKD model, fucoidan treatment inhibits the senescence of MSCs and increase cell proliferation via FAK-Akt-TWIST signal transduction. In addition, in a murine model of hind limb ischemia associated with CKD, fucoidan-treated MSCs show immunomodulatory activity and enhance cell proliferation, angiogenesis, and recovery of the damaged zone [99].

After administration of MSCs, their effects are limited by a poor environment. Anoikis is a general symptom of kidney disease that is characterized by a deficit of anchorage-dependent attachment to the extracellular matrix [100]. Therefore, to mimic the cellular microenvironment in vivo, a novel strategy is necessary to study the supply of extracellular matrix components. A thermosensitive hydrogel may supply a microenvironment similar to the environment in vivo and increase the survival rate of engrafted cells [101,102]. One study has shown that a chitosan-based hydrogel is a suitable carrier material to deliver MSCs into sites of IR-induced injury in a rat model of AKI. This hydrogel scaffold enhances the retention and survival of transplanted MSCs in harsh conditions. In another study, an IGF-1C domain-modified chitosan hydrogel was synthesized. This hydrogel scaffold was shown to protect cells from H_2O_2 treatment and reduce apoptosis [103] (Table 3).

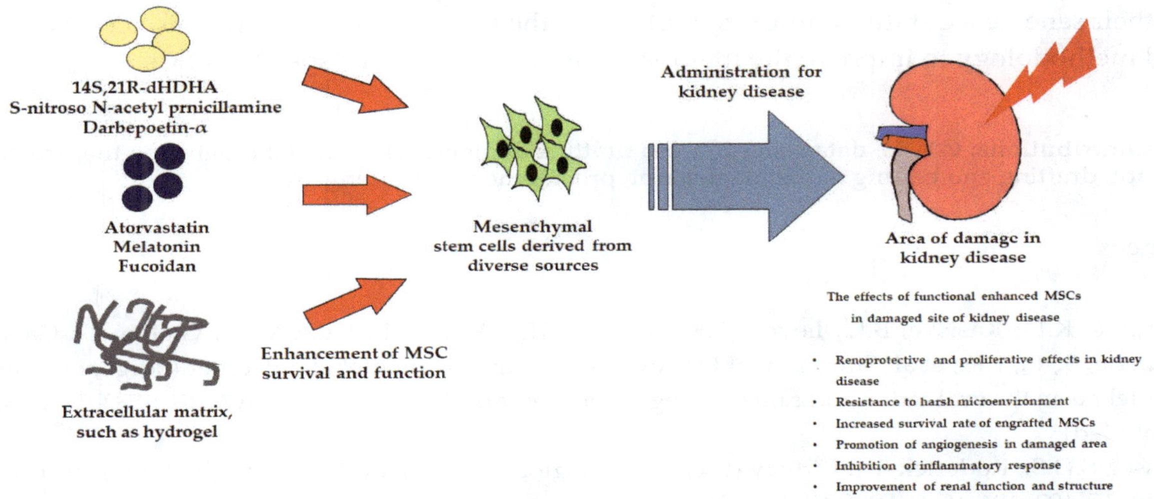

Figure 3. Schematic illustration of the use of active biological factors to enhance MSC functionality for the treatment of kidney disease.

Table 3. Effects of functionally enhanced MSCs in the treatment of kidney disease.

Pathological Condition	Type of Source	Findings	Reference
Renal IRI	14S,21R-dHDHA	Enhancement of MSC function, reduction of apoptosis and inflammatory response, improvement of renal function	[90]
Renal IRI	SNP	Cyto-protective and tissue-protective effects, promotion of MSC functionality (proliferation, survival)	[91]
Renal IRI	DPO	Protective and hematopoietic effects, reduction in kidney damage	[92]
Renal IRI	Ator	Improvement of renal function and survival of engrafted MSCs	[93]
Ischemic disease with CKD	Melatonin	Reduction in oxidative stress and senescence, increase in angiogenesis and injected MSC survival	[97]
CKD	Fucoidan	Inhibition of MSC senescence, increased cell proliferation, enhancement of immunomodulatory activity, recovery of damaged zone	[99]
AKI	chitosan-based hydrogel	Enhancement of transplanted MSC retention and survival, protection of MSC from oxidative stress, reduction of apoptosis	[103]

6. Conclusions

Experimental evidence and clinical trials have demonstrated the feasibility, safety, and efficacy of using MSCs for kidney disease therapy. However, there is still some doubt about the real effects of MSCs on kidney disease. This review has shown that MSCs can be used as therapeutic agents for acute and chronic kidney disease. However, despite the therapeutic potential of MSCs, their use is restricted due to the low survival rate in conditions of inflammation and oxidative stress at sites of injury. In addition, when MSCs are derived from patients with kidney disease for use as autologous MSCs, their function is compromised due to the poor health of the patient. Therefore, novel methods are required to improve the therapeutic efficacy of MSCs under pathophysiological conditions. In this review, we suggest various methods for improving the functionality of MSCs, to enhance their therapeutic potential for kidney disease. The characteristics of MSCs significantly differ depending on their site of origin, their senescence status, and the symptoms of the patient. Therefore, it is also critical to develop optimal methodology to improve the therapeutic efficacy of patient-specific MSCs.

Author Contributions: C.W.Y.: data collection and drafting of manuscript; S.H.L.: organizing the structure of the manuscript, drafting and editing of the manuscript, procurement of funding.

References

1. Lentine, K.L.; Kasiske, B.L.; Levey, A.S.; Adams, P.L.; Alberu, J.; Bakr, M.A.; Gallon, L.; Garvey, C.A.; Guleria, S.; Li, P.K.; et al. Summary of kidney disease: Improving global outcomes (kdigo) clinical practice guideline on the evaluation and care of living kidney donors. *Transplantation* **2017**, *101*, 1783–1792. [CrossRef] [PubMed]
2. Fraser, S.D.S.; Roderick, P.J. Kidney disease in the global burden of disease study 2017. *Nat. Rev. Nephrol.* **2019**, *15*, 193–194. [CrossRef] [PubMed]
3. Susantitaphong, P.; Cruz, D.N.; Cerda, J.; Abulfaraj, M.; Alqahtani, F.; Koulouridis, I.; Jaber, B.L.; Acute Kidney Injury Advisory Group of the American Society of Nephrology. World incidence of aki: A meta-analysis. *Clin. J. Am. Soc. Nephrol.* **2013**, *8*, 1482–1493. [CrossRef] [PubMed]
4. English, P.B. Acute renal failure in the dog and cat. *Aust. Vet. J.* **1974**, *50*, 384–392. [CrossRef] [PubMed]
5. Rahman, M.; Shad, F.; Smith, M.C. Acute kidney injury: A guide to diagnosis and management. *Am. Fam. Phys.* **2012**, *86*, 631–639.
6. Aghajani Nargesi, A.; Lerman, L.O.; Eirin, A. Mesenchymal stem cell-derived extracellular vesicles for kidney repair: Current status and looming challenges. *Stem Cell Res. Ther.* **2017**, *8*, 273. [CrossRef]
7. McFetridge, M.L.; Del Borgo, M.P.; Aguilar, M.I.; Ricardo, S.D. The use of hydrogels for cell-based treatment of chronic kidney disease. *Clin. Sci.* **2018**, *132*, 1977–1994. [CrossRef] [PubMed]
8. Chawla, L.S.; Kimmel, P.L. Acute kidney injury and chronic kidney disease: An integrated clinical syndrome. *Kidney Int.* **2012**, *82*, 516–524. [CrossRef]
9. Choi, J.R.; Yong, K.W.; Choi, J.Y. Effects of mechanical loading on human mesenchymal stem cells for cartilage tissue engineering. *J. Cell. Physiol.* **2018**, *233*, 1913–1928. [CrossRef]
10. Wan Safwani, W.K.Z.; Choi, J.R.; Yong, K.W.; Ting, I.; Mat Adenan, N.A.; Pingguan-Murphy, B. Hypoxia enhances the viability, growth and chondrogenic potential of cryopreserved human adipose-derived stem cells. *Cryobiology* **2017**, *75*, 91–99. [CrossRef]
11. Chamberlain, G.; Fox, J.; Ashton, B.; Middleton, J. Concise review: Mesenchymal stem cells: Their phenotype, differentiation capacity, immunological features, and potential for homing. *Stem Cells* **2007**, *25*, 2739–2749. [CrossRef] [PubMed]
12. Bruno, S.; Chiabotto, G.; Camussi, G. Concise review: Different mesenchymal stromal/stem cell populations reside in the adult kidney. *Stem Cells Transl. Med.* **2014**, *3*, 1451–1455. [CrossRef]
13. Choi, J.R.; Pingguan-Murphy, B.; Wan Abas, W.A.; Yong, K.W.; Poon, C.T.; Noor Azmi, M.A.; Omar, S.Z.; Chua, K.H.; Xu, F.; Wan Safwani, W.K. In situ normoxia enhances survival and proliferation rate of human adipose tissue-derived stromal cells without increasing the risk of tumourigenesis. *PLoS ONE* **2015**, *10*, e0115034. [CrossRef] [PubMed]
14. Kramann, R.; Humphreys, B.D. Kidney pericytes: Roles in regeneration and fibrosis. *Semin. Nephrol.* **2014**, *34*, 374–383. [CrossRef] [PubMed]
15. Jia, X.; Pan, J.; Li, X.; Li, N.; Han, Y.; Feng, X.; Cui, J. Bone marrow mesenchymal stromal cells ameliorate angiogenesis and renal damage via promoting pi3k-akt signaling pathway activation in vivo. *Cytotherapy* **2016**, *18*, 838–845. [CrossRef]
16. Casiraghi, F.; Perico, N.; Cortinovis, M.; Remuzzi, G. Mesenchymal stromal cells in renal transplantation: Opportunities and challenges. *Nat. Rev. Nephrol.* **2016**, *12*, 241–253. [CrossRef]
17. Villanueva, S.; Ewertz, E.; Carrion, F.; Tapia, A.; Vergara, C.; Cespedes, C.; Saez, P.J.; Luz, P.; Irarrazabal, C.; Carreno, J.E.; et al. Mesenchymal stem cell injection ameliorates chronic renal failure in a rat model. *Clin. Sci.* **2011**, *121*, 489–499. [CrossRef]

18. Idziak, M.; Pedzisz, P.; Burdzinska, A.; Gala, K.; Paczek, L. Uremic toxins impair human bone marrow-derived mesenchymal stem cells functionality in vitro. *Exp. Toxicol. Pathol.* **2014**, *66*, 187–194. [CrossRef] [PubMed]
19. Yoon, Y.M.; Han, Y.S.; Yun, C.W.; Lee, J.H.; Kim, R.; Lee, S.H. Pioglitazone protects mesenchymal stem cells against p-cresol-induced mitochondrial dysfunction via up-regulation of pink-1. *Int. J. Mol. Sci.* **2018**, *19*, 2898. [CrossRef] [PubMed]
20. Lira, R.; Oliveira, M.; Martins, M.; Silva, C.; Carvalho, S.; Stumbo, A.C.; Cortez, E.; Verdoorn, K.; Einicker-Lamas, M.; Thole, A.; et al. Transplantation of bone marrow-derived mscs improves renal function and na(+)+k(+)-atpase activity in rats with renovascular hypertension. *Cell Tissue Res.* **2017**, *369*, 287–301. [CrossRef]
21. Papazova, D.A.; Oosterhuis, N.R.; Gremmels, H.; van Koppen, A.; Joles, J.A.; Verhaar, M.C. Cell-based therapies for experimental chronic kidney disease: A systematic review and meta-analysis. *Dis. Models Mech.* **2015**, *8*, 281–293. [CrossRef]
22. Peired, A.J.; Sisti, A.; Romagnani, P. Mesenchymal stem cell-based therapy for kidney disease: A review of clinical evidence. *Stem Cells Int.* **2016**, *2016*, 4798639. [CrossRef] [PubMed]
23. Zou, X.; Gu, D.; Xing, X.; Cheng, Z.; Gong, D.; Zhang, G.; Zhu, Y. Human mesenchymal stromal cell-derived extracellular vesicles alleviate renal ischemic reperfusion injury and enhance angiogenesis in rats. *Am. J. Transl. Res.* **2016**, *8*, 4289–4299. [PubMed]
24. Ezquer, F.; Ezquer, M.; Simon, V.; Pardo, F.; Yanez, A.; Carpio, D.; Conget, P. Endovenous administration of bone-marrow-derived multipotent mesenchymal stromal cells prevents renal failure in diabetic mice. *Biol. Blood Marrow Transplant.* **2009**, *15*, 1354–1365. [CrossRef] [PubMed]
25. Fang, Y.; Tian, X.; Bai, S.; Fan, J.; Hou, W.; Tong, H.; Li, D. Autologous transplantation of adipose-derived mesenchymal stem cells ameliorates streptozotocin-induced diabetic nephropathy in rats by inhibiting oxidative stress, pro-inflammatory cytokines and the p38 mapk signaling pathway. *Int. J. Mol. Med.* **2012**, *30*, 85–92.
26. Ezquer, F.; Giraud-Billoud, M.; Carpio, D.; Cabezas, F.; Conget, P.; Ezquer, M. Proregenerative microenvironment triggered by donor mesenchymal stem cells preserves renal function and structure in mice with severe diabetes mellitus. *BioMed Res. Int.* **2015**, *2015*, 164703. [CrossRef]
27. Yu, B.; Zhang, X.; Li, X. Exosomes derived from mesenchymal stem cells. *Int. J. Mol. Sci.* **2014**, *15*, 4142–4157. [CrossRef]
28. Lai, R.C.; Chen, T.S.; Lim, S.K. Mesenchymal stem cell exosome: A novel stem cell-based therapy for cardiovascular disease. *Regen. Med.* **2011**, *6*, 481–492. [CrossRef]
29. Eirin, A.; Riester, S.M.; Zhu, X.Y.; Tang, H.; Evans, J.M.; O'Brien, D.; van Wijnen, A.J.; Lerman, L.O. Microrna and mrna cargo of extracellular vesicles from porcine adipose tissue-derived mesenchymal stem cells. *Gene* **2014**, *551*, 55–64. [CrossRef] [PubMed]
30. Koniusz, S.; Andrzejewska, A.; Muraca, M.; Srivastava, A.K.; Janowski, M.; Lukomska, B. Extracellular vesicles in physiology, pathology, and therapy of the immune and central nervous system, with focus on extracellular vesicles derived from mesenchymal stem cells as therapeutic tools. *Front. Cell. Neurosci.* **2016**, *10*, 109. [CrossRef]
31. Nargesi, A.A.; Lerman, L.O.; Eirin, A. Mesenchymal stem cell-derived extracellular vesicles for renal repair. *Curr. Gene Ther.* **2017**, *17*, 29–42. [CrossRef] [PubMed]
32. Wu, V.C.; Wu, C.H.; Huang, T.M.; Wang, C.Y.; Lai, C.F.; Shiao, C.C.; Chang, C.H.; Lin, S.L.; Chen, Y.Y.; Chen, Y.M.; et al. Long-term risk of coronary events after aki. *J. Am. Soc. Nephrol.* **2014**, *25*, 595–605. [CrossRef] [PubMed]
33. Kumate, J.; Sepulveda-Amor, J.; Valdespino, J.L.; de Mucha, J.; Diaz-Ortega, J.L.; Garcia-Sainz, J.A.; Ruiz-Puente, J.; Jimenez-Paredes, J.; Ruiz-Arriaga, A.; Gutierrez, G.; et al. Mexican contributions to vaccines. *Gac. Med. Mex.* **1988**, *124*, 73–97. [PubMed]
34. Malek, M.; Nematbakhsh, M. Renal ischemia/reperfusion injury; from pathophysiology to treatment. *J. Ren. Inj. Prev.* **2015**, *4*, 20–27. [PubMed]
35. Gatti, S.; Bruno, S.; Deregibus, M.C.; Sordi, A.; Cantaluppi, V.; Tetta, C.; Camussi, G. Microvesicles derived from human adult mesenchymal stem cells protect against ischaemia-reperfusion-induced acute and chronic kidney injury. *Nephrol. Dial. Transplant.* **2011**, *26*, 1474–1483. [CrossRef]
36. Lindoso, R.S.; Collino, F.; Bruno, S.; Araujo, D.S.; Sant'Anna, J.F.; Tetta, C.; Provero, P.; Quesenberry, P.J.; Vieyra, A.; Einicker-Lamas, M.; et al. Extracellular vesicles released from mesenchymal stromal cells modulate mirna in renal tubular cells and inhibit atp depletion injury. *Stem Cells Dev.* **2014**, *23*, 1809–1819.

[CrossRef]

37. Zhang, G.; Zou, X.; Miao, S.; Chen, J.; Du, T.; Zhong, L.; Ju, G.; Liu, G.; Zhu, Y. The anti-oxidative role of micro-vesicles derived from human wharton-jelly mesenchymal stromal cells through nox2/gp91(phox) suppression in alleviating renal ischemia-reperfusion injury in rats. *PLoS ONE* **2014**, *9*, e92129. [CrossRef]
38. Squillaro, T.; Peluso, G.; Galderisi, U. Clinical trials with mesenchymal stem cells: An update. *Cell Transplant.* **2016**, *25*, 829–848. [CrossRef]
39. Zeldich, E.; Chen, C.D.; Colvin, T.A.; Bove-Fenderson, E.A.; Liang, J.; Tucker Zhou, T.B.; Harris, D.A.; Abraham, C.R. The neuroprotective effect of klotho is mediated via regulation of members of the redox system. *J. Biol. Chem.* **2014**, *289*, 24700–24715. [CrossRef] [PubMed]
40. Oh, H.J.; Nam, B.Y.; Lee, M.J.; Kim, C.H.; Koo, H.M.; Doh, F.M.; Han, J.H.; Kim, E.J.; Han, J.S.; Park, J.T.; et al. Decreased circulating klotho levels in patients undergoing dialysis and relationship to oxidative stress and inflammation. *Perit. Dial. Int.* **2015**, *35*, 43–51. [CrossRef]
41. Geng, Y.; Zhang, L.; Fu, B.; Zhang, J.; Hong, Q.; Hu, J.; Li, D.; Luo, C.; Cui, S.; Zhu, F.; et al. Mesenchymal stem cells ameliorate rhabdomyolysis-induced acute kidney injury via the activation of m2 macrophages. *Stem Cell Res. Ther.* **2014**, *5*, 80. [CrossRef] [PubMed]
42. Lee, S.J.; Ryu, M.O.; Seo, M.S.; Park, S.B.; Ahn, J.O.; Han, S.M.; Kang, K.S.; Bhang, D.H.; Youn, H.Y. Mesenchymal stem cells contribute to improvement of renal function in a canine kidney injury model. *In Vivo* **2017**, *31*, 1115–1124.
43. Rodrigues, C.E.; Capcha, J.M.; de Braganca, A.C.; Sanches, T.R.; Gouveia, P.Q.; de Oliveira, P.A.; Malheiros, D.M.; Volpini, R.A.; Santinho, M.A.; Santana, B.A.; et al. Human umbilical cord-derived mesenchymal stromal cells protect against premature renal senescence resulting from oxidative stress in rats with acute kidney injury. *Stem Cell Res. Ther.* **2017**, *8*, 19. [CrossRef] [PubMed]
44. Togel, F.; Hu, Z.; Weiss, K.; Isaac, J.; Lange, C.; Westenfelder, C. Administered mesenchymal stem cells protect against ischemic acute renal failure through differentiation-independent mechanisms. *Am. J. Physiol. Ren. Physiol.* **2005**, *289*, F31–F42. [CrossRef]
45. Lai, R.C.; Yeo, R.W.; Lim, S.K. Mesenchymal stem cell exosomes. *Semin. Cell Dev. Biol.* **2015**, *40*, 82–88. [CrossRef]
46. Bellomo, R.; Kellum, J.A.; Ronco, C. Acute kidney injury. *Lancet* **2012**, *380*, 756–766. [CrossRef]
47. Togel, F.E.; Westenfelder, C. Kidney protection and regeneration following acute injury: Progress through stem cell therapy. *Am. J. Kidney Dis.* **2012**, *60*, 1012–1022. [CrossRef] [PubMed]
48. National Kidney, F. K/doqi clinical practice guidelines for chronic kidney disease: Evaluation, classification, and stratification. *Am. J. Kidney Dis.* **2002**, *39* (Suppl. 1), S1–S266.
49. Bruck, K.; Stel, V.S.; Fraser, S.; De Goeij, M.C.; Caskey, F.; Abu-Hanna, A.; Jager, K.J. Translational research in nephrology: Chronic kidney disease prevention and public health. *Clin. Kidney J.* **2015**, *8*, 647–655. [CrossRef]
50. Heywood, J.T.; Fonarow, G.C.; Costanzo, M.R.; Mathur, V.S.; Wigneswaran, J.R.; Wynne, J.; ADHERE Scientific Advisory Committee and Investigators. High prevalence of renal dysfunction and its impact on outcome in 118,465 patients hospitalized with acute decompensated heart failure: A report from the adhere database. *J. Card. Fail.* **2007**, *13*, 422–430. [CrossRef]
51. Tonelli, M.; Riella, M.C. Chronic kidney disease and the aging population. *Kidney Int.* **2014**, *85*, 487–491. [CrossRef]
52. Nugent, R.A.; Fathima, S.F.; Feigl, A.B.; Chyung, D. The burden of chronic kidney disease on developing nations: A 21st century challenge in global health. *Nephron. Clin. Pract.* **2011**, *118*, c269–c277. [CrossRef]
53. Thi Do, D.; Phan, N.N.; Wang, C.Y.; Sun, Z.; Lin, Y.C. Novel regulations of mef2-a, mef2-d, and cacna1s in the functional incompetence of adipose-derived mesenchymal stem cells by induced indoxyl sulfate in chronic kidney disease. *Cytotechnology* **2016**, *68*, 2589–2604. [CrossRef]
54. Meijers, B.K.; Claes, K.; Bammens, B.; de Loor, H.; Viaene, L.; Verbeke, K.; Kuypers, D.; Vanrenterghem, Y.; Evenepoel, P. P-cresol and cardiovascular risk in mild-to-moderate kidney disease. *Clin. J. Am. Soc. Nephrol.* **2010**, *5*, 1182–1189. [CrossRef]
55. Lee, S.R.; Lee, S.H.; Moon, J.Y.; Park, J.Y.; Lee, D.; Lim, S.J.; Jeong, K.H.; Park, J.K.; Lee, T.W.; Ihm, C.G. Repeated administration of bone marrow-derived mesenchymal stem cells improved the protective effects on a remnant kidney model. *Ren. Fail.* **2010**, *32*, 840–848. [CrossRef] [PubMed]
56. Wu, H.J.; Yiu, W.H.; Li, R.X.; Wong, D.W.; Leung, J.C.; Chan, L.Y.; Zhang, Y.; Lian, Q.; Lin, M.; Tse, H.F.; et al. Mesenchymal stem cells modulate albumin-induced renal tubular inflammation and fibrosis. *PLoS ONE* **2014**, *9*, e90883. [CrossRef]

57. Makhlough, A.; Shekarchian, S.; Moghadasali, R.; Einollahi, B.; Hosseini, S.E.; Jaroughi, N.; Bolurieh, T.; Baharvand, H.; Aghdami, N. Safety and tolerability of autologous bone marrow mesenchymal stromal cells in adpkd patients. *Stem Cell Res. Ther.* **2017**, *8*, 116. [CrossRef] [PubMed]
58. Camilleri, E.T.; Gustafson, M.P.; Dudakovic, A.; Riester, S.M.; Garces, C.G.; Paradise, C.R.; Takai, H.; Karperien, M.; Cool, S.; Sampen, H.J.; et al. Identification and validation of multiple cell surface markers of clinical-grade adipose-derived mesenchymal stromal cells as novel release criteria for good manufacturing practice-compliant production. *Stem Cell Res. Ther.* **2016**, *7*, 107. [CrossRef] [PubMed]
59. Saran, R.; Robinson, B.; Abbott, K.C.; Agodoa, L.Y.C.; Bhave, N.; Bragg-Gresham, J.; Balkrishnan, R.; Dietrich, X.; Eckard, A.; Eggers, P.W.; et al. Us renal data system 2017 annual data report: Epidemiology of kidney disease in the united states. *Am. J. Kidney Dis.* **2018**, *71*, A7. [CrossRef]
60. Gallagher, H.; Suckling, R.J. Diabetic nephropathy: Where are we on the journey from pathophysiology to treatment? *Diabetes Obes. Metab.* **2016**, *18*, 641–647. [CrossRef] [PubMed]
61. Abdel Aziz, M.T.; Wassef, M.A.; Ahmed, H.H.; Rashed, L.; Mahfouz, S.; Aly, M.I.; Hussein, R.E.; Abdelaziz, M. The role of bone marrow derived-mesenchymal stem cells in attenuation of kidney function in rats with diabetic nephropathy. *Diabetol. Metab. Syndr.* **2014**, *6*, 34. [CrossRef] [PubMed]
62. Ezquer, M.E.; Ezquer, F.E.; Arango-Rodriguez, M.L.; Conget, P.A. Msc transplantation: A promising therapeutic strategy to manage the onset and progression of diabetic nephropathy. *Biol. Res.* **2012**, *45*, 289–296. [CrossRef]
63. Srisawat, N.; Kellum, J.A. Acute kidney injury: Definition, epidemiology, and outcome. *Curr. Opin. Crit. Care* **2011**, *17*, 548–555. [CrossRef] [PubMed]
64. Zou, X.; Zhang, G.; Cheng, Z.; Yin, D.; Du, T.; Ju, G.; Miao, S.; Liu, G.; Lu, M.; Zhu, Y. Microvesicles derived from human wharton's jelly mesenchymal stromal cells ameliorate renal ischemia-reperfusion injury in rats by suppressing cx3cl1. *Stem Cell Res. Ther.* **2014**, *5*, 40. [CrossRef]
65. Perazella, M.A. Drug-induced renal failure: Update on new medications and unique mechanisms of nephrotoxicity. *Am. J. Med Sci.* **2003**, *325*, 349–362. [CrossRef] [PubMed]
66. Ghane Shahrbaf, F.; Assadi, F. Drug-induced renal disorders. *J. Ren. Inj. Prev.* **2015**, *4*, 57–60. [PubMed]
67. Nash, K.; Hafeez, A.; Hou, S. Hospital-acquired renal insufficiency. *Am. J. Kidney Dis.* **2002**, *39*, 930–936. [CrossRef]
68. Miller, R.P.; Tadagavadi, R.K.; Ramesh, G.; Reeves, W.B. Mechanisms of cisplatin nephrotoxicity. *Toxins* **2010**, *2*, 2490–2518. [CrossRef] [PubMed]
69. Silici, S.; Ekmekcioglu, O.; Kanbur, M.; Deniz, K. The protective effect of royal jelly against cisplatin-induced renal oxidative stress in rats. *World J. Urol.* **2011**, *29*, 127–132. [CrossRef]
70. Zhou, Y.; Xu, H.; Xu, W.; Wang, B.; Wu, H.; Tao, Y.; Zhang, B.; Wang, M.; Mao, F.; Yan, Y.; et al. Exosomes released by human umbilical cord mesenchymal stem cells protect against cisplatin-induced renal oxidative stress and apoptosis in vivo and in vitro. *Stem Cell Res. Ther.* **2013**, *4*, 34. [CrossRef] [PubMed]
71. Wang, B.; Jia, H.; Zhang, B.; Wang, J.; Ji, C.; Zhu, X.; Yan, Y.; Yin, L.; Yu, J.; Qian, H.; et al. Pre-incubation with hucmsc-exosomes prevents cisplatin-induced nephrotoxicity by activating autophagy. *Stem Cell Res. Ther.* **2017**, *8*, 75. [CrossRef] [PubMed]
72. Bruno, S.; Tapparo, M.; Collino, F.; Chiabotto, G.; Deregibus, M.C.; Soares Lindoso, R.; Neri, F.; Kholia, S.; Giunti, S.; Wen, S.; et al. Renal regenerative potential of different extracellular vesicle populations derived from bone marrow mesenchymal stromal cells. *Tissue Eng. Part A* **2017**, *23*, 1262–1273. [CrossRef]
73. Collino, F.; Bruno, S.; Incarnato, D.; Dettori, D.; Neri, F.; Provero, P.; Pomatto, M.; Oliviero, S.; Tetta, C.; Quesenberry, P.J.; et al. Aki recovery induced by mesenchymal stromal cell-derived extracellular vesicles carrying micrornas. *J. Am. Soc. Nephrol.* **2015**, *26*, 2349–2360. [CrossRef] [PubMed]
74. Grange, C.; Iampietro, C.; Bussolati, B. Stem cell extracellular vesicles and kidney injury. *Stem Cell Investig.* **2017**, *4*, 90. [CrossRef] [PubMed]
75. Ritchie, J.; Green, D.; Alderson, H.V.; Chiu, D.; Sinha, S.; Kalra, P.A. Risks for mortality and renal replacement therapy in atherosclerotic renovascular disease compared with other causes of chronic kidney disease. *Nephrology* **2015**, *20*, 688–696. [CrossRef]
76. Zhang, X.; Li, Z.L.; Woollard, J.R.; Eirin, A.; Ebrahimi, B.; Crane, J.A.; Zhu, X.Y.; Pawar, A.S.; Krier, J.D.; Jordan, K.L.; et al. Obesity-metabolic derangement preserves hemodynamics but promotes intrarenal adiposity and macrophage infiltration in swine renovascular disease. *Am. J. Physiol. Ren. Physiol.* **2013**, *305*, F265–F276. [CrossRef]
77. Eirin, A.; Zhu, X.Y.; Puranik, A.S.; Tang, H.; McGurren, K.A.; van Wijnen, A.J.; Lerman, A.; Lerman, L.O.

Mesenchymal stem cell-derived extracellular vesicles attenuate kidney inflammation. *Kidney Int.* **2017**, *92*, 114–124. [CrossRef] [PubMed]

78. Eirin, A.; Zhu, X.Y.; Jonnada, S.; Lerman, A.; van Wijnen, A.J.; Lerman, L.O. Mesenchymal stem cell-derived extracellular vesicles improve the renal microvasculature in metabolic renovascular disease in swine. *Cell Transplant.* **2018**, *27*, 1080–1095. [CrossRef]
79. Ucero, A.C.; Benito-Martin, A.; Izquierdo, M.C.; Sanchez-Nino, M.D.; Sanz, A.B.; Ramos, A.M.; Berzal, S.; Ruiz-Ortega, M.; Egido, J.; Ortiz, A. Unilateral ureteral obstruction: Beyond obstruction. *Int. Urol. Nephrol.* **2014**, *46*, 765–776. [CrossRef] [PubMed]
80. He, J.; Wang, Y.; Lu, X.; Zhu, B.; Pei, X.; Wu, J.; Zhao, W. Micro-vesicles derived from bone marrow stem cells protect the kidney both in vivo and in vitro by microrna-dependent repairing. *Nephrology* **2015**, *20*, 591–600. [CrossRef]
81. Choi, H.Y.; Lee, H.G.; Kim, B.S.; Ahn, S.H.; Jung, A.; Lee, M.; Lee, J.E.; Kim, H.J.; Ha, S.K.; Park, H.C. Mesenchymal stem cell-derived microparticles ameliorate peritubular capillary rarefaction via inhibition of endothelial-mesenchymal transition and decrease tubulointerstitial fibrosis in unilateral ureteral obstruction. *Stem Cell Res. Ther.* **2015**, *6*, 18. [CrossRef]
82. Nassar, W.; El-Ansary, M.; Sabry, D.; Mostafa, M.A.; Fayad, T.; Kotb, E.; Temraz, M.; Saad, A.N.; Essa, W.; Adel, H. Umbilical cord mesenchymal stem cells derived extracellular vesicles can safely ameliorate the progression of chronic kidney diseases. *Biomater. Res.* **2016**, *20*, 21. [CrossRef] [PubMed]
83. Martinez-Castelao, A.; Navarro-Gonzalez, J.F.; Gorriz, J.L.; de Alvaro, F. The concept and the epidemiology of diabetic nephropathy have changed in recent years. *J. Clin. Med.* **2015**, *4*, 1207–1216. [CrossRef] [PubMed]
84. Ebrahim, N.; Ahmed, I.A.; Hussien, N.I.; Dessouky, A.A.; Farid, A.S.; Elshazly, A.M.; Mostafa, O.; Gazzar, W.B.E.; Sorour, S.M.; Seleem, Y.; et al. Mesenchymal stem cell-derived exosomes ameliorated diabetic nephropathy by autophagy induction through the mtor signaling pathway. *Cells* **2018**, *7*, 226. [CrossRef] [PubMed]
85. Jiang, Z.Z.; Liu, Y.M.; Niu, X.; Yin, J.Y.; Hu, B.; Guo, S.C.; Fan, Y.; Wang, Y.; Wang, N.S. Exosomes secreted by human urine-derived stem cells could prevent kidney complications from type i diabetes in rats. *Stem Cell Res. Ther.* **2016**, *7*, 24. [CrossRef] [PubMed]
86. Burst, V.R.; Gillis, M.; Putsch, F.; Herzog, R.; Fischer, J.H.; Heid, P.; Muller-Ehmsen, J.; Schenk, K.; Fries, J.W.; Baldamus, C.A.; et al. Poor cell survival limits the beneficial impact of mesenchymal stem cell transplantation on acute kidney injury. *Nephron Exp. Nephrol.* **2010**, *114*, e107–e116. [CrossRef] [PubMed]
87. He, N.; Zhang, L.; Cui, J.; Li, Z. Bone marrow vascular niche: Home for hematopoietic stem cells. *Bone Marrow Res.* **2014**, *2014*, 128436. [CrossRef] [PubMed]
88. Mias, C.; Trouche, E.; Seguelas, M.H.; Calcagno, F.; Dignat-George, F.; Sabatier, F.; Piercecchi-Marti, M.D.; Daniel, L.; Bianchi, P.; Calise, D.; et al. Ex vivo pretreatment with melatonin improves survival, proangiogenic/mitogenic activity, and efficiency of mesenchymal stem cells injected into ischemic kidney. *Stem Cells* **2008**, *26*, 1749–1757. [CrossRef]
89. Manning, B.D.; Toker, A. Akt/pkb signaling: Navigating the network. *Cell* **2017**, *169*, 381–405. [CrossRef] [PubMed]
90. Tian, H.; Lu, Y.; Shah, S.P.; Wang, Q.; Hong, S. 14s,21r-dihydroxy-docosahexaenoic acid treatment enhances mesenchymal stem cell amelioration of renal ischemia/reperfusion injury. *Stem Cells Dev.* **2012**, *21*, 1187–1199. [CrossRef] [PubMed]
91. Masoud, M.S.; Anwar, S.S.; Afzal, M.Z.; Mehmood, A.; Khan, S.N.; Riazuddin, S. Pre-conditioned mesenchymal stem cells ameliorate renal ischemic injury in rats by augmented survival and engraftment. *J. Transl. Med.* **2012**, *10*, 243. [CrossRef]
92. Altun, B.; Yilmaz, R.; Aki, T.; Akoglu, H.; Zeybek, D.; Piskinpasa, S.; Uckan, D.; Purali, N.; Korkusuz, P.; Turgan, C. Use of mesenchymal stem cells and darbepoetin improve ischemia-induced acute kidney injury outcomes. *Am. J. Nephrol.* **2012**, *35*, 531–539. [CrossRef]
93. Cai, J.; Yu, X.; Zhang, B.; Zhang, H.; Fang, Y.; Liu, S.; Liu, T.; Ding, X. Atorvastatin improves survival of implanted stem cells in a rat model of renal ischemia-reperfusion injury. *Am. J. Nephrol.* **2014**, *39*, 466–475. [CrossRef]
94. Fernandez, A.; Ordonez, R.; Reiter, R.J.; Gonzalez-Gallego, J.; Mauriz, J.L. Melatonin and endoplasmic reticulum stress: Relation to autophagy and apoptosis. *J. Pineal Res.* **2015**, *59*, 292–307. [CrossRef] [PubMed]
95. Reiter, R.J.; Mayo, J.C.; Tan, D.X.; Sainz, R.M.; Alatorre-Jimenez, M.; Qin, L. Melatonin as an antioxidant: Under promises but over delivers. *J. Pineal Res.* **2016** *61*, 253–278. [CrossRef]

96. Mauriz, J.L.; Collado, P.S.; Veneroso, C.; Reiter, R.J.; Gonzalez-Gallego, J. A review of the molecular aspects of melatonin's anti-inflammatory actions: Recent insights and new perspectives. *J. Pineal Res.* **2013**, *54*, 1–14. [CrossRef] [PubMed]
97. Han, Y.S.; Kim, S.M.; Lee, J.H.; Jung, S.K.; Noh, H.; Lee, S.H. Melatonin protects chronic kidney disease mesenchymal stem cells against senescence via prp(c)-dependent enhancement of the mitochondrial function. *J. Pineal Res.* **2019**, *66*, e12535. [CrossRef]
98. Lee, J.H.; Yun, C.W.; Hur, J.; Lee, S.H. Fucoidan rescues p-cresol-induced cellular senescence in mesenchymal stem cells via fak-akt-twist axis. *Mar. Drugs* **2018**, *16*, 121. [CrossRef] [PubMed]
99. Han, Y.S.; Lee, J.H.; Jung, J.S.; Noh, H.; Baek, M.J.; Ryu, J.M.; Yoon, Y.M.; Han, H.J.; Lee, S.H. Fucoidan protects mesenchymal stem cells against oxidative stress and enhances vascular regeneration in a murine hindlimb ischemia model. *Int. J. Cardiol.* **2015**, *198*, 187–195. [CrossRef]
100. Taddei, M.L.; Giannoni, E.; Fiaschi, T.; Chiarugi, P. Anoikis: An emerging hallmark in health and diseases. *J. Pathol.* **2012**, *226*, 380–393. [CrossRef] [PubMed]
101. Christman, K.L.; Vardanian, A.J.; Fang, Q.; Sievers, R.E.; Fok, H.H.; Lee, R.J. Injectable fibrin scaffold improves cell transplant survival, reduces infarct expansion, and induces neovasculature formation in ischemic myocardium. *J. Am. Coll. Cardiol.* **2004**, *44*, 654–660. [CrossRef] [PubMed]
102. Davis, M.E.; Motion, J.P.; Narmoneva, D.A.; Takahashi, T.; Hakuno, D.; Kamm, R.D.; Zhang, S.; Lee, R.T. Injectable self-assembling peptide nanofibers create intramyocardial microenvironments for endothelial cells. *Circulation* **2005**, *111*, 442–450. [CrossRef] [PubMed]
103. Feng, G.; Zhang, J.; Li, Y.; Nie, Y.; Zhu, D.; Wang, R.; Liu, J.; Gao, J.; Liu, N.; He, N.; et al. Igf-1 c domain-modified hydrogel enhances cell therapy for aki. *J. Am. Soc. Nephrol.* **2016**, *27*, 2357–2369. [CrossRef] [PubMed]

LPS-Binding Protein Modulates Acute Renal Fibrosis by Inducing Pericyte-to-Myofibroblast Trans-Differentiation through TLR-4 Signaling

Giuseppe Castellano [1,*,†], Alessandra Stasi [1,†], Rossana Franzin [1], Fabio Sallustio [1,2], Chiara Divella [1], Alessandra Spinelli [1], Giuseppe Stefano Netti [3], Enrico Fiaccadori [4], Vincenzo Cantaluppi [5], Antonio Crovace [6], Francesco Staffieri [6], Luca Lacitignola [6], Giuseppe Grandaliano [3], Simona Simone [1], Giovanni Battista Pertosa [1] and Loreto Gesualdo [1]

1 Nephrology, Dialysis and Transplantation Unit, Department of Emergency and Organ Transplantation, University of Bari, 70124 Bari, Italy
2 Department of Basic Medical Sciences, Neuroscience and Sense Organs, University of Bari, 70124 Bari, Italy
3 Nephrology, Dialysis and Transplantation Unit, Department of Medical and Surgical Sciences, University of Foggia, 71122 Foggia, Italy
4 Nephrology Unit, Department of Medicine and Surgery, University of Parma, 43121 Parma, Italy
5 Department of Translational Medicine, University of Piemonte Orientale, 28100 Novara, Italy
6 Veterinary Surgery Unit, Department of Emergency and Organ Transplantation, University of Bari, 70010 Bari, Italy
* Correspondence: giuseppe.castellano@uniba.it
† These two authors equally contributed to the present study.

Abstract: During sepsis, the increased synthesis of circulating lipopolysaccharide (LPS)-binding protein (LBP) activates LPS/TLR4 signaling in renal resident cells, leading to acute kidney injury (AKI). Pericytes are the major source of myofibroblasts during chronic kidney disease (CKD), but their involvement in AKI is poorly understood. Here, we investigate the occurrence of pericyte-to-myofibroblast trans-differentiation (PMT) in sepsis-induced AKI. In a swine model of sepsis-induced AKI, PMT was detected within 9 h from LPS injection, as evaluated by the reduction of physiologic PDGFRβ expression and the dysfunctional α-SMA increase in peritubular pericytes. The therapeutic intervention by citrate-based coupled plasma filtration adsorption (CPFA) significantly reduced LBP, TGF-β, and endothelin-1 (ET-1) serum levels, and furthermore preserved PDGFRβ and decreased α-SMA expression in renal biopsies. In vitro, both LPS and septic sera led to PMT with a significant increase in Collagen I synthesis and α-SMA reorganization in contractile fibers by both SMAD2/3-dependent and -independent TGF-β signaling. Interestingly, the removal of LBP from septic plasma inhibited PMT. Finally, LPS-stimulated pericytes secreted LBP and TGF-β and underwent PMT also upon TGF-β receptor-blocking, indicating the crucial pro-fibrotic role of TLR4 signaling. Our data demonstrate that the selective removal of LBP may represent a therapeutic option to prevent PMT and the development of acute renal fibrosis in sepsis-induced AKI.

Keywords: LPS-binding protein; fibrosis; pericyte; myofibroblast; endotoxemia-induced oliguric kidney injury

---

1. Introduction

Sepsis is a multi-organ disease and represents a systemic immune response to a bacterial infection. In critically ill patients, sepsis is the major cause of acute kidney injury (AKI) and is associated with high mortality or risk of chronic kidney disease (CKD) [1]. The pathophysiology of sepsis-induced AKI is complex and characterized by an overwhelming inflammatory response that leads to metabolic dysfunction, tubular damage, and microvascular dysfunction [2,3]. The most common bacteria involved in sepsis-induced

AKI are gram-negative, since their outer wall component, named lipopolysaccharide (LPS) or endotoxin, can activate a wide variety of cells through interaction with specific pattern recognition receptors (PRR), such as TLRs (toll-like receptors) [4]. In the kidney, LPS is mainly recognized by TLR4, which is expressed by tubular, endothelial cells [2,5] and pericytes [6]. The cellular response to endotoxin requires a shuttle protein—LPS-binding protein (LBP)—that brings LPS to TLR4 and maximizes intracellular signaling [7–12].

Renal pericytes are a large population of resident stromal cells lining the peritubular capillaries that stabilize the endothelium. Recently, Heng Zeng et al. evaluated the critical role of capillary pericytes in sepsis-associated vascular destabilization and leakage, which is crucial in the pathogenesis of end-organ dysfunction and septic shock [13,14]. Indeed, sepsis may cause microvascular hyper-permeability via disruption of pericyte/endothelial cell (EC) interactions. Furthermore, renal pericytes represent a major source of the pathological extracellular matrix [6]. Although pericytes do not have specific markers, the receptor tyrosin kinase PDGFRβ is considered a constitutive marker for renal pericyte isolation and characterization [15,16]. It has been extensively shown that after injury, PDGFRβ$^+$ pericytes are able to detach from the endothelium, and after migration and differentiation into α-SMA$^+$ myofibroblasts, may lead to interstitial fibrosis [17–21].

Renal fibrosis is the common, final process directed to repair tissue injury; however during sepsis-induced AKI overwhelming and persistent inflammation can lead to renal AKI. Despite recent developments in understanding the immunopathology of sepsis, therapeutic advances have been slow. Further protective therapies are based on the concept that increased levels of pro-inflammatory mediators or endotoxin are associated with the development of AKI, whereby their elimination can prevent sepsis-induced AKI. Indeed, elimination of cytokines and endotoxin is feasible by purification of blood in extracorporeal circuit, through a device (membrane, sorbent) where solute (toxins, cytokines) and fluid can be removed [22,23]. In a previous study, we observed a protective effect of coupled plasma filtration adsorption (CPFA) treatment on EC dysfunction and renal fibrosis; we demonstrated that this beneficial effect was due to the clearance of LBP, a soluble carrier of LPS [11,12].

Here, we investigate the involvement of LBP and TLR4 signalling in pericyte activation. We demonstrate the occurrence of pericyte-to-myofibroblast trans-differentiation (PMT) in a swine model of LPS-induced oliguric kidney. We elucidate that PMT is regulated by the cross-talk between TLR4 and TGF-β signaling and is mediated by common effectors (as SMADs proteins). We also show that CPFA treatment reduces PMT through a mechanism mediated by LBP removal, which might represent a potential strategy to prevent the occurrence of early fibrosis in patients with sepsis-induced AKI.

2. Results

2.1. Acute Induction of PMT in Endotoxemia-Induced Oliguric Kidney Injury

First, we analyzed the activation of renal pericytes in our model of LPS-induced AKI by immunohistochemistry analysis for PDGFRβ. In healthy and CPFA-treated healthy pigs (T9 CTR, T9 CPFA, Figure 1A), PDGFRβ$^+$ expression was detected in interstitial peritubular capillaries, in mesangial cells, and Bowman's capsule. 9 h after LPS infusion, we found a significant reduction of PDGFRβ expression in endotoxemic pigs at peritubular capillary level (T9 LPS) (Figure 1C); on the contrary, PDGFRβ expression of mesangial cells was not significantly down-regulated, as expected [21]. Interestingly, CPFA treatment significantly inhibited PDGFRβ downregulation (Figure 1A, T9 LPS CPFA and Figure 1C).

To investigate whether the PDGFRβ decrease could be associated with occurrence of PMT, we performed a double immunofluorescence for both PDGFRβ and α-SMA marker. In the CTR and CPFA groups (Figure 1B, T9 CTR, and T9 CPFA), PDGFRβ$^+$ pericytes were weakly positive for α-SMA, as expected. As shown in Figure 1B and calculated in Figure 1E, α-SMA positivity was predominately found on larger arterial wall (Figure 1B, T9 CTR, white arrow). In the septic pigs, 9 h after LPS infusion (T9 LPS), the phenotype of renal pericytes dramatically changed with a significant increase in α-SMA (Figure 1B, T9 LPS). The co-localization of these two markers (PDGFRβ/α-SMA) was more evident in arterioles, peritubular capillaries and mesangial cells (Figure 1B, T9 LPS), indicating that these cells acquired myofibroblast characteristics. After 9 h of adsorption treatment with CPFA, the number of PDGFRβ$^+$/α-SMA$^+$ cells in the peritubular capillaries was significantly reduced (Figure 1D), concurrent with the restoring of a physiological cellular phenotype (Figure 1B, T9 LPS CPFA).

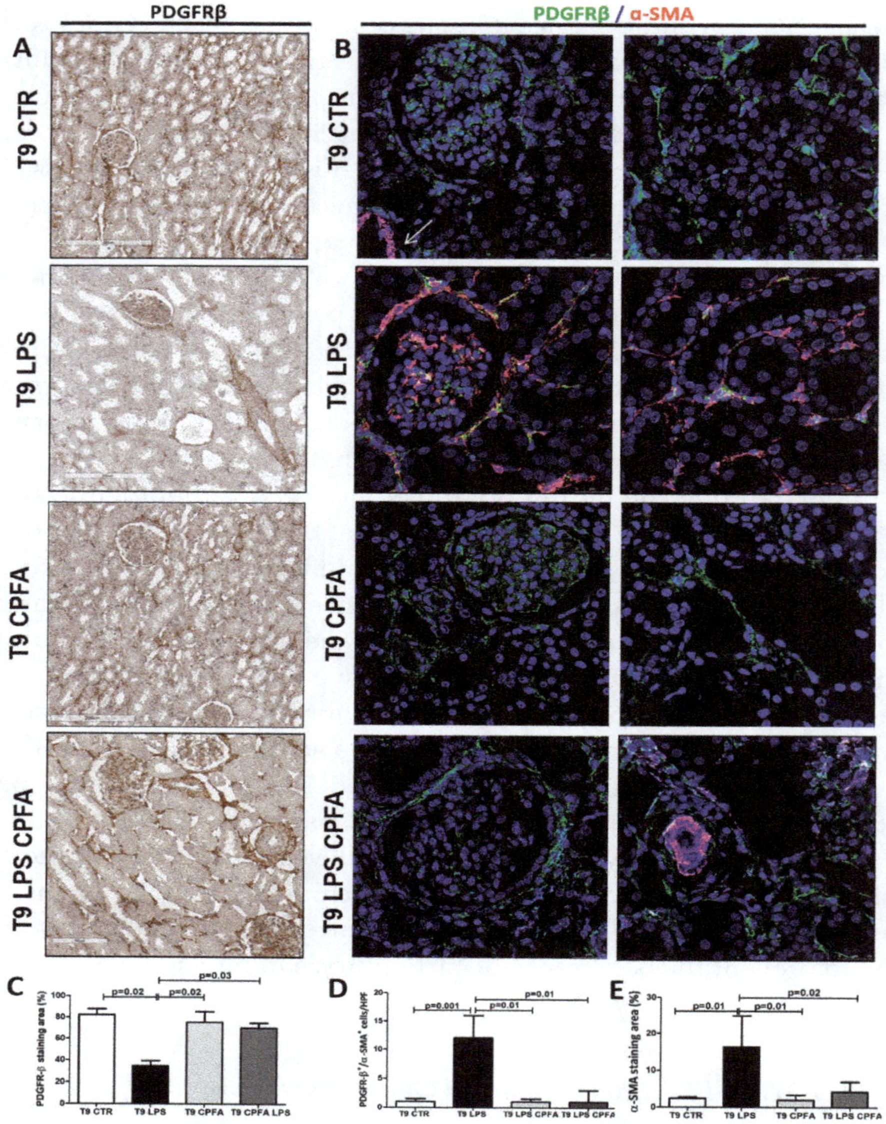

Figure 1. CPFA inhibited LPS-induced PDGFRβ down-regulation and pericyte-to-myofibroblast trans-differentiation (PMT) in endotoxemic pigs. (**A**) IHC (Immunohistochemistry) revealed a strong decrease in PDGFRβ expression at perivascular level after 9 h from LPS infusion (T9 LPS) compared to control (T9 CTR) and CPFA-treated healthy pigs (T9 CPFA). Renal biopsies of endotoxemic animals after CPFA treatment showed a preservation of PDGFRβ$^+$ cells (T9 LPS CPFA) Magnification 10x. (**B**) Pericytes were double-stained for PDGFRβ (green) and α-SMA marker (red) to further demonstrate the occurrence of PMT. In the interstitium of T9 CTR and T9 CPFA pigs, PDGFRβ$^+$/α-SMA$^+$ cells were rarely detectable. Nine h after LPS infusion, the number of these cells dramatically increased (T9 LPS). CPFA treatment reversed LPS-induced PMT, decreasing the number of these transitioning cells (T9 LPS CPFA) Magnification 630×. The fluorescent dye To-pro 3 was used to counterstain nuclei (blue)Quantitative analyses of PDGFRβ (**C**), PDGFRβ/ α-SMA double positive cells (**D**) and α-SMA staining (**E**) were obtained as described in the Methods section and expressed as median ± interquartile range (IQR) of five independent pigs for each group. (**D**) Results are expressed as median ± IQR of the numbers of PDGFRβ$^+$/α-SMA$^+$ cells/ high-power (×630) fields (HPF) of five independent pigs for each group. Results were statistically analyzed in GraphPad Prism. Statistically significant differences were assessed by the Mann–Whitney test. (**E**) Moreover, α-SMA expression (red-stained area) significantly increased in endotoxemic pigs (T9 LPS) and was reduced by CPFA treatment (T9 LPS CPFA). Magnification 630×.

2.2. LPS-Mediated Early Pericyte-to-Myofibroblast Trans-Differentiation (PMT)

To test whether LPS was directly involved in the trans-differentiation of pericytes in myofibroblast, we cultured human pericytes in presence of LPS. A significant increase of α-SMA protein expression was detected after 9 h from LPS stimulation compared to basal condition (LPS:3.9 ± 1.27 vs. basal:1.08 ± 0.5, $p = 0.03$) (Figure 2A).

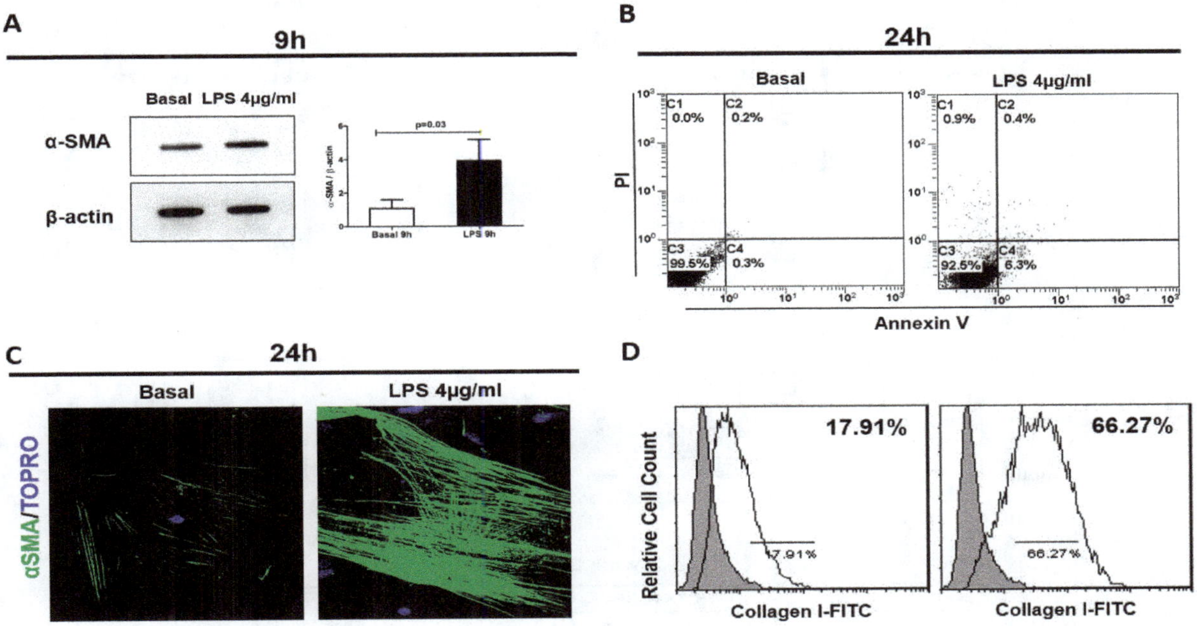

Figure 2. LPS mediated early PMT. Cultured pericytes were incubated with LPS 4 μg/mL, for 9 and 24 h. (**A**) WB analysis revealed a significant increase of α-SMA expression after 9 h of LPS stimulation, compared to basal level. β-actin protein expression was used for normalization. Data are expressed as mean ± standard deviation (SD) of three independent experiments and compared with the Student t test. 24 h of LPS exposure did not affect pericyte viability (**B**) and induced a remodeling of contractile α-SMA-stress fibers (**C**) and a protein increase of Collagen I (**D**). Results are representative of three independent experiments.

Moreover, we found that endotoxin exposure did not affect pericyte viability (Figure 2B) and LPS-stimulated pericytes changed their morphology to an elongated and spindle-like cell shape similar to that of fibroblasts. Under immunofluorescence analysis, pericytes showed high α-SMA expression localized in stress fibers, indicating the acquirement of a contractile phenotype (Figure 2C). Finally, flow cytometry analysis revealed that these changes were accompanied by increased Collagen I protein expression (Figure 2D). Collectively, these findings showed that LPS triggered PMT in vitro, indicating the differentiation towards a pro-fibrotic phenotype (Figure 2C,D).

2.3. LPS Binding Protein (LBP) Was Critical in LPS-Mediated PMT

Next, we investigated whether LPS/TLR4 signaling may be critical in mediating PMT during endotoxemia-induced AKI. Recently, we demonstrated in the same animal model that CPFA treatment prevented an LBP serum increase and that the removal of LBP drastically reduced the binding of LPS to TLR4 receptor [11]. We cultured pericytes in the presence of different swine sera for 9 h and 24 h (CTR, CPFA, LPS, and LPS CPFA). Firstly, we examined whether LBP and swine sera could affect pericyte viability. After 24 h of LBP-activation and incubation with swine sera, flow cytometry analysis showed that pericytes did not undergo apoptosis (Figure 3A).

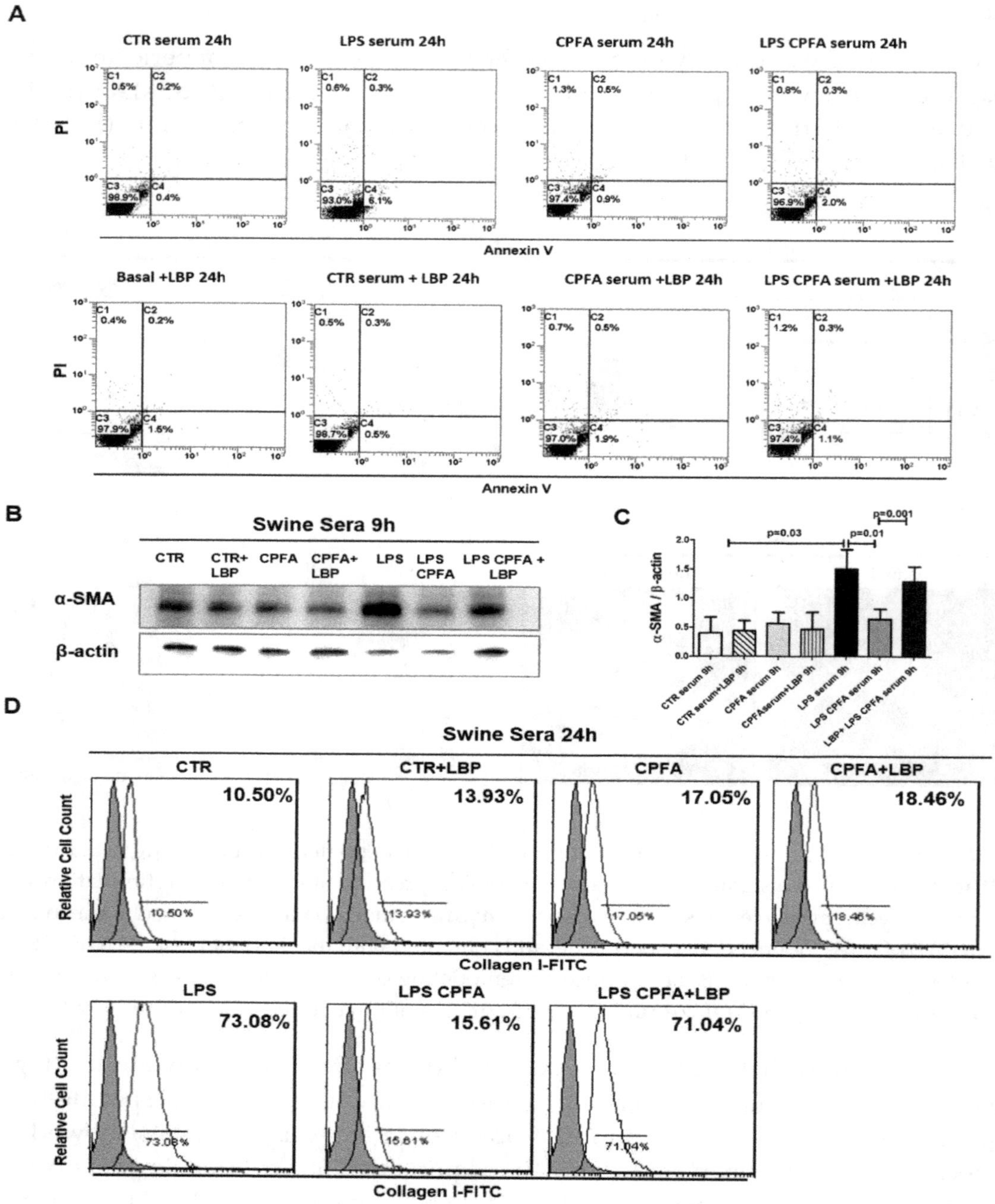

Figure 3. LBP was critical in LPS-mediated early PMT. Cultured pericytes were stimulated with LPS 4 μg/Ml or LBP 9 μg/Ml, or cultured in presence of different swine sera with/without LBP for the indicated time period. (**A**) Pericyte viability was evaluated by flow cytometry analysis (AnnV/PI). Cells did not undergo apoptosis. (**B**,**C**) WB analysis revealed a significant increase of α-SMA expression after 9 h of endotoxemic sera incubation. CPFA-treated septic sera (LPS CPFA) maintained the expression of α-SMA at low level as CPFA-treated healthy sera (CPFA group). Both in CTR and CPFA sera, the addition of exogenous LBP did not increase α-SMA expression. Remarkably, the addition of LBP in CPFA-treated endotoxemic sera (LPS CPFA) induced PMT like the untreated endotoxemic sera. β-actin protein expression was used for normalization. Data were shown as mean ± standard deviation (SD) and compared with the Student t test. (**D**) FACS (Fluorescence Activated Cell Sorting) showed a strong increase of Collagen I after 24 h of endotoxemic sera incubation compared to control. In accordance, CPFA-treated endotoxemic sera maintained Collagen I expression at basal level as CTR and CPFA group. Exogenous LBP supplementation in CTR and CPFA group did not stimulate Collagen I synthesis in pericytes. The LBP addition in LPS CPFA group completely reversed the effects of CPFA treatment, leading to PMT. Results are representative of three independent experiments.

Western blot analysis revealed a significant increase of α-SMA expression after incubation with LPS group sera compared to CTR group sera (data LPS vs. CTR) (Figure 3B,C). CPFA treatment restored the expression of α-SMA at CTR group level in pericytes (LPS CPFA: 0.6 ± 0.21 vs. LPS: 1.02 ± 0.22, $p = 0.001$). Moreover, CPFA-treated healthy sera maintained α-SMA expression at basal level as CTR group.

Flow cytometry analysis also showed a strong increase of Collagen I after 24 h of endotoxemic sera incubation compared to control, indicating that PMT resulted in active contribution to the synthesis of extracellular matrix components (Figure 3D). CPFA-healthy sera did not affect pericyte phenotype. In accordance, CPFA-treated endotoxemic sera maintained Collagen I expression at basal level.

In order to understand the molecular mechanism involved in the CPFA anti-fibrotic function on human pericyte, we reconstituted the swine group sera with LBP. Both in CTR and CPFA sera, the addition of exogenous LBP did not influence α-SMA and Collagen I expression. Remarkably, the addition of exogenous LBP in sera of LPS CPFA pigs completely reverted the CPFA protective effect. We detected that after LBP sera reconstitution, LPS CPFA group sera re-acquired the capacity to induce PMT in vitro, as shown by the increase of α-SMA and Collagen I protein expression (Figure 3B,D).

2.4. *TLR4 Signaling Mediates PMT via Enhanced Canonical and Non-Canonical TGF-β Signaling*

Next, to identify the signaling involved in PMT and directly activated by LBP/LPS/TLR4 we analyzed the early extracellular signal-regulated kinase 1 (ERK1) phosphorylation, a mediator that is common to TLR4 and pro-fibrotic TGF-β pathways. Regarding TGF-β pathway, we assessed the level of activation of the two different SMAD 2/3-dependent and SMAD2/3- independent signaling.

Pericytes were cultured with or without LPS or sera from LPS group for 5, 30, and 60 min. To analyze the intracellular signaling activated during the incubation, we studied pERK1 and pSMAD2/3 protein expression. Both LPS and endotoxemic sera significantly increased phosphorylation of SMAD2/3 and ERK1, demonstrating the involvement of both canonical SMAD2/3-dependent and non-canonical SMAD2/3-independent signaling, respectively. (Figure 4A–D).

Because we found the maximum increase of pERK1 and pSMAD2/3 level after 30 min of activation by LPS or incubation with septic serum, we decided to further analyze at this time point the potential effect of CPFA treatment on this signaling activation (Figure 4E,F). Compared to LPS group sera, the LPS CPFA group sera led to a significant downregulation of ERK1 and SMAD2/3. In line with the previous findings regarding α-SMA and collagen I protein expression (Figure 3B,D), the restoration of LBP serum significantly increased the phosphorylation of ERK1 and SMAD2/3. Otherwise, the addition of LBP in CTR and CPFA-treated healthy sera did not modify the phosphorylation of SMAD2/3 and ERK1 (Figure 4E,F, quantization in Figure 4G,H). All together, these data indicated that CPFA treatment was able to remove the serum components capable to induce the rapid ERK1 and SMAD2/3 phosphorylation during endotoxemia, and that LBP may be considered a key factor not only in LPS/TLR4 signaling but also in the pro-fibrotic activity of TGF-β pathway.

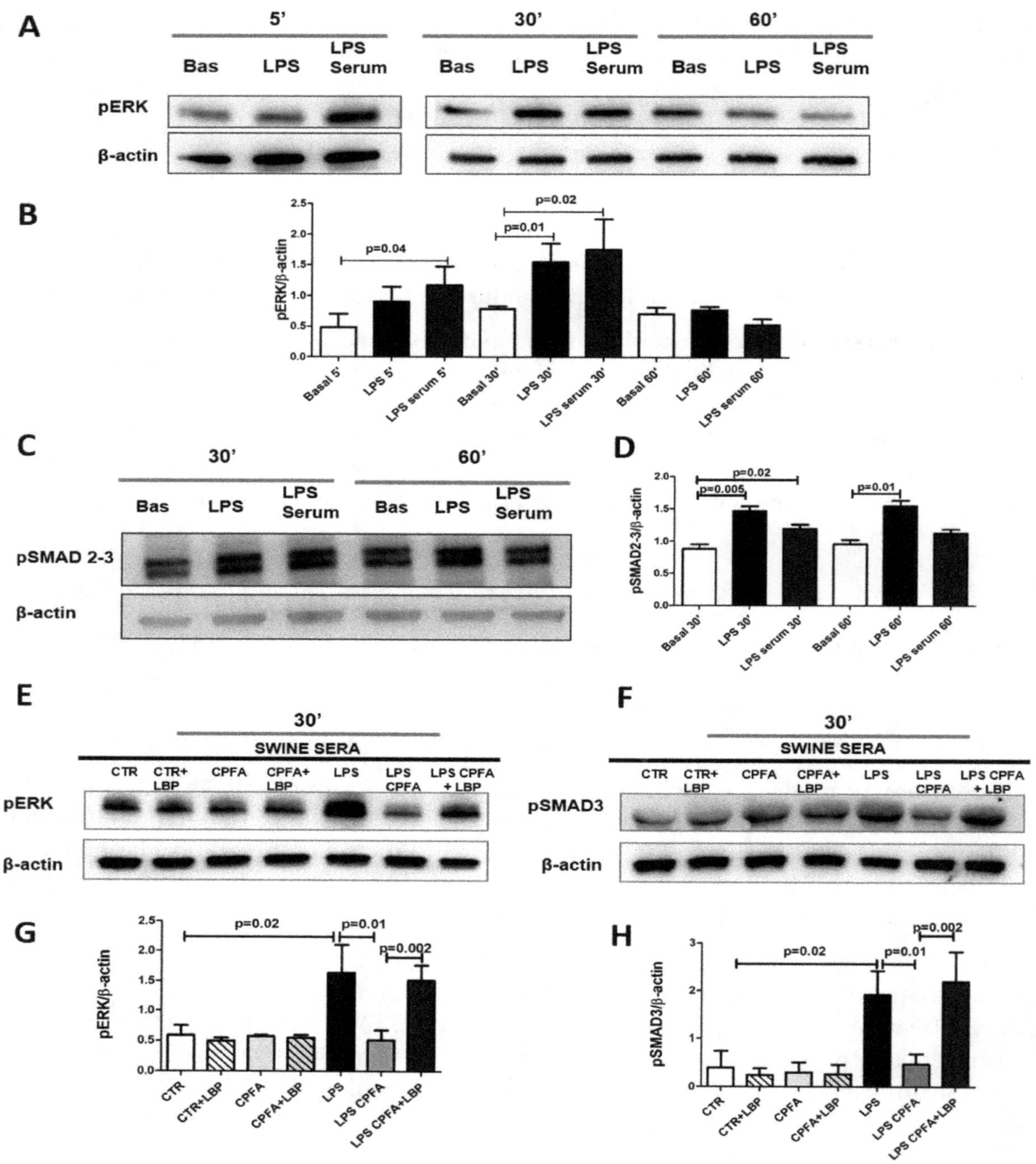

Figure 4. LPS and endotoxemic sera induced PMT by canonical TGF-β-SMAD2/3-dependent and non-canonical TGF-β-SMAD-independent signaling. (**A–D**) Pericytes were cultured with LPS or endotoxemic sera for 5, 30, and 60 min. Cell extracts were then used for WB analysis for pERK1 and pSMAD2/3. Both LPS and endotoxemic sera augmented SMAD2/3 and ERK1 phosphorylation, demonstrating the involvement of both canonical TGF-β-SMAD2/3-dependent and non-canonical TGF-β-SMAD-independent signaling. (**E–H**) Cultured pericytes were incubated in the presence of 1% of different swine sera for 30 min, with/without LBP (pre-treatment 1 h). CTR and CPFA-treated healthy sera maintained the phosphorylation of SMAD2/3 and ERK1 at basal level. Endotoxemic sera significantly increased phosphorylation of SMAD2/3 and ERK1. CPFA-treated endotoxemic sera reduced the phosphorylation of SMAD2/3 and ERK1 at basal level. The addition of LBP in CTR and CPFA-treated healthy sera did not augment phosphorylation of SMAD2/3 and ERK1. Otherwise, the addition of LBP in LPS CPFA sera reversed CPFA effects, increasing the activation of SMAD2/3 and ERK1. Results are representative of three independent experiments. Data are shown as mean ± standard deviation (SD) and compared with the Student t test.

2.5. CPFA Treatment Significantly Decreased Pro-Fibrotic Factors in Endotoxemic Pigs

Several reports have referred to an increase of circulating TGF-β in septic patients [24] and the involvement of Endothelin-1 (ET-1) in the pathogenesis of sepsis [25]. In addition, it is also known that TGF-β can amplify and further enhance LPS signaling [26] and ET-1 promotes the induction of the myofibroblast phenotype from vascular pericytes [27].

In line with these findings, in LPS group sera we found an increase of the TGF-β and ET-1 levels compared to CTR group after 9 h from LPS infusion. Interestingly, CPFA-treated endotoxemic pigs presented a significant reduction in TGF-β and ET-1 serum levels (Figure 5A,B).

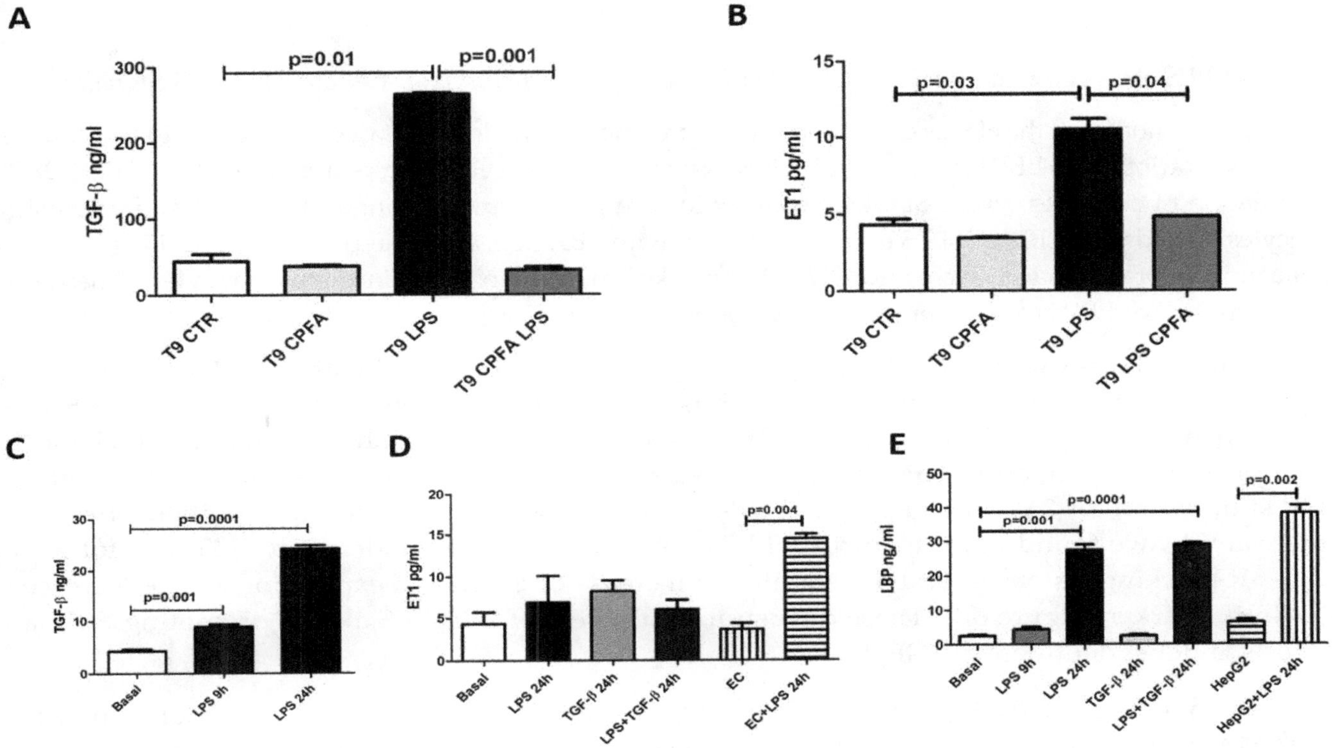

Figure 5. CPFA treatment modulated serum levels of TGF-β and ET-1, and LPS-stimulated pericytes secreted TGF-β and LBP. (**A**,**B**) Serum levels of TGF-β and ET-1 significantly increased after 9 h of LPS infusion compared to healthy pigs. Interestingly, CPFA-treated pigs presented a dramatic reduction in serum TGF-β and ET-1 levels. Data are expressed as median ± IQR of five independent pigs for each group. Statistically significant differences were assessed by the Mann–Whitney test. (**C**–**E**) cultured pericytes were stimulated with LPS and/or TGF-β, and their supernatants were analyzed by ELISA. Human endothelial cells (EC) and human liver hepatocellular cells (HepG2) were used as control positive for ET-1 and LBP synthesis, respectively.(**C**) LPS augmented TGF-β production in pericytes, particularly at 24 h. (**D**) LPS and/or TGF-β stimulation did not increase ET-1 production compared with EC treated with LPS for 24 h (positive control). (**E**) After 24 h from LPS stimulation, pericytes significantly increased LBP synthesis. Stimulation of pericytes with TGF-β alone did not influence LBP production. HepG2 stimulated with LPS for 24 h were used as positive control. Data were shown as mean ± standard deviation (SD) and compared with the Student t test.

In order to clarify the contribution of pericytes to circulating TGF-β, ET-1, and LBP serum release, we evaluated whether LPS exposition could influence their production in culture (Figure 5C–E).

Thereby, we stimulated pericytes with LPS and/or TGF-β for 9 h and 24 h and analyzed the pericyte culture supernatants by ELISA. Interestingly, LPS augmented TGF-β production, particularly at 24 h (LPS 24 h: 24.20 ± 1.51 vs. basal: 4.22 ± 0.88, $p = 0.001$) (Figure 5C). Otherwise, LPS and TGF- β, alone or in combination, did not induce ET-1 production by pericytes.

Because we have already demonstrated [11], in the same animal model, the increase of circulating LBP in endotoxemic pigs, we also evaluated the contribution of pericytes to LBP secretion. 24 h after LPS stimulation, we observed a significant increase of LBP with respect to basal level. Otherwise, TGF-β did not induce LBP synthesis in pericytes.

2.6. LBP-LPS Axis-Induced PMT was Characterized by Canonical and Non-Canonical TGF-β Signaling

First, we analyzed the effects of LBP alone or in presence of LPS. In vitro, we observed that LPS-stimulated pericytes contributed to LBP synthesis, which is known to maximize cellular response to endotoxin [11,12,28,29]. Stimulation of pericytes with LBP alone did not induce phenotypical changes in pericytes. Interestingly, pericytes treated with LBP and LPS in combination or with LBP, LPS, and TGF-β mixture additively increased Collagen I expression and decreased PDGFRβ marker more than LPS-stimulated pericytes. These data demonstrate that LBP is a cofactor of LPS that contributes to LPS signaling (Figure 6A).

Moreover, we observed that LPS-stimulated pericytes are associated with TGF-β secretion, which, in turn, can trigger or enhance PMT [19,21]. Thus, in order to selectively analyze the role of LPS/TLR4 signaling in inducing PMT, we blocked the TGF-β pathway by TGF-βR inhibition (Figure 6B). Pericytes were pre-treated with anti-TGF-βR -specific neutralizing antibody for 1 h followed by LPS and/or LBP stimulation for 24 h. As expected, LBP-stimulated pericytes did not modify their phenotype. Interestingly, we found that LPS or LBP/LPS-stimulated pericytes underwent PMT also following TGF-βR-blocking, as observed by a significant increase of collagen I expression and a decrease of PDGFRβ marker (Figure 6B). These data support the role of LBP-LPS axis in promoting PMT and fibrosis, independently from TGF-β.

Moreover, the anti-TGF-βR neutralizing antibody did not reduce phosphorylation of both ERK1/2 and SMAD3 (Figure 6C–F) mediated by LPS alone or in combination with LBP at 30 min. Stimulation of pericytes with LBP alone did not modify phosphorylation of both ERK1/2 and SMAD3. Collectively, these data indicated that in vitro LPS alone or in combination with LBP can promote both TGF-β canonical and non-canonical pathways, leading to fibrosis and collagen release independently from TGF-β receptor activation.

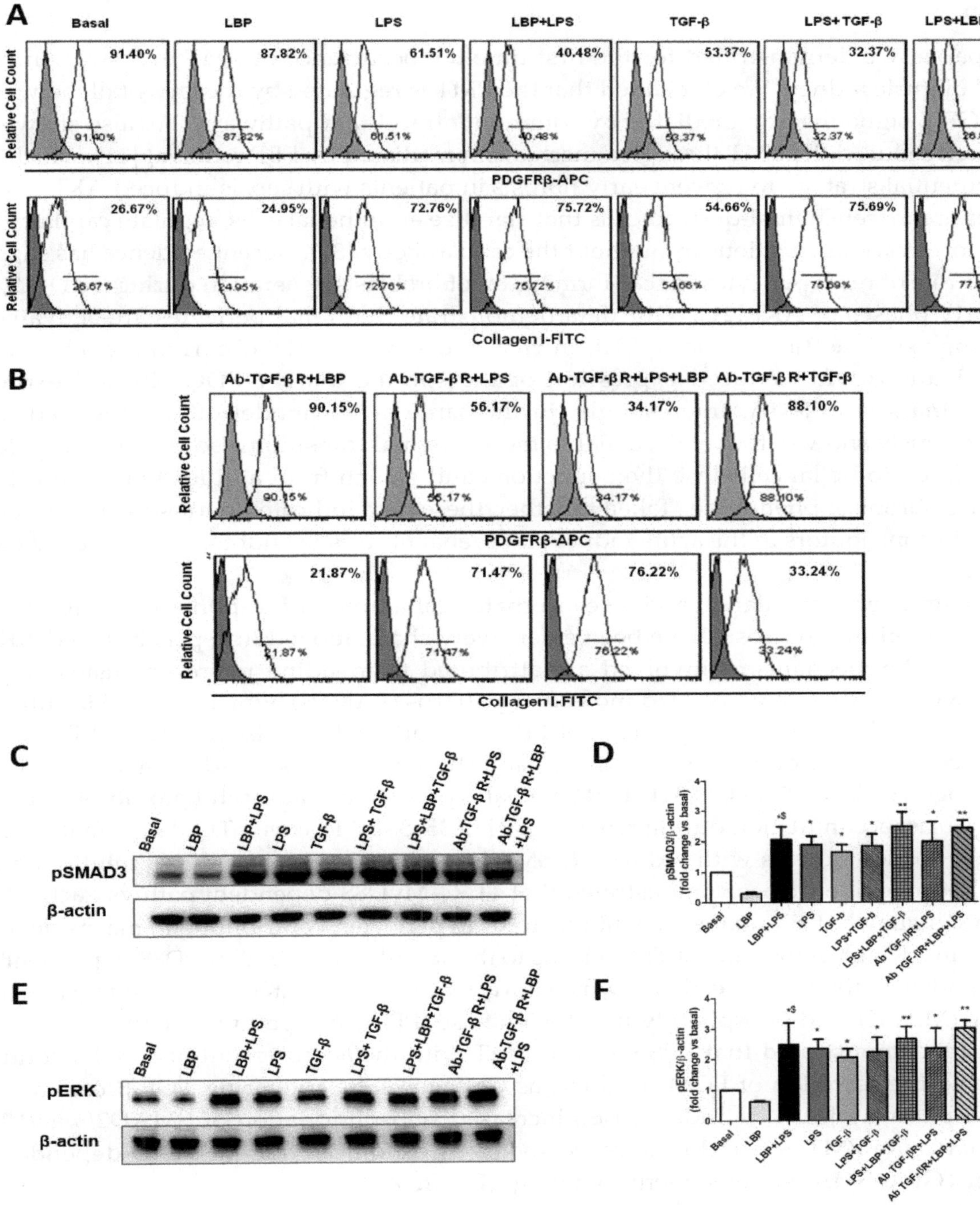

Figure 6. LBP-LPS axis induced PMT upon blocking TGF-βR. (**A**) Cultured pericytes were treated with LBP and/or LPS or TGF- β and with LBP, LPS, and TGF-β mixture for 24 h. LBP alone did not induce phenotypical changes in pericytes. Pericytes treated with LBP and LPS in combination or with LBP, LPS, and TGF-β mixture additively increased Collagen I expression and decreased PDGFRβ marker. (**B**) Pericytes were pretreated with anti-TGF-Br-specific neutralizing antibody for 1 h followed by LPS and/or LBP stimulation for 24 h. FACS analysis showed that pericytes acquired phenotypic change also upon TGF-βR-blocking. Results are representative of three independent experiments. (**C–F**) Pericytes were pretreated with anti-TGF-βR specific neutralizing antibody for 1 h followed by LPS and/or LBP for short stimulation time (30 min). Pretreatment of pericytes with anti-TGF-βR antibody did not reduce LPS and LPS/LBP-induced phosphorylation of both SMAD3 (**C**,**D**) and ERK1/2 (**E**,**F**) at 30 min. Results are representative of three independent experiments. Data are shown as mean ± standard deviation (SD) and compared with the Student t test (**D**,**F**: * $p < 0.05$, ** $p \leq 0.005$, versus basal level; $^{\$}$ $p < 0.05$ versus LBP).

3. Discussion

In this paper, we demonstrated for the first time the occurrence of PMT in a swine model of LPS-induced oliguric kidney. We elucidated that the PMT is regulated by the cross-talk between the TLR-4 and TGF-β signaling and mediated by common intracellular pathways. We also showed that CPFA treatment reduced the PMT through a mechanism mediated by LBP removal [11], which might represent a potential strategy to prevent early fibrosis in patients with sepsis-induced AKI.

Pericytes are mesenchymal-derived cells that stabilize endothelial cells, regulate capillary blood flow, and perform various functions throughout the cellular body [30]. Recent evidence has suggested the prominent role of renal pericytes in scar-forming myofibroblasts generation during CKD [17,18,31] as well as early phases of AKI [21]. Our data demonstrate that renal pericytes are activated also in acute settings such as LPS induced AKI; in vivo and in vitro PMT occurred already after 9 h from LPS activation, with reduced expression of the specific marker PDGFRβ and expression myofibroblast markers α-SMA. Interestingly, in the same swine model of LPS-induced kidney injury, we previously showed that endothelial to mesenchymal transition also contributes to kidney fibrosis [11,12]. Endothelial cells lose their functions and switch from a quiescent to an activated state, acquiring fibroblast phenotype. Taken together, these data indicated pericytes and endothelial cells as the main contributors in the acute induction of renal fibrosis in endotoxemia-induced oliguric kidney injury.

Hyperdinamic renal circulation and an exacerbated inflammatory response without significant evidence of acute tubular necrosis have been extensively characterized in sepsis-induced AKI [32]. In this scenario, the mechanisms involved are attributed to invading microorganisms and their products, known as pathogen-associated molecular patterns (PAMPs), which activate immune cells and renal resident cells by a broad spectrum of PPRs, including TLRs. In particular, LPS, a critical structural component of the outer wall of gram-negative bacteria, is considered the main PAMP and is specifically recognized by TLR-4 [4,33,34]. TLR4 mediates pro-inflammatory and pro-fibrotic pathways, leading to fibroblast accumulation during renal injury [15,35–38]. Moreover, TLR4-deficient mice were protected from kidney fibrosis with reduced α-SMA protein expression and less tubulointerstitial fibrosis [39]. Recent evidence has demonstrated that TLR4-MyD88-dependent pathway activates not only immune signaling but simultaneously fibrogenesis in pericytes, contributing to matrix deposition and pathology in AKI [6]. Activation of TLR-4 leads to the stimulation of both MyD88-dependent and a MyD88-indipendent pathway that lead to downstream activation of the IKK complex, mitogen-activated protein kinase (MAPK), and phosphatidylinositol 3-kinase (PI3K)/Akt pathways [40].

Our results demonstrated that LPS induced PMT with the acquirement of α-SMA contractile stress fibers and the secretion of ECM products as Collagen I, by triggering TGF-β canonical and non-canonical pathway [41–47]. Indeed, LPS increased phosphorylation of SMAD2/3 and ERK1, suggesting that acute PMT was induced, respectively, by canonical TGF-β-SMAD-dependent and non-canonical TGF-β-SMAD-independent signaling. (Figure A1)

Moreover, our study showed that LPS can directly induce SMAD2/3 phosphorylation in a TGF-β independent manner. LPS-stimulated pericytes secreted TGF-β and underwent PMT also following TGF-β receptor-blocking, pointing out the pro-fibrotic role of TLR4 signaling. Since LPS may modulate TGF-β synthesis in pericytes, we speculated that LPS/TLR4 signaling contributes to further accumulation of TGF-β, amplifying LPS signaling and developing a self-sustaining positive feedback loop that initiates collagen accumulation and leads to renal fibrosis progression. As LPS and TGF-β additively triggered PMT process in vitro, we suggest that this endotoxin can amplify the responsiveness of pericytes to TGF-β stimulation. Our data are in line with other papers showing that the activation of TLR4 signaling enhanced the sensitivity of fibroblasts to the stimulatory effect of TGF-β, activating SMAD signaling and down-regulating anti-fibrotic antagonist BAMBI [48].

Among the different factors involved in TLR-4 signaling, LBP seems to be crucial in enhancing and amplifying cellular response to endotoxin [11,12,28,29]. In vivo, the binding of LPS to TLR-4 requires a carrier protein—LBP—an acute phase protein, synthesized by hepatocytes and released into the bloodstream after gram-negative infection. During the acute inflammatory response, LBP blood levels increase and amplify the host response to infection, even at low concentrations of endotoxin [7,9,10,49]. LBP alone has no effect on the development of tissue injury but serves as a key modulator of cellular and systemic responses to LPS. Moreover, many different types of cells in several organs such as lungs, kidneys, and liver contribute to LBP synthesis, maximizing the local parenchymal inflammation [50]. Here, we showed that pericytes release LBP, as well as TGF-β, in response to LPS. These secretory capacities of pericytes in response to LPS may be particularly important for their contribution to kidney fibrosis.

Moreover, pericytes treated with LBP in combination with LPS and TGF-β significantly amplified PMT process respect to LPS-stimulated pericytes. Our findings are consistent with published data showing that LBP functions as a "biological taxi service" [51] for transporting endotoxin in blood and facilitating LPS binding to TLR-4 maximizing inflammatory response on host cells.

Accordingly with our previous study, in the same swine model of LPS-induced oliguric kidney injury, endotoxemic pigs with high levels of LBP were prone to inflammation, endothelial dysfunction, early development of fibrosis, and increased risk of mortality [11].

Thus, targeting TLR signaling may confer a novel therapeutic strategy for renal fibrosis in early and end-stage renal disease. Until now, soluble receptors and monoclonal antibodies used to block the interaction of LPS and other ligands with TLR-4 did not have any efficacy [52]. Extracorporeal elimination techniques have been proposed as a possible approach for cytokine elimination to improve the clinical conditions of septic patients. Recently, we have demonstrated the beneficial effects of CPFA treatment in LPS-induced oliguric kidney injury. CPFA is a technique of blood purification in which systemic blood circulates through a plasmafilter that separates plasma from whole blood, allowing the non-selective removal of inflammatory mediators through the adsorption resin cartridge [53]. In our previous study, in the same swine model, we demonstrated that the removal of LBP by CPFA, rather than endotoxin, impaired the development of endothelial to mesenchymal transition and prevented the acute development of tubulo-interstitial fibrosis [11]. Accordingly, here we have found that the in vivo removal of LBP strongly reduces LPS binding to TLR4 and the subsequent pericyte activation; moreover, in vitro supplementation of exogenous LBP in treated endotoxemic sera induced the early development of PMT through the activation of TLR-4 signaling and both SMAD dependent and independent TGF-β- signal transduction. On the basis of our results, the in vivo blocking of LBP, rather than endotoxin, may significantly reduce the intracellular signaling regulating pericyte dysfunction and kidney fibrosis (Figure A2). Other studies with knockout mice for LBP are needed to underline the potential benefit of LBP blockade in endotoxemic kidney injury.

Furthermore, we observed that CPFA treatment was critical in modulating TGF-β serum level in endotoxemic pigs, suggesting the efficacy of adsorption treatments in preventing kidney fibrosis and the subsequent progression to CKD.

ET-1 is also of interest, since it is able to promote the induction of myofibroblast differentiation from vascular pericytes contributing to fibrotic disorders in several organs and tissues. It has been described as an important factor both in renal pathophysiology and kidney diseases. Accordingly, we showed a significant increase of ET-1 in endotoxemic pigs that could contribute to phenotypical changes in pericytes. We also demonstrated for the first time that CPFA treatment reduced ET-1 sera levels, thus regulating the pro-fibrotic process. However, pericytes did not contribute to ET-1 synthesis, and we supposed that other cells like glomerular endothelial cells [27] could be the main source for this factor.

In conclusion, our data suggest that in the early phase of LPS-induced AKI, renal pericytes contribute to renal fibrosis and kidney failure. Extracorporeal treatment by CPFA decrease PMT and might affect fibrosis progression, thereby counteracting the long-term effect of sepsis-induced AKI.

4. Materials and Methods

4.1. Animal Model

Animal studies were carried out under protocol approved by Ethical Committee of the Italian Ministry of Health, Prot. N823/2016-PR (2016, approved on 2 September 2016). Briefly, endotoxemia was induced in pig by intravenous infusion of a saline solution containing 300 μg/kg of LPS (lipopolisaccharide membrane of escherichia coli), as described previously [11]. Pigs were divided into four groups: control (CTR, healthy pigs, $n = 7$), CPFA (CPFA-treated healthy pigs, $n = 7$), LPS (endotoxemic pigs, $n = 7$), and LPS CPFA (CPFA-treated endotoxemic pigs, $n = 7$). CTR and CPFA pigs received 10 mL of sterile saline solution.

CPFA treatment was performed for 6 h, as previously described [11]. Animals were sacrified after 9 h from LPS/saline infusion or after 6 h CPFA treatment (T9).

4.2. Collection of Samples

Renal biopsies were performed at the start of experimental procedure (T0) and at different intervals from saline or LPS infusion until death (T9). A portion of each biopsy was fixed in buffered formalin (4%) for 12 h and embedded in paraffin by using standard procedures as previously described [11]. Swine sera were collected at T0, at intermediate time points, and at T9 from an arterial blood catheter.

4.3. Cell Culture

Human placental-derived pericytes (PromoCell, Heidelberg, Germany) were grown in Serum-Free Pericyte Growth Medium (PromoCell) at 5% CO2 and 37 °C [21]. Human umbilical vein endothelial cells (HUVEC, EC) and Human Hepato Cancer cells (HepG2) were purchased from American Type Culture Collection (ATCC-LGC Standards S.r.l., Sesto San Giovanni, Milan, Italy). EC and HepG2 were maintained in their recommended medium, EndGro (Merck Millipore, Darmstadt, Germany) and DMEM high-glucose medium supplemented with 10% Fetal Bovine serum (FBS), 100 U/mL penicillin, 0.1 mg/mL streptomycin, 2 mM L-glutamine (Sigma Aldrich, Milan, Italy), respectively. When cells became confluent, they were stimulated with LPS 4 μg/mL (E. Coli O111:B4, Sigma-Aldrich, Milan, Italy), LPS Binding Protein (LBP, HycultBiotech, Uden, The Netherlands) 9 μg/mL [11], and TGF-β1 10 ng/mL (Biovision, San Francisco, CA, USA). Moreover cells were incubated in the presence of 1% of different swine sera with/without LPS Binding Protein (LBP), 9 μg/mL [11], for the indicated time period. All experiments were performed at early P3–P5 passages. For TGF-βR inhibition assay, pericytes were pre-treated with mouse monoclonal anti-TGF-βR (Abcam, Cambridge, UK) at 5–10–20–25–30 μg/mL for 1 h before the TGF-β (10 ng/mL) exposition (Figure A2). The concentration used for TGF-βR blocking before LPS (4 μg/mL) and/or LBP (9 μg/mL) stimulation was 20 μg/mL.

4.4. Immunohistochemistry (IHC)

Renal sections underwent deparaffination and heat-mediated antigen retrieval as previously described [11]. Sections were incubated with the primary antibody PDGFRβ (Abcam, Cambridge, MA, USA) and detected by the Peroxidase/DAB Dako Real EnVision Detection System ((Dako, Glostrup, Denmark). Negative controls were obtained by incubation with a control irrelevant antibody. Images were acquired by Aperio ScanScope CS2 device, and signals were analyzed with the ImageScope V12.1.0.5029 (Aperio Technologies, Vista, CA, USA).

4.5. Confocal Laser Scanning Microscopy

Swine paraffin-embedded renal sections and cultured pericytes were stained or double stained for α-SMA (Santa Cruz Biotechnologies, Santa Cruz, CA, USA) and PDGFRβ (Abcam, Cambridge,

MA, USA) as previously described [21]. All the antibodies cross-reacted with pig tissue. For immunofluorescence microscopy on cultured pericytes, 5×10^4 cells were seeded on a cover slip, grown to 70% confluence, and then stimulated with LPS 4 μg/mL. After stimulation, cells were fixed in 3.7% paraformaldehyde for 5 min. To counterstain nuclei of renal tissue and cells, we used the fluorescent dye TO-PRO-3 (Molecular Probes, Eugene, OR, USA). Image acquisition was performed with confocal microscope Leica TCS SP2 (Leica, Wetzlar, Germany). The number of PDGFRβ+/α-SMA+ cells was quantified in at least 10 high-power (×630) fields (HPF)/sections by two independent observers. The final counts were the mean of the two measures. In no case was interobserver variability higher than 20%.

4.6. *Detection of Viable and Apoptotic Pericytes by Flow Cytometry Analysis (FACS)*

Apoptotic and viable pericytes were evaluated with Annexin V(Ann V)–fluorescein isothiocyanate (FITC) and propidium iodide (PI) according to manufacturers' instructions (Beckman Coulter, Brea, CA, USA). Three independent experiments were performed. Data were obtained using a FC500 flow cytometer (Beckman Coulter, Brea, CA, USA) and analyzed by Kaluza software.

4.7. *Immunophenotypic Analysis*

After stimulations, pericytes were permeabilized with IntraPrep kit (Instrumentation Laboratory) and incubated with APC-conjugated anti-PDGFRβ (LSBio, Seattle, WA, USA) and FITC-conjugated anti-collagen I (Millipore, Millimarck, Germany) as previously described [21]. Data were analyzed with FC500 (Beckman Coulter, Brea, CA, USA) and Kaluza software. This assay was done in triplicate. The area of positivity was determined by using an isotype-matched mAb, and, in total, 10^4 events for each sample were acquired. Data were obtained by using a FC500 (Beckman Coulter) flow cytometer and analyzed with Kaluza software. Three independent experiments were performed.

4.8. *ELISA for TGF-β, ET-1, and LBP*

TGF-β (ELISA; Enzo Life Sciences, Farmingdale, NY, USA) and ET-1 (ELISA; R&D Systems, Minneapolis, MN, USA) levels in swine sera and in cell culture supernatants were measured by a commercially available enzyme-linked immunosorbent assay (ELISA).

LBP levels were revealed in cell culture supernatants were measured by ELISA kit from HycultBiotech (Uden, The Netherlands).

4.9. *Protein Extraction and Western Blotting*

The cell monolayer was rapidly rinsed twice with ice-cold PBS and lysed in RIPA buffer (1 mM PMSF, 5 mM EDTA, 1 mM sodium orthovanadate, 150 mM sodium chloride, 8 μg/mL leupeptin, 1.5% Nonidet P-40, and 20 mM tris-HCl (pH 7.4)) with phosphatase and protease inhibitors. The samples (30 μg of proteins) were separated in 4–15% polyacrylamide gel and then transferred to PVDF membrane (0.2 mM) by Trans-Blot Turbo (BioRad, Hercules, CA, USA). After blocking in BSA at 5%, the membranes were probed with the following primary antibodies: pSMAD2/3 (Abcam), pSMAD3 (Cell Signaling, Danvers, MA, USA), and pERK (Cell Signaling) extracellular signal regulated kinases (ERK) α-SMA (Santa Cruz Biotechnology, Inc.), and then with secondary antibody (hrp-conjugated, Abcam). The same membranes were incubated with mouse monoclonal anti-βactin antibody (1:20,000; Sigma). Immune complexes were detected by the ECL chemiluminescence system (Amersham Pharmacia, Little Chalfont, UK), according to the manufacturer's instructions. The chemiluminescent blots were acquired by Chemidoc and analyzed using Image J software. Each experiments was repeated three times.

4.10. Statistical Analysis

Animal data were expressed as median±interquartile range (IQR) and compared with a Mann–Whitney test. For FACS analysis and western blot, data were shown as mean ± standard deviation (SD) and compared with the Student t test. A p value < 0.05 was considered statistically significant. All analyses were performed by using GraphPad Prism 5.0 (GraphPad software, Inc., San Diego, CA, USA).

Author Contributions: G.C. and A.S. (Alessandra Stasi). are equal first authors. G.C. provided new analytic tools, designed and supervised the research and drafted the manuscript. A.S. (Alessandra Stasi) planned the research, coordinated the study, performed most experiments, and drafted the manuscript. R.F. contributed to design most experiments, analyzed the respective data, and drafted the manuscript. F.S. (Fabio Sallustio) participated in the design of the study and assisted in vitro experiments and in manuscript preparation. C.D. participated in the immunolabeling and confocal microscopy of renal sections and contributed to data analysis. A.S. (Alessandra Spinelli). participated in the coordination of the study and assisted in in vitro experiments. G.S.N. contributed to the in vivo swine model and performed statistical analysis of clinical parameters. E.F. participated in the design of the study and helped to draft the manuscript. V.C. participated in the coordination of the study and assisted in manuscript preparation. A.C., F.S. (Francesco Staffieri), and L.L. carried out all surgical procedures of the animal model and helped to revise the manuscript. G.G., S.S., and G.B.P. participated in the design of the study and critically revised the manuscript. L.G. participated in the coordination of the study and assisted in manuscript preparation.

Acknowledgments: We thank Eustacchio Montemurno for technical assistance in image editing.

Abbreviations

PMT	Pericyte-to-Myofibroblast Trans-differentiation
LBP	LPS Binding Protein
AKI	Acute Kidney Injury
HepG2	Human Hepato Cancer Cells
CKD	Chronic Kidney Disease
CPFA	Citrate-Based Coupled Plasma Filtration Adsorption
EC	Endothelial Cell
WB	Western Blot
TLR-4	Toll Like Receptor-4
ET-1	Endothelin-1
LPS	Lipopolysaccharide
PRR	Pattern Recognition Receptors
Ab	Antibody
TGF-βR	TGF-βReceptor
Ab-TGF-βR	Antibody Anti-TGF-βReceptor

Appendix A

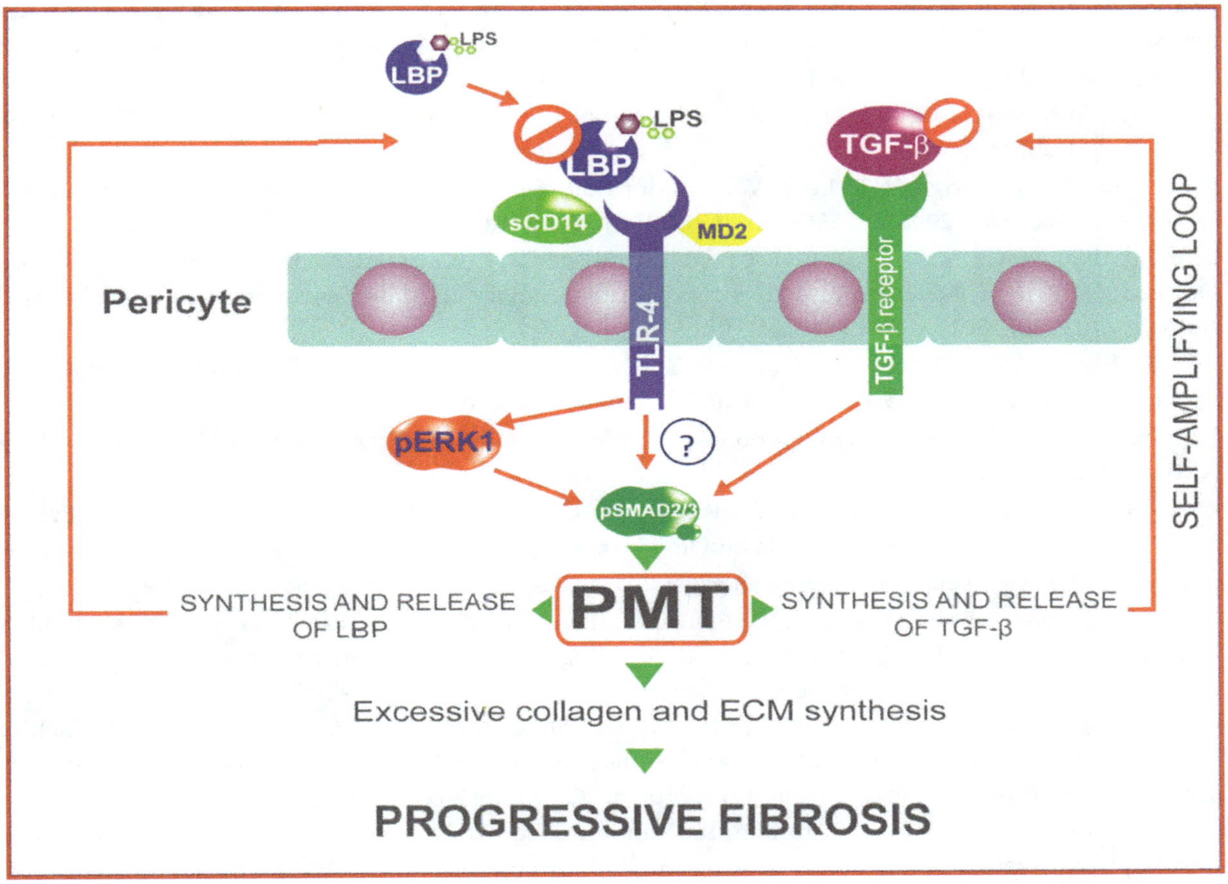

Figure A1. CPFA reduced activation of pericytes and PMT by LBP and TGF-β removal from septic sera. Pericyte TLR4 signaling might contribute to further accumulation of TGF-β and LBP, developing a self-sustaining feed-forward loop that amplifies and maintains renal fibrosis. Disrupting persistent TLR4 signaling activation by the removal of LBP and other molecules as TGF-β represents a potential novel strategy for breaking the cycle of progressive fibrosis.

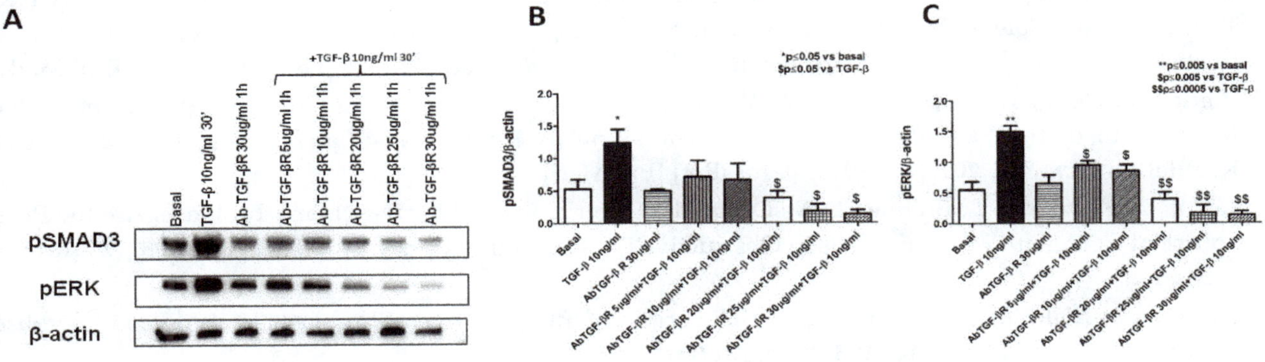

Figure A2. TGF-βR inhibition assay. (**A–C**) Pericytes were pre-treated with mouse monoclonal anti-TGF-βR at 5-10-20-25-30 μg/mL for 1 h before the TGF-β (10 ng/mL) exposition for 30 min. Pretreatment of pericytes with anti-TGF-βR antibody at 20 μg/mL is sufficient to significantly reduce TGF-β-induced phosphorylation of SMAD3 and ERK.

References

1. Gómez, H.; Kellum, J.A. Sepsis-induced acute kidney injury. *Curr. Opin. Crit. Care* **2016**, *22*, 546–553. [CrossRef] [PubMed]

2. Zarbock, A.; Gomez, H.; Kellum, J.A. Sepsis-induced acute kidney injury revisited: Pathophysiology, prevention and future therapies. *Curr. Opin. Crit. Care* **2014**, *20*, 588–595. [CrossRef] [PubMed]
3. Fenhammar, J.; Rundgren, M.; Hultenby, K.; Forestier, J.; Taavo, M.; Kenne, E.; Weitzberg, E.; Eriksson, S.; Ozenci, V.; Wernerson, A.; et al. Renal effects of treatment with a TLR4 inhibitor in conscious septic sheep. *Crit. Care* **2014**, *18*, 488. [PubMed]
4. Lu, Y.-C.; Yeh, W.-C.; Ohashi, P.S. LPS/TLR4 signal transduction pathway. *Cytokine* **2008**, *42*, 145–151. [CrossRef] [PubMed]
5. Schouten, M.; Wiersinga, W.J.; Levi, M.; van der Poll, T. Inflammation, endothelium, and coagulation in sepsis. *J. Leukoc. Biol.* **2008**, *83*, 536–545. [CrossRef] [PubMed]
6. Leaf, I.A.; Nakagawa, S.; Johnson, B.G.; Cha, J.J.; Mittelsteadt, K.; Guckian, K.M.; Gomez, I.G.; Altemeier, W.A.; Duffield, J.S. Pericyte MyD88 and IRAK4 control inflammatory and fibrotic responses to tissue injury. *J. Clin. Investig.* **2017**, *127*, 321–334. [CrossRef] [PubMed]
7. Peri, F.; Piazza, M.; Calabrese, V.; Damore, G.; Cighetti, R. Exploring the LPS/TLR4 signal pathway with small molecules. *Biochem. Soc. Trans.* **2010**, *38*, 1390–1395. [CrossRef] [PubMed]
8. Park, B.S.; Lee, J.-O. Recognition of lipopolysaccharide pattern by TLR4 complexes. *Exp. Mol. Med.* **2013**, *45*, e66. [CrossRef] [PubMed]
9. Opal, S.M.; Scannon, P.J.; Vincent, J.L.; White, M.; Carroll, S.F.; Palardy, J.E.; Parejo, N.A.; Pribble, J.P.; Lemke, J.H. Relationship between plasma levels of lipopolysaccharide (LPS) and LPS-binding protein in patients with severe sepsis and septic shock. *J. Infect. Dis.* **1999**, *180*, 1584–1589. [CrossRef]
10. Villar, J.; Pérez-Méndez, L.; Espinosa, E.; Flores, C.; Blanco, J.; Muriel, A.; Basaldúa, S.; Muros, M.; Blanch, L.; Artigas, A.; et al. Serum lipopolysaccharide binding protein levels predict severity of lung injury and mortality in patients with severe sepsis. *PLoS ONE* **2009**, *4*, e6818. [CrossRef]
11. Castellano, G.; Stasi, A.; Intini, A.; Gigante, M.; Di Palma, A.M.; Divella, C.; Netti, G.S.; Prattichizzo, C.; Pontrelli, P.; Crovace, A.; et al. Endothelial dysfunction and renal fibrosis in endotoxemia-induced oliguric kidney injury: Possible role of LPS-binding protein. *Crit. Care* **2014**, *18*, 520. [CrossRef] [PubMed]
12. Stasi, A.; Intini, A.; Divella, C.; Franzin, R.; Montemurno, E.; Grandaliano, G.; Ronco, C.; Fiaccadori, E.; Pertosa, G.B.; Gesualdo, L.; et al. Emerging role of Lipopolysaccharide binding protein in sepsis-induced acute kidney injury. *Nephrol. Dial. Transplant.* **2016**, *32*, 24–31. [CrossRef] [PubMed]
13. Goldenberg, N.M.; Steinberg, B.E.; Slutsky, A.S.; Lee, W.L. Broken barriers: A new take on sepsis pathogenesis. *Sci. Transl. Med.* **2011**, *3*, 88ps25. [CrossRef]
14. Page, A.V.; Liles, W.C. Biomarkers of endothelial activation/dysfunction in infectious diseases. *Virulence* **2013**, *4*, 507–516. [CrossRef] [PubMed]
15. Chen, Y.-T.; Chang, F.-C.; Wu, C.-F.; Chou, Y.-H.; Hsu, H.-L.; Chiang, W.-C.; Shen, J.; Chen, Y.-M.; Wu, K.-D.; Tsai, T.-J.; et al. Platelet-derived growth factor receptor signaling activates pericyte–myofibroblast transition in obstructive and post-ischemic kidney fibrosis. *Kidney Int.* **2011**, *80*, 1170–1181. [CrossRef] [PubMed]
16. Wang, N.; Deng, Y.; Liu, A.; Shen, N.; Wang, W.; Du, X.; Tang, Q.; Li, S.; Odeh, Z.; Wu, T.; et al. Novel Mechanism of the Pericyte-Myofibroblast Transition in Renal Interstitial Fibrosis: Core Fucosylation Regulation. *Sci. Rep.* **2017**, *7*, 16914. [CrossRef] [PubMed]
17. Lin, S.-L.; Kisseleva, T.; Brenner, D.A.; Duffield, J.S. Pericytes and Perivascular Fibroblasts Are the Primary Source of Collagen-Producing Cells in Obstructive Fibrosis of the Kidney. *Am. J. Pathol.* **2008**, *173*, 1617–1627. [CrossRef]
18. Grgic, I.; Duffield, J.S.; Humphreys, B.D. The origin of interstitial myofibroblasts in chronic kidney disease. *Pediatr. Nephrol.* **2012**, *27*, 183–193. [CrossRef]
19. Wu, C.-F.; Chiang, W.-C.; Lai, C.-F.; Chang, F.-C.; Chen, Y.-T.; Chou, Y.-H.; Wu, T.-H.; Linn, G.R.; Ling, H.; Wu, K.-D.; et al. Transforming growth factor β-1 stimulates profibrotic epithelial signaling to activate pericyte-myofibroblast transition in obstructive kidney fibrosis. *Am. J. Pathol.* **2013**, *182*, 118–131. [CrossRef]
20. Kuppe, C.; Kramann, R. Role of mesenchymal stem cells in kidney injury and fibrosis. *Curr. Opin. Nephrol. Hypertens.* **2016**, *25*, 372–377. [CrossRef]
21. Castellano, G.; Franzin, R.; Stasi, A.; Divella, C.; Sallustio, F.; Pontrelli, P.; Lucarelli, G.; Battaglia, M.; Staffieri, F.; Crovace, A.; et al. Complement activation during ischemia/reperfusion injury induces pericyte-to-myofibroblast transdifferentiation regulating peritubular capillary Lumen Reduction Through pERK Signaling. *Front. Immunol.* **2018**, *9*, 1002. [CrossRef] [PubMed]

22. Ronco, C.; D'Intini, V.; Bellomo, R.; Ricci, Z.; Bonello, M.; Ratanarat, R.; Salvatori, G.; Bordoni, V.; Andricos, E.; Brendolan, A. Rationale for the use of extracorporeal treatments for sepsis. *Anesteziol. Reanimatol.* **2005**, *2*, 87–91.
23. Ronco, C.; Brendolan, A.; Dan, M.; Piccinni, P.; Bellomo, R.; De Nitti, C.; Inguaggiato, P.; Tetta, C. Adsorption in sepsis. *Kidney Int. Suppl.* **2000**, *76*, S148–S155. [CrossRef] [PubMed]
24. de Pablo, R.; Monserrat, J.; Reyes, E.; Díaz, D.; Rodríguez-Zapata, M.; de la Hera, A.; Prieto, A.; Alvarez-Mon, M. Sepsis-induced acute respiratory distress syndrome with fatal outcome is associated to increased serum transforming growth factor beta-1 levels. *Eur. J. Intern. Med.* **2012**, *23*, 358–362. [CrossRef] [PubMed]
25. Freeman, B.D.; Machado, F.S.; Tanowitz, H.B.; Desruisseaux, M.S. Endothelin-1 and its role in the pathogenesis of infectious diseases. *Life Sci.* **2014**, *118*, 110–119. [CrossRef] [PubMed]
26. Bhattacharyya, S.; Kelley, K.; Melichian, D.S.; Tamaki, Z.; Fang, F.; Su, Y.; Feng, G.; Pope, R.M.; Budinger, G.R.S.; Mutlu, G.M.; et al. Toll-Like Receptor 4 Signaling Augments Transforming Growth Factor-β Responses. *Am. J. Pathol.* **2013**, *182*, 192–205. [CrossRef] [PubMed]
27. Rodríguez-Pascual, F.; Busnadiego, O.; González-Santamaría, J. The profibrotic role of endothelin-1: Is the door still open for the treatment of fibrotic diseases? *Life Sci.* **2014**, *118*, 156–164. [CrossRef]
28. Dunzendorfer, S.; Lee, H.-K.; Soldau, K.; Tobias, P.S. Toll-like receptor 4 functions intracellularly in human coronary artery endothelial cells: Roles of LBP and sCD14 in mediating LPS responses. *FASEB J.* **2004**, *18*, 1117–1119. [CrossRef]
29. Tran, M.; Tam, D.; Bardia, A.; Bhasin, M.; Rowe, G.C.; Kher, A.; Zsengeller, Z.K.; Akhavan-Sharif, M.R.; Khankin, E.V.; Saintgeniez, M.; et al. PGC-1α promotes recovery after acute kidney injury during systemic inflammation in mice. *J. Clin. Investig.* **2011**, *121*, 4003–4014. [CrossRef]
30. Kennedy-Lydon, T.M.; Crawford, C.; Wildman, S.S.P.; Peppiatt-Wildman, C.M. Renal pericytes: Regulators of medullary blood flow. *Acta Physiol.* **2013**, *207*, 212–225. [CrossRef]
31. Kramann, R.; Schneider, R.K.; DiRocco, D.P.; Machado, F.; Fleig, S.; Bondzie, P.A.; Henderson, J.M.; Ebert, B.L.; Humphreys, B.D. Perivascular Gli1+ progenitors are key contributors to injury-induced organ fibrosis. *Cell Stem Cell* **2015**, *16*, 51–66. [CrossRef] [PubMed]
32. Langenberg, C.; Wan, L.; Egi, M.; May, C.N.; Bellomo, R. Renal blood flow in experimental septic acute renal failure. *Kidney Int.* **2006**, *69*, 1996–2002. [CrossRef] [PubMed]
33. Anders, H.-J.; Banas, B.; Schlöndorff, D. Signaling danger: Toll-like receptors and their potential roles in kidney disease. *J. Am. Soc. Nephrol.* **2004**, *15*, 854–867. [CrossRef] [PubMed]
34. Dauphinee, S.M.; Karsan, A. Lipopolysaccharide signaling in endothelial cells. *Lab. Investig.* **2006**, *86*, 9–22. [CrossRef] [PubMed]
35. Bonventre, J.V.; Yang, L. Cellular pathophysiology of ischemic acute kidney injury. *J. Clin. Investig.* **2011**, *121*, 4210–4221. [CrossRef] [PubMed]
36. Souza, A.C.P.; Tsuji, T.; Baranova, I.N.; Bocharov, A.V.; Wilkins, K.J.; Street, J.M.; Alvarez-Prats, A.; Hu, X.; Eggerman, T.; Yuen, P.S.T.; et al. TLR4 mutant mice are protected from renal fibrosis and chronic kidney disease progression. *Physiol. Rep.* **2015**, *3*, e12558. [CrossRef]
37. Zhang, Y.; Su, X.; Zou, F.; Xu, T.; Pan, P.; Hu, C. Toll-like receptor-4 deficiency alleviates chronic intermittent hypoxia-induced renal injury, inflammation, and fibrosis. *Sleep Breath.* **2019**, *23*, 503–513. [CrossRef]
38. Jiang, H.; Qu, P.; Wang, J.-W.; Li, G.-H.; Wang, H.-Y. Effect of NF-κB inhibitor on Toll-like receptor 4 expression in left ventricular myocardium in two-kidney-one-clip hypertensive rats. *Eur. Rev. Med. Pharmacol. Sci.* **2018**, *22*, 3224–3233.
39. Campbell, M.T.; Hile, K.L.; Zhang, H.; Asanuma, H.; Vanderbrink, B.A.; Rink, R.R.; Meldrum, K.K. Toll-Like Receptor 4: A Novel Signaling Pathway During Renal Fibrogenesis. *J. Surg. Res.* **2011**, *168*, e61–e69. [CrossRef]
40. Tanimura, N.; Saitoh, S.; Matsumoto, F.; Akashi-Takamura, S.; Miyake, K. Roles for LPS-dependent interaction and relocation of TLR4 and TRAM in TRIF-signaling. *Biochem. Biophys. Res. Commun.* **2008**, *368*, 94–99. [CrossRef]
41. Sato, M.; Muragaki, Y.; Saika, S.; Roberts, A.B.; Ooshima, A. Targeted disruption of TGF-beta1/Smad3 signaling protects against renal tubulointerstitial fibrosis induced by unilateral ureteral obstruction. *J. Clin. Investig.* **2003**, *112*, 1486–1494. [CrossRef] [PubMed]
42. Carthy, J.M. TGFβ signaling and the control of myofibroblast differentiation: Implications for chronic inflammatory disorders. *J. Cell. Physiol.* **2018**, *233*, 98–106. [CrossRef] [PubMed]

43. Derynck, R.; Zhang, Y.E. Smad-dependent and Smad-independent pathways in TGF-β family signalling. *Nature* **2003**, *425*, 577–584. [CrossRef]
44. Li, J.H.; Huang, X.R.; Zhu, H.-J.; Oldfield, M.; Cooper, M.; Truong, L.D.; Johnson, R.J.; Lan, H.Y. Advanced glycation end products activate Smad signaling via TGF-beta-dependent and independent mechanisms: Implications for diabetic renal and vascular disease. *FASEB J.* **2004**, *18*, 176–178. [CrossRef] [PubMed]
45. Mori, Y.; Ishida, W.; Bhattacharyya, S.; Li, Y.; Platanias, L.C.; Varga, J. Selective inhibition of activin receptor-like kinase 5 signaling blocks profibrotic transforming growth factor beta responses in skin fibroblasts. *Arthritis Rheum.* **2004**, *50*, 4008–4021. [CrossRef]
46. Meng, X.-M.; Huang, X.R.; Xiao, J.; Chung, A.C.K.; Qin, W.; Chen, H.; Lan, H.Y. Disruption of Smad4 impairs TGF-β/Smad3 and Smad7 transcriptional regulation during renal inflammation and fibrosis in vivo and in vitro. *Kidney Int.* **2012**, *81*, 266–279. [CrossRef]
47. Gu, H.; Mickler, E.A.; Cummings, O.W.; Sandusky, G.E.; Weber, D.J.; Gracon, A.; Woodruff, T.; Wilkes, D.S.; Vittal, R. Crosstalk between TGF-β1 and complement activation augments epithelial injury in pulmonary fibrosis. *FASEB J.* **2014**, *28*, 4223–4234. [CrossRef]
48. Bhattacharyya, S.; Midwood, K.S.; Yin, H.; Varga, J. Toll-Like Receptor-4 Signaling Drives Persistent Fibroblast Activation and Prevents Fibrosis Resolution in Scleroderma. *Adv. Wound Care* **2017**, *6*, 356–369. [CrossRef]
49. Jerala, R. Structural biology of the LPS recognition. *Int. J. Med. Microbiol.* **2007**, *297*, 353–363. [CrossRef]
50. Wang, S.C.; Klein, R.D.; Wahl, W.L.; Alarcon, W.H.; Garg, R.J.; Remick, D.G.; Su, G.L. Tissue Coexpression of LBP and CD14 mRNA in a Mouse Model of Sepsis. *J. Surg. Res.* **1998**, *76*, 67–73. [CrossRef]
51. Stromberg, L.R.; Mendez, H.M.; Kubicek-Sutherland, J.Z.; Graves, S.W.; Hengartner, N.W.; Mukundan, H. Presentation matters: Impact of association of amphiphilic LPS with serum carrier proteins on innate immune signaling. *PLoS ONE* **2018**, *13*, e0198531. [CrossRef] [PubMed]
52. Webster, N.R.; Galley, H.F. Immunomodulation in the critically ill. *Br. J. Anaesth.* **2009**, *103*, 70–81. [CrossRef] [PubMed]
53. Bellomo, R.; Wan, L.; Langenberg, C.; May, C. Septic Acute Kidney Injury: New Concepts. *Nephron Exp. Nephrol.* **2008**, *109*, e95–e100. [CrossRef] [PubMed]

10

Kidney Injury by Variants in the *COL4A5* Gene Aggravated by Polymorphisms in Slit Diaphragm Genes Causes Focal Segmental Glomerulosclerosis

Jenny Frese [1,†], Matthias Kettwig [2,†], Hildegard Zappel [2], Johannes Hofer [3], Hermann-Josef Gröne [4], Mato Nagel [5], Gere Sunder-Plassmann [6], Renate Kain [7], Jörg Neuweiler [8] and Oliver Gross [1,*]

1 Clinic of Nephrology and Rheumatology, University Medical Center Goettingen, 37075 Goettingen, Germany; jenny.frese@dpdhl.com
2 Clinic of Pediatrics and Adolescent Medicine, University Medical Center Goettingen, 37075 Goettingen, Germany; matthias.kettwig@med.uni-goettingen.de (M.K.); hzappel@med.uni-goettingen.de (H.Z.)
3 Department of Pediatrics, Pediatrics I, Innsbruck Medical University, 6020 Innsbruck, Austria; Johannes.Hofer@i-med.ac.at
4 Department of Cellular and Molecular Pathology, German Cancer Research Center, 69120 Heidelberg, Germany; h.-j.groene@dkfz-heidelberg.de
5 Center for Nephrology and Metabolic Disorders, Molecular Diagnostics, 02943 Weißwasser, Germany; nagel@moldiag.de
6 Division of Nephrology and Dialysis, Department of Medicine III, Medical University of Vienna, 1090 Vienna, Austria; Gere.Sunder-Plassmann@meduniwien.ac.at
7 Department of Pathology, Medical University of Vienna, 1090 Vienna, Austria; renate.kain@meduniwien.ac.at
8 Institute of Pathology, Kantonsspital, 9007 St. Gallen, Switzerland; joerg.neuweiler@kssg.ch
* Correspondence: gross.oliver@med.uni-goettingen.de
† These authors contributed equally to this work.

Abstract: Kidney injury due to focal segmental glomerulosclerosis (FSGS) is the most common primary glomerular disorder causing end-stage renal disease. Homozygous mutations in either glomerular basement membrane or slit diaphragm genes cause early renal failure. Heterozygous carriers develop renal symptoms late, if at all. In contrast to mutations in slit diaphragm genes, hetero- or hemizygous mutations in the X-chromosomal *COL4A5* Alport gene have not yet been recognized as a major cause of kidney injury by FSGS. We identified cases of FSGS that were unexpectedly diagnosed: In addition to mutations in the X-chromosomal *COL4A5* type IV collagen gene, nephrin and podocin polymorphisms aggravated kidney damage, leading to FSGS with ruptures of the basement membrane in a toddler and early renal failure in heterozygous girls. The results of our case series study suggest a synergistic role for genes encoding basement membrane and slit diaphragm proteins as a cause of kidney injury due to FSGS. Our results demonstrate that the molecular genetics of different players in the glomerular filtration barrier can be used to evaluate causes of kidney injury. Given the high frequency of X-chromosomal carriers of Alport genes, the analysis of genes involved in the organization of podocyte architecture, the glomerular basement membrane, and the slit diaphragm will further improve our understanding of the pathogenesis of FSGS and guide prognosis of and therapy for hereditary glomerular kidney diseases.

Keywords: kidney injury; alport syndrome; modifier gene; nephrin; podocin; glomerular basement membrane; slit diaphragm; focal segmental glomerulosclerosis

---

1. Introduction

Focal segmental glomerulosclerosis (FSGS) is the most common primary glomerular disorder causing end-stage renal disease (ESRD) in the United States [1]. Podocyte injury plays a critical role in the pathogenesis of proteinuric kidney diseases, as podocytes are important for maintaining the glomerular filtration barrier [2]. They restore crucial components of the glomerular basement membrane (GBM), such as $\alpha3/\alpha4/\alpha5$ type IV collagen chains (*COL4A3/4/5*), and of the slit diaphragm, such as nephrin (*NPHS1*) and podocin (*NPHS2*). Homozygous or hemizygous mutations in glomerular filtration barrier genes, such as the *COL4A3/4/5* genes, result in Alport syndrome (AS) [3–5], while homozygous mutations in the *NPHS1* and *NPHS2* genes result in congenital nephrotic syndrome [6,7]. The development of these syndromes leads to early ESRD. Few heterozygous carriers develop late changes, and they rarely (or never, in the case of *NPHS1/2* heterozygotes) develop ESRD. Polymorphisms in these genes are thought to result in an even milder phenotype or no phenotype.

The typical clinical signs of FSGS are marked proteinuria and podocyte injury. FSGS often manifests as nephrotic syndrome and frequently leads to renal failure. As FSGS is much less responsive to steroid therapy than minimal change disease, its prognosis for preserving renal function is (much) worse, with a high recurrence rate after renal transplantation [8].

The initial injuries leading to FSGS vary widely from monogenetic forms to secondary forms, which can be triggered by maladaptation of the podocyte to hyperfiltration, virus infections, drug use, or (unknown) circulating factors [8]. Primary (monogenetic) FSGS is caused by variants in the structural genes of the podocyte or the extracellular matrix (GBM). Primary FSGS typically results in in early onset of disease during childhood or adolescence.

Approximately 80% of adult cases of FSGS are primary (idiopathic) [1]. Up to 10% of familial FSGS can be explained by autosomal *COL4A3/4* mutations [9]; however, *COL4A5* mutations leading to X-linked Alport syndrome (XLAS) are much more common. Here, we describe three families with FSGS, which was unexpectedly diagnosed in toddlers with XLAS and in adolescent XLAS carriers with renal failure. In addition to mutations in the XLAS-related *COL4A5* gene, nephrin and podocin polymorphisms seem to have aggravated kidney damage, including severe FSGS with GBM ruptures in a toddler and unusually early renal failure in heterozygous girls.

2. Results

Patient 1 (case 1) was the index patient, in whom a severe kidney phenotype and GBM ruptures led to the discovery that in FSGS due to genetic GBM diseases, such as AS, polymorphisms in slit diaphragm genes can aggravate kidney damage. Subsequently, two other families with X-chromosomal AS were found to have FSGS, which was aggravated by slit diaphragm gene polymorphisms (Table 1).

Table 1. Summary of patient phenotypes and genotypes.

Patient	Sex	First Clinical Presentation > Symptoms	Genotype *COL4A5*	Genotype *Nphs-1/-2*	Ear/Eye	Dialysis/Tx	Medication	Affected Family Members
Case 1 A.N. II-1	♂	27 months macrohematuria acanthocytes proteinuria urinary tract infection	*COL4A5* p.W1538X (TGG>TGA) hemizygous	*Nphs1*: p.R408Q (CGG>CAG) polymorphism heterozygous *Nphs1*:p.S1105S(TCG>TCA) polymorphism homozygous *Nphs2*: p.G34G (GGA>GGG) polymorphism homozygous	no pathological findings	none	2012–today ACEi	no kidney diseases known mother without symptoms: *Nphs1*: p.R408Q (CGG>CAG) polymorphism heterozygous
Case 2 C.V. II-4	♀	11 years macrohematuria proteinuria urinary tract infection	*COL4A5* Exon 49, Codon 1510, IVS49+3A>G heterozygous	*Nphs2*: p.R229Q (CGA>CAA) polymorphism heterozygous	no pathological findings	Tx age: 15	/refused treatment	no other family members affected
S.V. III-1	♀	1 year macrohematuria Proteinuria	*COL4A5* Exon 49, Codon 1510, IVS49+3A>G heterozygous	*Nphs2*: p.R229Q (CGA>CAA) polymorphism heterozygous	no pathological findings	none	/refused treatment	
M.V. III-2	♂	4 months macrohematuria proteinuria	*COL4A5* Exon 49, Codon 1510, IVS49+3A>G hemizygous	none	no pathological findings	none	/refuse treatment	
Case 3 L.U. II-3	♀	27 years hematuria proteinuria	*COL4A5* p.G624D (GGT>GAT) heterozygous	*Nphs2*: p.R229Q (CGA>CAA) polymorphism heterozygous *Nphs2*: p.G34G(GGA>GGG) polymorphism homozygous	minimal high-frequency hearing loss (2013)	Tx age: 51	Before Tx: ACEi from 33 years	see pedigree of family (Figure 3)
W.T. II-7	♀	40 years: microhematuria 42 years: proteinuria	*COL4A5* p.G624D (GGT>GAT) heterozygous	none	retinal detachment	none	02/2013: ACEi (discontinued due to angioedema)	
T.O. II.4	♀	microhematuria	*COL4A5* p.G624D (GGT>GAT) heterozygous	none	high-frequency hearing loss (2013)	none	none	
S.O. III-7	♂	microhematuria	*COL4A5* p.G624D (GGT>GAT) heterozygous	none	no pathological findings (2013)	none	none	
O.T. III-12	♀	no symptoms	*COL4A5* p.G624D (GGT>GAT) heterozygous	not investigated	not investigated	none	none	

2.1. Clinical Presentation

Patient 1 was a 27-month-old boy with persistent macrohematuria, proteinuria (1300 mg/L), active sediment, and normal renal function. His older sister and his non-consanguineous Lithuanian parents were healthy, with no family history of kidney diseases (Figure 1a). Post-infectious glomerulonephritis was excluded. Due to the initial suspicion of an infection and normal renal morphology on ultrasound examination, a cystoscopy was performed, which revealed hemorrhagic cystitis. However, common causes of hemorrhagic cystitis in childhood [10,11], such as cytomegalovirus or BK-polyomavirus infection, were ruled out. Consequently, a renal biopsy was performed. Light microscopy and immunohistochemistry (Figure 1b,c) revealed profound FSGS, IgM-positive deposits, and slight mesangial expansion. Ultrastructurally, the GBM presented with diffuse splitting, thinning, and ruptures (Figure 1d–f). The podocytes showed foot process effacement, with partial loss of the slit diaphragm (Figure 1d). These structural changes led to the diagnosis of AS. Hearing and eye evaluations did not reveal any abnormalities. Nephroprotective angiotensin-converting enzyme (ACE)-inhibitor therapy with ramipril was started [12,13], and the proteinuria slowly decreased from 1300 mg/L to less than 400 mg/L (Figure 1g). No further macrohematuria was reported.

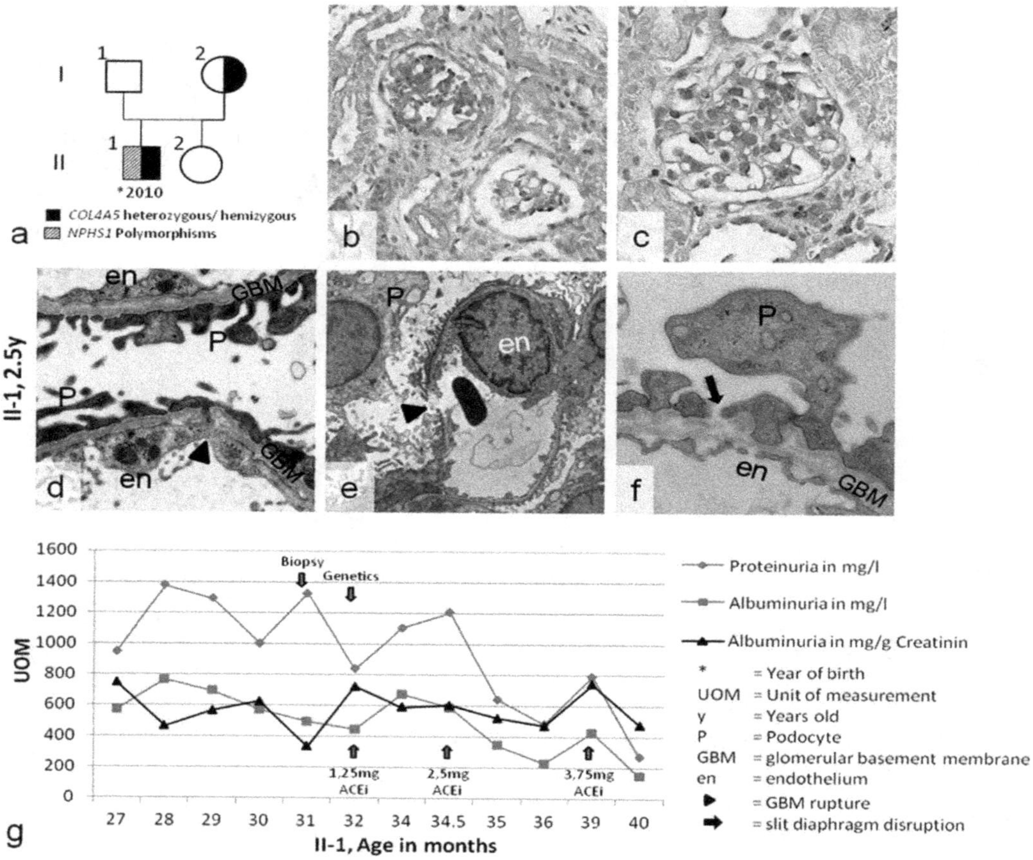

Figure 1. (**a**) Pedigree of case 1. (**b–f**) Nephropathological evaluation of the kidney biopsy of patient II-1. (**b**,**c**) Light microscopy showing focal segmental glomerulosclerosis (FSGS) and slight mesangial matrix expansion. (**d–f**) Ultrastructural analysis showing gross broadening of the podocyte foot processes; partial loss of the slit diaphragm (black arrow); and splitting, thinning, and ruptures of the glomerular basement membrane (GBM) (arrowhead). (**g**) The course of disease during ACE-inhibitor therapy: proteinuria constantly decreased (arrow). The diagnostic timescale is indicated by the blue arrows. Magnification: (**b**,**c**) 400×, (**d**) 20,000×, (**e**) 8000×, (**f**) 25,000×.

Case 2 was an Austrian family with severe kidney disease in the mother, daughter, and son (Figure 2). The mother presented with hematuria and proteinuria in childhood. She soon developed ESRD and received a kidney transplant from her father at the age of 15. Her kidney biopsy at 11 years of age revealed advanced FSGS, hyalinosis, tubulointerstitial foam cells, podocyte effacement, splitting, lamellations, and partial thinning of the GBM. AS was considered; however, due to the unusual nature of a severe manifestation in a girl with healthy parents, she was diagnosed as having FSGS and nephrotic syndrome, with secondary structural changes in the GBM (Figure 2b,c).

Her daughter and son both presented with hematuria and progressive proteinuria during the first year of life. A kidney biopsy performed when the daughter was two years old appeared relatively normal under light microscopy, although ultrastructural analysis showed advanced pathology, with podocyte effacement and splitting and thinning of the GBM, similar to the mother's biopsy (Figure 2d–g). Hearing and eye evaluations did not reveal any pathological abnormalities in any family member. The family refused therapeutic intervention, leading to progressive proteinuria in both siblings (Figure 2h). Currently, the daughter and son have reached stage 3 of chronic kidney disease.

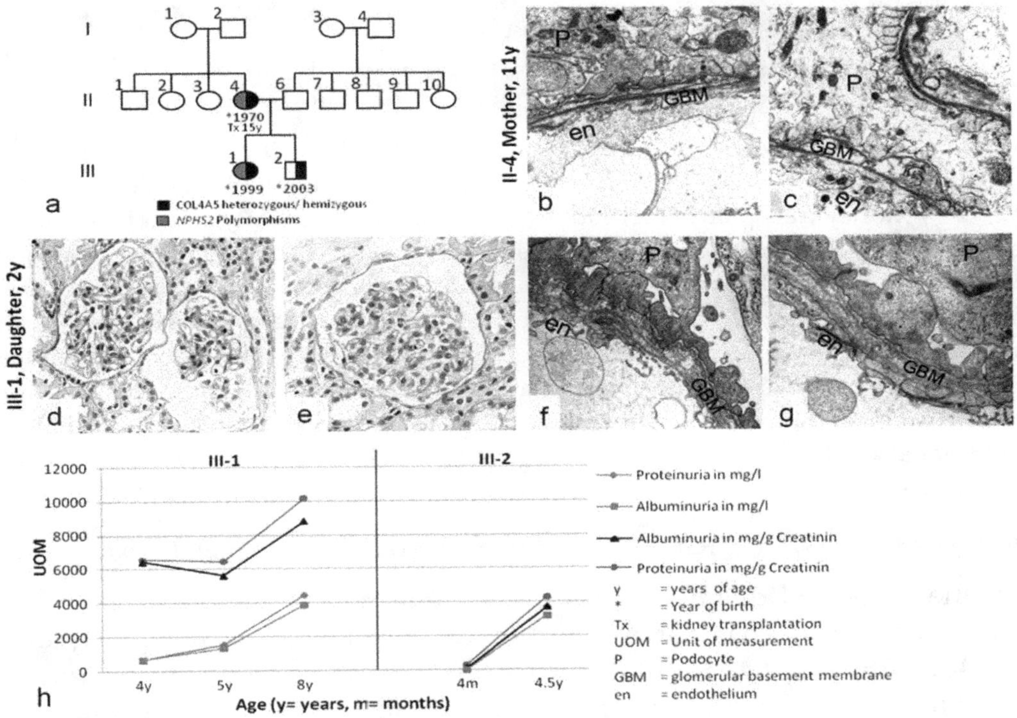

Figure 2. (**a**) Pedigree of case 2. (**b**,**c**) Kidney biopsy of the mother (11 y) revealing partial GBM thinning, splitting, and laminations in the lamina densa, with plump podocyte (P) foot processes. (**d**–**g**) Kidney biopsy of the daughter (3 y). (**d**,**e**) Light microscopy showing relatively normal glomerular and tubulointerstitial structures. Electron microscopy uncovered GBM pathology with splitting and thinning, similar to the mother's nephropathology. (**h**) The course of disease without therapy in this X-chromosomal *COL4A5* genotype was unexpectedly very similar in the heterozygous girl (III-1) and her hemizygous brother (III-2): proteinuria constantly increased into the nephrotic range. Magnification: (**b**,**c**) 10,000×, (**d**,**e**) 400×, (**f**,**g**) 12,500×.

Case 3 was a family originating from Austria and Poland (Figure 3a). A kidney biopsy performed in a 27-year-old female (II-3) with hematuria and proteinuria showed advanced FSGS (Figure 3b,c). The biopsied material was not sufficient for ultrastructural analysis. A definite diagnosis was not possible; however, FSGS was suspected. The patient developed ESRD at approximately 40 years of age and received a kidney transplant at 51 years of age. Kidney disease progressed more slowly in her sister (II-7), who first presented with microhematuria at the age of 40. Further evaluation of several other affected family members (Figure 3a) revealed moderate hearing loss in patients II-3 and II-4 and eye involvement in patient II-7. Therefore, a complex hereditary kidney disease was considered.

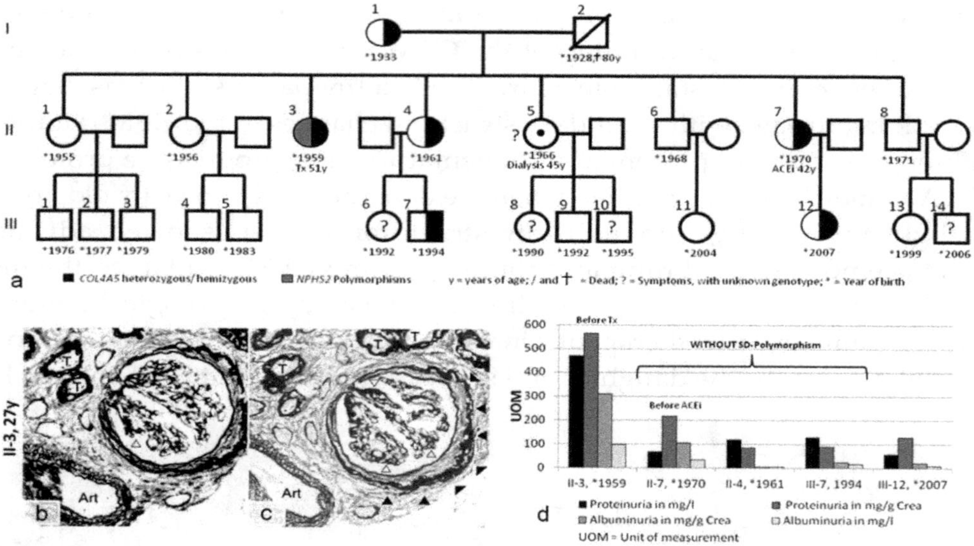

Figure 3. (**a**) Pedigree of case 3, with I-1 and family members (II-1, II-2, II-5, II-6, and II-8) living in Poland. Further evaluation was performed on family members living in Vienna (II-3, II-4, II-7, III-7, and III-12). Tx = kidney transplant. (**b**,**c**) Kidney biopsy in case II-3. Only a small core of renal tissue could be obtained for light microscopy. This tissue contained only one relatively intact glomerulus and three glomerular scars. The pathology was described as nonspecific and dominated by sclerosis. The glomerulus showed segmental scarring of the capillary loops (open arrowheads) and pronounced periglomerular fibrosis (solid arrowheads). The tubules (T) were dissociated by interstitial fibrosis, and thickening of the tubular basement membranes confirmed advanced atrophy. One small artery (Art) exhibited minimal intimal fibrosis. (**d**) Proteinuria and albuminuria in family members with and without additional slit diaphragm (SD) polymorphisms. Methenamine silver (**b**) and PAS staining (**c**); magnification: 400×.

2.2. Genetic Analyses of COL4A3/4/5 GBM Genes and NPHS1/2 Slit Diaphragm Genes

In case 1, the suspected diagnosis of AS was confirmed by genetic testing. A hemizygous X-chromosomal *COL4A5* de novo mutation was discovered in the boy but not in his parents: p.W1538X (TGG>TGA), c.4614 G>A. *COL4A5* mutations are typically associated with microhematuria in the first few years of life, slowly progressing to microalbuminuria below 300 mg [14], but not with high levels of proteinuria such as the 1300 mg/L observed in the two-year-old boy. Therefore, the severe phenotype of the two-year-old boy, an origin close to Scandinavia, and unusually severe FSGS led to the exploration of the slit diaphragm genes *NPHS1* and *NPHS2*. A polymorphism (p.R408Q (CGG>CAG), c.1223G>A) in *NPHS1* (nephrin) was identified in the boy and in his mother, who was not affected by the *COL4A5* mutation. Furthermore, homozygous silent polymorphisms in *NPHS1* (p.S1105S (TCG>TCA), c.102A>G) and *NPHS2* (p.G34G (GGA>GGG) c.3315G>A) were discovered in the boy (Table 1).

In case 2, a *COL4A5* splice mutation (exon 49, codon 1510, IVS49+3A>G) was hemizygous in the boy and heterozygous in the girl and the mother. No other family members were affected, suggesting that this was a de novo mutation in the mother (Figure 2 and Table 1). The heterozygous mother and daughter were both severely affected; however, proteinuria is usually mild or absent in young heterozygous *COL4A5* females, and early progression to ESRD before the third decade of life has never been described [14,15]. As in case 1, the severe phenotype of the heterozygous carriers led to an exploration of the slit diaphragm genes. Both heterozygous females, but not the hemizygous son, had a heterozygous *NPHS2* polymorphism (p.R229Q (CGA>CAA), c.686G>A; Table 1) that has been described as a modifier gene in thin basement membrane disease [16,17]. The clinical course of the son, who lacked the *NPHS2* polymorphism, was consistent with X-chromosomal AS in males. In contrast, the clinical courses of his heterozygous sister and mother, who had the *NPHS2* polymorphism, were very unusual.

In case 3, patient II-3 had a heterozygous *COL4A5* mutation (p.G624D (GGT>GAT), c.1871 G>A) that generally results in benign hematuria in females and late-onset ESRD in hemizygous males (in the 4th decade of life) [16]. Again, the severe phenotype resulted in further evaluation, and a polymorphism in *NPHS2* (p.R229Q (CGA>CAA), c.686G>A) in addition to a silent single-nucleotide polymorphism (SNP) in *NPHS2* (p.G34G (GGA>GGG), c.102A>G) were identified. Importantly, the G34G variant was found independently in case 1 and case 3, but represents a polymorphism of unknown relevance. All other family members presented only the *COL4A5* mutation (Figure 3a), and their clinical courses were consistent with benign hematuria (in females) and slowly progressing renal disease (in males) (Table 1). The heterozygous female with the *NPHS2* polymorphism (II-3) had higher proteinuria compared with her heterozygous sisters (II-7 and II-4) at the same age, who did not have the *NPHS2* polymorphism (Figure 3d).

2.3. Slit Diaphragm Gene Polymorphisms Aggravate Glomerular Architecture towards FSGS in Patients with GBM Mutations

Morphological analysis of case 1 further underscored the evidence that a *COL4A5* mutation in a basement membrane component can be aggravated by polymorphisms in slit diaphragm genes: (1) pronounced FSGS has not been previously described in toddlers with AS (Figure 1b,c); however, (2) initial thinning (and splitting) of the GBM is a common feature in children with AS (Figure 1d). GBM ruptures have not been previously described in patients with AS (Figure 1e). (3) Gross broadening of the podocyte foot processes, with partial loss of the slit diaphragm (Figure 1d), is a very notable and unusual finding in toddlers with AS, and (4) a high level of proteinuria (1300 mg/l with persistent macrohematuria) is unusual for a toddler with AS. The last feature and the FSGS were judged as being indicative of additional podocyte pathology. The structural changes led to the presumptive diagnosis of AS, though with the differential diagnosis of mutations in podocyte genes, as the atypically progressive structural changes could not be attributed to the patient's age and his primary diagnosis of AS.

In case 2, the mother was diagnosed in childhood as having nephrotic-range FSGS with secondary GBM changes (Figure 2b,c). Kidney pathology in the 3-year-old daughter, with gross broadening of the podocyte foot processes (Figure 2f,g), was similar to that of her mother. In both individuals, despite their "merely" heterozygous AS status, the *NPHS2* polymorphism aggravated GBM pathology toward FSGS and early ESRD. Despite X-inactivation, ESRD has not been previously described in heterozygous AS carriers during adolescence. Notably, the hemizygous son, who had full-pattern AS but lacked the *NPHS2* polymorphism, had a clinical course that was identical to that of his "merely" heterozygous sister with the *NPHS2* polymorphism.

In case 3, the kidney pathology of the *COL4A5* carrier (II-3) was dominated by sclerosis (Figure 3b,c). This finding is a clear contradiction to the thin GBM that one would have expected in a young female with a heterozygous p.G624D mutation. This glomerulosclerosis may be due to the *NPHS2* polymorphism, as proteinuria was much lower in all other p.G624D-affected family members without the *NPHS2* polymorphism (e.g., the sister (II-4) at the same age). Even the *COL4A5* hemizygous adult male presented with less than 20% of the proteinuria of his aunt (II-3).

3. Discussion

It has been predicted that next-generation sequencing will identify most of the monogenic disease-causing genes by the year 2020 [18]. Next-generation sequencing has recently been shown to improve mutation screening in familial hematuric nephropathies [19]. However, the increasing knowledge of human genetic pathology will be associated with major challenges. Here, we show that for personalized medical care, physicians need all (1) a careful clinical evaluation of their patients,

(2) close cooperation with the pathologist interpreting (kidney) specimens, and (3) genetic information about mutations and polymorphisms that might influence disease. Remarkably, thorough clinical exploration and its correlation with the kidney histology by the pathologist were essential tools guiding disease-focused genetic evaluation in the three families that we described. Without clinical and histological assessment preceding mutation analysis, physicians would not be able to understand and interpret the pathology of the glomerular filtration barrier [20].

As a limitation of our study, phenotyping of all family members and the extension of genetic correlation to other slit diaphragm genes was restricted by regional barriers, as family members originated from four different countries. The use of Sanger sequencing limited our search for possible disease-causing mutations to only five genes, whereas mutations in other podocyte genes could be contributory [21]. Additional regional legal barriers hindered us from extending the genetic analysis beyond the *COL4A3/4/5* and *NPHS1/2* genes. Still, our study was able to correlate the phenotype to the genetic changes in most members of a large three-generation pedigree, with a less severe phenotype in patients II-4, II-7, and III-7 without polymorphisms in slit diaphragm genes (Figure 3).

Podocytes evolve into crucial cells that maintain the glomerular filtration barrier in renal diseases. Because of their need to withstand permanent filtration pressure, these cells adhere tightly to the underlying GBM [22]. The dynamic control of their cytoskeleton is affected by the slit diaphragm [22]. As a consequence, podocyte dedifferentiation, effacement, and FSGS are very common features in renal diseases [23]. Reducing the filtration pressure and thus protecting podocytes is a crucial therapeutic goal, even in children with congenital renal diseases [24].

Malone and coworkers demonstrated that up to 10% of familial FSGS can be explained by autosomal *COL4A3/4* mutations [9]. Our investigations expand previous findings that FSGS can also be caused by *COL4A5* mutations, the most common cause of AS, aggravated by polymorphisms in slit diaphragm genes [20,25]. $\alpha3/\alpha4/\alpha5$ type IV collagen chains stabilize the GBM against filtration pressure [26]. Loss of any of the $\alpha3/\alpha4/\alpha5$ type IV collagen chains results in a weaker GBM and increased podocyte cytoskeleton vulnerability [27]. As the cell–cell adhesions of the slit diaphragm are closely linked to the podocyte cytoskeleton, any polymorphism in slit diaphragm genes [28–31], as demonstrated in our study, might result in further damage in the histological picture of FSGS. This hypothesis should be tested in animal models using heterozygous $NPHS2^{+/R140Q}$ mice, which correspond to the most common p.R138Q mutation found in humans and $COL4A3^{+/-}$ mice [32–35]. $NPHS2^{+/R140Q}$ mice develop no phenotype [32], while $COL4A3^{+/-}$ mice develop benign familial hematuria [33,34]. The mature GBM with the $\alpha3/4/5$ (IV) collagen chains can solely be built by podocytes, which sense the integrity of the GBM via their type IV collagen receptors, such as discoidin receptor 1 (DDR1) and integrins [4]. On the other hand, the crosstalk between the collagen receptor and the podocyte actin cytoskeleton, which also interacts with the slit diaphragm, might be the crucial link between the GBM and slit diaphragm that causes FSGS in our patients [4].

In conclusion, our findings demonstrate that after thorough clinical evaluation, the molecular genetics of different players in the glomerular filtration barrier can be used to evaluate FSGS. The analysis of genes involved in the organization of podocyte architecture, the GBM, and the slit diaphragm will further our understanding of the histological picture of FSGS. Our increasing knowledge of genes, arising from next-generation sequencing, will help to personalize the diagnosis and prognosis of and therapy for glomerular kidney diseases. Experienced physicians and pathologists are still needed to classify genetic results for the benefit of the patient.

4. Methods

4.1. Ethical Considerations

Written informed consent was given by the families for the publication of their cases. ICH-GCP data acquisition and storage of the European Alport registry was approved by the IRB of the University Medicine Goettingen, Germany (AZ 10/11/06; updated version from 2014).

The European Alport registry has been registered at ClinicalTrials.gov (NCT 02378805) and as EudraCT number 2014-003533-25.

4.2. Genetic Analyses

EDTA-treated blood was obtained after written informed consent was provided. Genomic DNA was extracted from peripheral blood leukocytes. The coding regions of *COL4A3*, *COL4A4*, *COL4A5*, *NPHS1*, and *NPHS2* were analyzed: The entire coding regions and splice sites of the *NPHS1* (transcript NM_004646.3; 29 exons), *NPHS2* (transcript NM_014625.2; 8 exons), *COL4A3* (transcript NM_000091.4; 52 exons), *COL4A4* (transcript NM_000092.4; 48 exons), and *COL4A5* (transcript NM_033380.2; 53 exons) genes were sequenced using unidirectional tagged primer Sanger sequencing in a 96-well format. Polymerase chain reaction (PCR) primers were designed using Primer-BLAST® from the NCBI (National Center for Biotechnology Information, Bethesda, MD, USA). PCR products were generated using Buffer HOT Fire Polymerase® (Solis Biodyne Solis, Tartu, Estonia) at an annealing temperature of 60 °C and were cleaned up using an Illustra ExoProStar One-Step® kit (GE Healthcare, Freiburg, Germany). Sequencing was performed using a BigDye® Terminator v1.1 cycle kit (Applied Biosystems®, Life Technologies GmbH, Darmstadt, Germany), and products were cleaned up using a CentriSep ABI® kit (Applied Biosystems®, Life Technologies GmbH, Darmstadt, Germany). The sequences were read with an ABI Prism® 3130XL DNA analyzer (Applied Biosystems®, Life Technologies GmbH, Darmstadt, Germany) and were analyzed using our in-house sequence analysis software (SeqEdit).

4.3. Morphological Analyses

Kidney biopsies were analyzed by light microscopy, immunohistochemistry, and electron microscopy.

Author Contributions: H.-J.G., R.K. and J.N. analyzed and interpreted the kidney biopsies, including the interpretation of the clinical and genetic data, and co-wrote the manuscript. M.N. analyzed and interpreted all mutations and polymorphisms, including the interpretation of the clinical and histological data, and co-wrote the manuscript. M.K., H.Z., J.H. and G.S.-P. took care of the patients, analyzed and interpreted the clinical data, including the interpretation of the genetic and histological data, and co-wrote the manuscript. J.F. collected all data, was involved in all data analysis and interpretation, and wrote the primary version of the manuscript. O.G. conceived the study design and concept, was involved in all data analysis and interpretation, and wrote the final version of the manuscript. All authors read and approved the manuscript.

Acknowledgments: We thank all families for their contribution and consent for the publication of their cases.

References

1. D'Agati, V.D.; Kaskel, F.J.; Falk, R.J. Focal segmental glomerulosclerosis. *N. Engl. J. Med.* **2011**, *365*, 2398–2411. [CrossRef] [PubMed]
2. Brinkkoetter, P.T.; Ising, C.; Benzing, T. The role of the podocyte in albumin filtration. *Nat. Rev. Nephrol.* **2013**, *9*, 328–336. [CrossRef] [PubMed]
3. Hudson, B.G.; Tryggvason, K.; Sundaramoorthy, M.; Neilson, E.G. Alport's syndrome, Goodpasture's syndrome, and type IV collagen. *N. Engl. J. Med.* **2003**, *348*, 2543–2556. [CrossRef] [PubMed]
4. Kruegel, J.; Rubel, D.; Gross, O. Alport syndrome—Insights from basic and clinical research. *Nat. Rev. Nephrol.* **2013**, *9*, 170–178. [CrossRef] [PubMed]
5. Storey, H.; Savige, J.; Sivakumar, V.; Abbs, S.; Flinter, F.A. COL4A3/COL4A4 mutations and features in individuals with autosomal recessive Alport syndrome. *J. Am. Soc. Nephrol.* **2013**, *24*, 1945–1954. [CrossRef] [PubMed]
6. Gubler, M.C. Podocyte differentiation and hereditary proteinuria/nephrotic syndromes. *J. Am. Soc. Nephrol.* **2003**, *14* (Suppl. 1), S22–S26. [CrossRef] [PubMed]
7. Niaudet, P. Genetic forms of nephrotic syndrome. *Pediatr. Nephrol.* **2004**, *19*, 1313–1318. [CrossRef]

8. Fogo, A.B. Causes and pathogenesis of focal segmental glomerulosclerosis. *Nat. Rev. Nephrol.* **2015**, *11*, 76–87. [CrossRef]
9. Malone, A.F.; Phelan, P.J.; Hall, G.; Cetincelik, U.; Homstad, A.; Alonso, A.S.; Jiang, R.; Lindsey, T.B.; Wu, G.; Sparks, M.A.; et al. Rare hereditary COL4A3/COL4A4 variants may be mistaken for familial focal segmental glomerulosclerosis. *Kidney Int.* **2014**, *86*, 1253–1259. [CrossRef]
10. Megged, O.; Stein, J.; Ben-Meir, D.; Shulman, L.M.; Yaniv, I.; Shalit, I.; Levy, I. BK-virus-associated hemorrhagic cystitis in children after hematopoietic stem cell transplantation. *J. Pediatr. Hematol. Oncol.* **2011**, *33*, 190–193. [CrossRef]
11. Kloos, R.Q.; Boelens, J.J.; de Jong, T.P.; Versluys, B.; Bierings, M. Hemorrhagic cystitis in a cohort of pediatric transplantations: Incidence, treatment, outcome, and risk factors. *Biol. Blood Marrow Transplant.* **2013**, *19*, 1263–1266. [CrossRef] [PubMed]
12. Gross, O.; Licht, C.; Anders, H.J.; Hoppe, B.; Beck, B.; Tönshoff, B.; Höcker, B.; Wygoda, S.; Ehrich, J.H.; Pape, L.; et al. Early angiotensin-converting enzyme inhibition in Alport syndrome delays renal failure and improves life expectancy. *Kidney Int.* **2012**, *81*, 494–501. [CrossRef] [PubMed]
13. Gross, O.; Friede, T.; Hilgers, R.; Görlitz, A.; Gavénis, K.; Ahmed, R.; Dürr, U. Safety and Efficacy of the ACE-Inhibitor Ramipril in Alport Syndrome: The Double-Blind, Randomized, Placebo-Controlled, Multicenter Phase III EARLY PRO-TECT Alport Trial in Pediatric Patients. *ISRN Pediatr.* **2012**, *2012*, 436046. [CrossRef] [PubMed]
14. Gross, O.; Netzer, K.O.; Lambrecht, R.; Seibold, S.; Weber, M. Meta-analysis of genotype-phenotype correlation in X-linked Alport syndrome: Impact on clinical counselling. *Nephrol. Dial. Transplant.* **2002**, *17*, 1218–1227. [CrossRef] [PubMed]
15. Jais, J.P.; Knebelmann, B.; Giatras, I.; De Marchi, M.; Rizzoni, G.; Renieri, A.; Weber, M.; Gross, O.; Netzer, K.O.; Flinter, F.; et al. X-linked Alport syndrome: Natural history and genotype-phenotype correlations in girls and women belonging to 195 families: A "European Community Alport Syndrome Concerted Action" study. *J. Am. Soc. Nephrol.* **2003**, *14*, 2603–2610. [CrossRef] [PubMed]
16. Knebelmann, B.; Breillat, C.; Forestier, L.; Arrondel, C.; Jacassier, D.; Giatras, I.; Drouot, L.; Deschênes, G.; Grünfeld, J.P.; Broyer, M.; et al. Spectrum of mutations in the COL4A5 collagen gene in X-linked Alport syndrome. *Am. J. Hum. Genet.* **1996**, *59*, 1221–1232. [PubMed]
17. Voskarides, K.; Arsali, M.; Athanasiou, Y.; Elia, A.; Pierides, A.; Deltas, C. Evidence that NPHS2-R229Q predisposes to proteinuria and renal failure in familial hematuria. *Pediatr. Nephrol.* **2012**, *27*, 675–679. [CrossRef]
18. Boycott, K.M.; Vanstone, M.R.; Bulman, D.E.; MacKenzie, A.E. Rare-disease genetics in the era of next-generation sequencing: Discovery to translation. *Nat. Rev. Genet.* **2013**, *14*, 681–691. [CrossRef]
19. Morinière, V.; Dahan, K.; Hilbert, P.; Lison, M.; Lebbah, S.; Topa, A.; Bole-Feysot, C.; Pruvost, S.; Nitschke, P.; Plaisier, E.; et al. Improving Mutation Screening in Familial Hematuric Nephropathies through Next Generation Sequencing. *J. Am. Soc. Nephrol.* **2014**, *25*, 2740–2751. [CrossRef]
20. Gibson, J.; Gilbert, R.D.; Bunyan, D.J.; Angus, E.M.; Fowler, D.J.; Ennis, S. Exome analysis resolves differential diagnosis of familial kidney disease and uncovers a potential confounding variant. *Genet. Res.* **2014**, *28*, 1–9. [CrossRef]
21. Bullich, G.; Trujillano, D.; Santín, S.; Ballarín, J.; Torra, R.; Estivill, X.; Ars, E. Targeted next-generation sequencing in steroid-resistant nephrotic syndrome: Mutations in multiple glomerular genes may influence disease severity. *Eur. J. Hum. Genet.* **2014**, *23*, 1192. [CrossRef] [PubMed]
22. Cravedi, P.; Kopp, J.B.; Remuzzi, G. Recent progress in the pathophysiology and treatment of FSGS recurrence. *Am. J. Transplant.* **2013**, *13*, 266–274. [CrossRef] [PubMed]
23. Sachs, N.; Sonnenberg, A. Cell-matrix adhesion of podocytes in physiology and disease. *Nat. Rev. Nephrol.* **2013**, *9*, 200–210. [CrossRef] [PubMed]
24. Ingelfinger, J.R. Blood-pressure control and delay in progression of kidney disease in children. *N. Engl. J. Med.* **2009**, *361*, 1701–1703. [CrossRef] [PubMed]
25. Adam, J.; Connor, T.M.; Wood, K.; Lewis, D.; Naik, R.; Gale, D.P.; Sayer, J.A. Genetic testing can resolve diagnostic confusion in Alport syndrome. *Clin. Kidney J.* **2014**, *7*, 197–200. [CrossRef] [PubMed]
26. Fidler, A.L.; Vanacore, R.M.; Chetyrkin, S.V.; Pedchenko, V.K.; Bhave, G.; Yin, V.P.; Stothers, C.L.; Rose, K.L.; McDonald, W.H.; Clark, T.A.; et al. A unique covalent bond in basement membrane is a primordial innovation for tissue evolution. *Proc. Natl. Acad. Sci. USA* **2014**, *111*, 331–336. [CrossRef] [PubMed]

27. Welsh, G.I.; Saleem, M.A. The podocyte cytoskeleto—Key to a functioning glomerulus in health and disease. *Nat. Rev. Nephrol.* **2011**, *8*, 14–21. [CrossRef]
28. Tsukaguchi, H.; Sudhakar, A.; Le, T.C.; Nguyen, T.; Yao, J.; Schwimmer, J.A.; Schachter, A.D.; Poch, E.; Abreu, P.F.; Appel, G.B.; et al. NPHS2 mutations in late-onset focal segmental glomerulosclerosis: R229Q is a common disease-associated allele. *J. Clin. Invest.* **2002**, *110*, 1659–1666. [CrossRef]
29. Ozaltin, F.; Ibsirlioglu, T.; Taskiran, E.Z.; Baydar, D.E.; Kaymaz, F.; Buyukcelik, M.; Kilic, B.D.; Balat, A.; Iatropoulos, P.; Asan, E.; et al. Disruption of PTPRO causes childhood-onset nephrotic syndrome. *Am. J. Hum. Genet.* **2011**, *89*, 139–147. [CrossRef]
30. Tory, K.; Menyhárd, D.K.; Woerner, S.; Nevo, F.; Gribouval, O.; Kerti, A.; Stráner, P.; Arrondel, C.; Huynh Cong, E.; Tulassay, T.; et al. Mutation-dependent recessive inheritance of NPHS2-associated steroid-resistant nephrotic syndrome. *Nat. Genet.* **2014**, *46*, 299–304. [CrossRef]
31. Kerti, A.; Csohány, R.; Wagner, L.; Jávorszky, E.; Maka, E.; Tory, K. NPHS2 homozygous p.R229Q variant: Potential modifier instead of causal effect in focal segmental glomerulosclerosis. *Pediatr. Nephrol.* **2013**, *28*, 2061–2429. [CrossRef] [PubMed]
32. Philippe, A.; Weber, S.; Esquivel, E.L.; Houbron, C.; Hamard, G.; Ratelade, J.; Kriz, W.; Schaefer, F.; Gubler, M.C.; Antignac, C. A missense mutation in podocin leads to early and severe renal disease in mice. *Kidney Int.* **2008**, *73*, 1038–1047. [CrossRef] [PubMed]
33. Tonna, S.; Wang, Y.Y.; Wilson, D.; Rigby, L.; Tabone, T.; Cotton, R.; Savige, J. The R229Q mutation in NPHS2 may predispose to proteinuria in thin-basement-membrane nephropathy. *Pediatr. Nephrol.* **2008**, *23*, 2201–2207. [CrossRef] [PubMed]
34. Beirowski, B.; Weber, M.; Gross, O. Chronic renal failure and shortened lifespan in COL4A3$^{+/-}$ mice: An animal model for thin basement membrane nephropathy. *J. Am. Soc. Nephrol.* **2006**, *17*, 1986–1994. [CrossRef] [PubMed]
35. Cosgrove, D.; Meehan, D.T.; Grunkemeyer, J.A.; Kornak, J.M.; Sayers, R.; Hunter, W.J.; Samuelson, G.C. Collagen COL4A3 knockout: A mouse model for autosomal Alport syndrome. *Genes Dev.* **1996**, *10*, 2981–2992. [CrossRef] [PubMed]

11

Glomerular Hematuria: Cause or Consequence of Renal Inflammation?

Juan Antonio Moreno [1,2,*], Ángel Sevillano [3], Eduardo Gutiérrez [3], Melania Guerrero-Hue [1,2], Cristina Vázquez-Carballo [1], Claudia Yuste [3], Carmen Herencia [1], Cristina García-Caballero [1], Manuel Praga [3] and Jesús Egido [1,4,*]

1 Renal, Vascular and Diabetes Research Laboratory. Fundacion Jimenez Diaz University Hospital-Health Research Institute (FIIS-FJD), Autonoma University of Madrid (UAM), 28040 Madrid, Spain; mel10anie@gmail.com (M.G.-H.); cvazqu01@ucm.es (C.V.-C.); carmen_herencia@hotmail.com (C.H.); crisgcomplutense@gmail.com (C.G.-C.)

2 Department of Cell Biology, Physiology, and Immunology, Maimonides Biomedical Research Institute of Cordoba (IMIBIC), University of Cordoba, 14014 Cordoba, Spain

3 Department of Nephrology, Hospital 12 de Octubre, 28040 Madrid, Spain; sevillano.am@gmail.com (Á.S.); eduardogutmat90@hotmail.com (E.G.); claudiayustelozano@yahoo.es (C.Y.); mpragat@senefro.org (M.P.)

4 Spanish Biomedical Research Centre in Diabetes and Associated Metabolic Disorders (CIBERDEM), 28040 Madrid, Spain

* Correspondence: juan.moreno@uco.es (J.A.M.); jegido@quironsalud.es (J.E.)

Abstract: Glomerular hematuria is a cardinal symptom of renal disease. Glomerular hematuria may be classified as microhematuria or macrohematuria according to the number of red blood cells in urine. Recent evidence suggests a pathological role of persistent glomerular microhematuria in the progression of renal disease. Moreover, gross hematuria, or macrohematuria, promotes acute kidney injury (AKI), with subsequent impairment of renal function in a high proportion of patients. In this pathological context, hemoglobin, heme, or iron released from red blood cells in the urinary space may cause direct tubular cell injury, oxidative stress, pro-inflammatory cytokine production, and further monocyte/macrophage recruitment. The aim of this manuscript is to review the role of glomerular hematuria in kidney injury, the role of inflammation as cause and consequence of glomerular hematuria, and to discuss novel therapies to combat hematuria.

Keywords: hematuria; inflammation; oxidative stress; tubular injury; AKI; chronic kidney disease (CKD)

---

1. Introduction

Hematuria is described as the presence of red blood cells (RBCs) in the urine. Dysmorphic (abnormally shaped) RBCs in the urine are the consequence of RBC egression through the glomerular filtration barrier, and indicate hematuria of glomerular origin. Glomerular hematuria is a frequent manifestation of many renal diseases, and may be classified as microscopic or macroscopic according to its intensity. Recent evidence suggests a negative repercussion of glomerular hematuria on kidney function. In addition, gross hematuria promotes acute kidney injury (AKI), with a subsequent impairment of renal function by different pathological mechanisms, including an exacerbated inflammatory response. In the next sections, we will fully address the role of glomerular hematuria on kidney injury, emphasizing the causes as well as the pathophysiological consequences.

2. Glomerular Hematuria: An Important and Often-Neglected Clinical Sign

2.1. *Prevalence of Glomerular Hematuria*

The prevalence of hematuria in the general population is certainly unsettled. Screening programs show hematuria in 0.18–16.1% of healthy adults [1–5] and in between 0.03% and 3.9% of children [6–9]. This broad range reflects a relative lack of interest in hematuria, based in its traditionally benign consideration, the absence of standardized methods to detect and quantify hematuria [10,11], or even the difficulties in distinguishing non-glomerular from glomerular hematuria. Moreover, there is striking limited data on the prevalence and severity of glomerular hematuria in renal biopsy registries [12–16]. In these studies, the occurrence of glomerular hematuria ranged between 63.7% and 75.8% of cases. Glomerular hematuria seems to be more frequent in males than in females, regardless of age [17]. Children present more frequent macroscopic hematuria bouts than adults, whereas microhematuria is more common in adults [12,17].

2.2. *Common Causes of Glomerular Hematuria*

IgA nephropathy (IgAN), the commonest primary glomerulonephritis (GN), is the most frequent cause of glomerular hematuria (Table 1) [12,17]. Approximately half of patients can present with outbreaks of macroscopic gross hematuria (MGH), while the other half can do so with microhematuria. Macroscopic bouts of hematuria are more common in the early stages of IgAN and in children, concomitant with mucosal infections, usually in the respiratory tract and occasionally in the gastrointestinal tract [18].

Table 1. Significance of hematuria in glomerular disease.

Disease	Significance
Lupus nephritis	Classical symptom Marker of activity [19]
ANCA-associated vasculitis	Classical symptom Marker of activity Marker of risk to relapse after response to therapy [20]
Disorders of collagen IV $\alpha345$	Classical symptom
IgAN	Classical symptom Marker of activity Probable implicated in progression of the disease Implicated in AKI associated to gross hematuria [21] Probable risk factor to progression to ESRD [22]
Other primary glomerulopathies	Classical symptom Marker of activity [19]

Rapidly progressive glomerulonephritis (RPGN), vasculitis, and acute glomerular inflammation, as observed in postinfectious GN or lupus, may also be associated with glomerular hematuria. Although hematuria is a usual urinalysis feature in endocapillary GN [23], extracapillary GN [12], and membranoproliferative GN [24], the real prevalence of hematuria in these diseases is mainly based in observational cohorts [25–27]. Data from the Spanish renal biopsy registry [17] reported an unexpectedly high rate of hematuria (50%) among patients that were traditionally considered as not hematuric GN, including minimal change disease, membranous GN, or focal and segmental glomerulosclerosis. In the recently characterized C3 glomerulonephritis (C3GN), hematuria—mainly microhematuria—was also present in 87% of the patients [28]. Interestingly, macrohematuria bouts have been also described in C3GN concurrently with upper respiratory tract infections, mimicking IgAN [29].

Current advances in genetic testing have allowed the condition previously known "benign familial hematuria" to be split into several type-IV collagen-associated diseases, such as Alport syndrome, thin basement membrane disease (TBMN), and the hereditary angiopathy, nephropathy, aneurysms and muscle cramps syndrome (HANAC) [30]. These type IV collagen-related disorders show persistent microscopic hematuria in the early stages, which progress over the years to proteinuria and chronic kidney disease (CKD), dependent on individual genetic background [31]. Further, infections have been reported as a trigger of macroscopic bouts of hematuria in collagen-associated disorders [32,33]. Finally, anticoagulant-related nephropathy (ARN) is a recently described entity characterized by gross glomerular hematuria and AKI in patients receiving warfarin [34] or other types of anticoagulant therapy [35,36]. ARN is secondary to a profuse glomerular hemorrhage as a consequence of over-anticoagulation (INR > 3) [37]. ARN shows a disease rate of 2–26 cases per year of follow-up [38–40] and a prevalence of the entity of 20% in over-coagulated patients (INR > 3) [41]. Unpublished data from our group shows that anticoagulant therapy is associated with AKI related to hematuria bouts in patients with IgAN. This could be a link between ARN and IgAN.

3. Hematuria and Renal Damage: Cause or Consequence?

3.1. Hematuria as a Sign of Glomerular Inflammation and Disease Progression

Although hematuria is a cardinal symptom of renal disease, it has occupied very little relevance as a negative prognostic factor, unlike proteinuria that continues to play a central role in the diagnosis and treatment of kidney diseases. This lack of interest in hematuria is surprising because it is a defining symptom of IgAN and other pathologies. New evidence suggests a link between inflammation and the genesis of glomerular hematuria. In an experimental model of IgAN, treatment with an IgA1 protease decreased IgA1 deposition—a fact that correlated with a decrease in inflammation, mesangial expansion, and from a clinical point of view, with a very significant reduction in hematuria without a significant influence on proteinuria [42]. In IgAN patients, macroscopic hematuria coincides with aero-digestive infections [43], indicating that dysregulation of the mucosal immune system may play an important role in the pathogenesis of hematuria through a mucosa–kidney axis [44]. In fact, the activation of Toll-like receptors (TLRs) by bacterial or viral antigens causes polyclonal lymphocyte proliferation [45,46] and the formation of circulating immune complex [43,47]. Another possible mechanism involved in the exacerbation of macrohematuria by inflammation includes the CX3CL1/CX3CR1 axis. The peripheral mononuclear cells of patients with IgAN have a higher expression of CX3CR1 during the episode of macrohematuria, as well as increased serum and urinary levels of CX3CL1, the unique ligand of CX3CR1 [48]. The CX3CL1/CX3CR1 axis may play a primordial role through its chemotactic activity to recruit infiltrating cells that can modify the glomerular filtration barrier. Increased CXC3CL1 expression is not exclusive to IgAN, and can be increased in other glomerular diseases associated with hematuria, such as lupus nephritis [49].

Recent data have shown the value of hematuria as a possible marker of relapse in antineutrophil cytoplasmic antibody (ANCA)-associated vasculitis. The authors found a significant positive association between the persistence of hematuria and subsequent nephritis relapse, although this association was not significant with the persistence of proteinuria [20]. One of the great future challenges is the establishment of a clear association between the glomerular damage and its potential utility to decide if it is necessary to increase the immunosuppressive treatment. Following these studies, the question arises as to whether hematuria is a simple marker of major renal damage. Hematuria could be an early indicator of recurrence, particularly if we consider that this is the first study examining the value of the level of hematuria in the relapse of vasculitis. Hematuria was previously demonstrated as a marker of flare in patients with systematic lupus erythematosus (SLE). Ding et al. suggested that alterations in the sediment, either in the form of isolated microhematuria or associated with sterile pyuria, were associated with the activity of the SLE, being able to serve as a marker of activity phase [19]. This hypothesis was confirmed in an analysis based on a prospective study of urine sediment changes in the Ohio SLE study [50].

3.2. *Pathophysiological Consequences of Hematuria (AKI and CKD)*

3.2.1. Hematuria and AKI

Renal findings in pathologies related to glomerular hematuria usually include tubules filled with RBC casts and acute tubular necrosis, mainly during the gross hematuria bouts. Massive hematuria of glomerular origin produces AKI and damage in tubular cells through different mechanisms: (a) direct tubular damage due to intratubular obstruction of the blood casts, (b) direct tubular toxic effect of hemoglobin (Hb) and heme produced after rupture of the erythrocytes in the tubular lumen, and (c) processes of erythrophagocytosis by the renal tubular cells. Taking all these aspects into account, the duration of macrohematuria bouts becomes a crucial phenomenon for the recovery of renal function. This may be especially relevant in elderly patients and patients with previous chronic renal failure, who may not be able to recover their full functional capacity, especially if the insult is prolonged [21,51].

From a physiopathological point of view, red blood cells in the urine in patients with hematuria release Hb and heme-related products, which are further taken up by tubular cells (Figure 1). Once inside the cell, Hb dissociates, releasing the globins and the heme group, which induces several pathological effects, including oxidative stress, cell death, inflammation, and fibrosis [51,52]. Recent data from our group show that, in addition to the tubular cells, podocytes may be the cellular target of Hb-mediated kidney damage. Thus, Hb induces oxidative damage, podocyte dysfunction, and finally apoptosis, with the detachment of the podocyte from the glomerular capillary [53]. The traffic of Hb through the capillary wall can damage the podocyte, and consequently originate an alteration of the glomerular filtration barrier in patients with glomerular diseases with outbreaks of macroscopic hematuria, such as IgAN. This could explain, at least in part, the deterioration of renal function suffered by those patients after a hematuria bout, especially in elderly patients [21]. However, this hypothesis has not yet been tested. The injury suffered by erythrocytes during their pass throughout the glomerular filtration barrier may promote the release of microvesicles containing microRNA (miRNA). miRNA can be swallowed by nearly all cells, playing an important role in the regulation of oxidative stress and intercellular communication by regulating gene expression. The more prevalent miRNA present in the urinary sediment of IgAN patients with hematuria were mainly derived from urinary erythrocytes, such as miR-25-3p, miR-144-3p, and miR-486-5p [54]. That implies that miRNA delivered by hematuria could act over renal parenchymal cells, changing their gene expression, and could be involved in the pathogenesis and evolution of kidney disease [55]. In other words, the presence of specific miRNA in the sediment could be a marker of the activity of hematuric disease, and may be a useful diagnostic tool. Thus, miR-215-5p and miR-378i appear more frequently in IgAN patients [54,56].

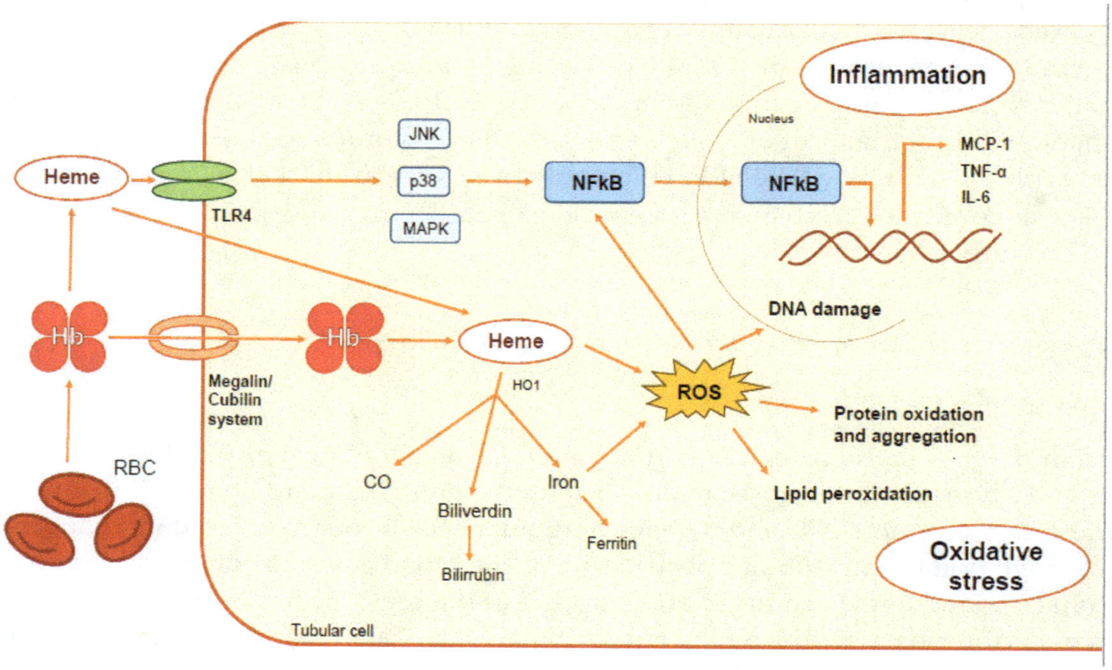

Figure 1. Pathophysiological mechanisms involved in renal damage associated with hematuria. Hemoglobin released by intratubular degradation of erythrocytes may be incorporated into proximal tubules through the megalin-cubilin receptor system or degraded in the tubular lumen, releasing heme. Hb, heme and iron accumulation within tubular cells triggers oxidative stress (lipid peroxidation, protein oxidation and aggregation and DNA damage) and inflammatory cytokine secretion (MCP-1 (monocyte chemoattractant protein 1), TNF-alpha (tumor necrosis factor-alpha), and interleukin 6 (IL-6)) throughout NF-κB transcription factor activation. The heme group may be recognized by the Toll-Like Receptor 4 (TLR4), resulting in the activation of the pro-inflammatory downstream signaling pathways like c-Jun kinases, p38, MAPK and NF-κB.

3.2.2. Hematuria as a Risk Factor for CKD

For many years, hematuria has been considered as only a symptom of some renal disorders. However, multiple studies have challenged this concept, pointing out that the presence of hematuria is associated with an increased risk of developing end-stage renal disease (ESRD). Glomerular diseases, specially IgAN, constitute the scenario where the association between hematuria and long-term renal dysfunction have been best analyzed. In this way, the persistence of hematuria in IgAN has been related to a greater probability of developing ESRD compared to patients with minimal or negative hematuria [22]. In fact, in that disease mild hematuria is associated with an increased risk of ESRD after 10 years of follow-up [57].

In an epidemiological study, the presence of isolated microhematuria significantly increased the risk for ESRD after 22 years of follow-up in a young Israeli population [6]. The presence of hematuria was also associated with a faster decline in renal function in advanced CKD patients compared with those without hematuria [58]. Similar findings emerged from the Chronic Renal Insufficiency Cohort (CRIC) Study [59] and the EPPIC (Evaluating Prevention of Progression In Chronic kidney disease) trials [60]. These studies evidenced an increase of the risk of ESRD after two years of follow-up among patients with baseline hematuria and a decrease of the risk to develop ESRD in those without hematuria. Finally, a recent report showed a significant association of hematuria with an increased risk of ESDR in a group of patients with diabetic nephropathy—the first cause of CKD in developed countries [61]. Based on these pieces of evidence, we consider that hematuria should be added to the traditional risk factor of CKD progression.

4. Should Hematuria be Included as a Surrogate Marker in Clinical Trials of Renal Diseases?

The search for adequate surrogate markers of disease progression, including the progression of renal diseases, is a key issue in many clinical conditions. However, the doubling of serum creatinine is currently the only validated marker associated with renal outcome [62]. Some evidence indicates that proteinuria disappearance could also be a good candidate as a surrogate marker, but further studies are necessary before its acceptance [62]. Hematuria is considered a marker of activity in ANCA vasculitis, lupus nephritis, or IgAN [19,20,63], and recent data indicate that the persistence of hematuria in IgAN is associated with increased risk of the development of ESRD [21,64,65]. For that reason, hematuria disappearance could be a surrogate marker of renal outcome in different diseases, such as vasculitis or glomerulonephritis. However, additional studies are necessary to validate this hypothesis.

5. Hematuria at the Crossroads of Inflammation and Oxidative Stress

The lysis of RBC in the urinary space releases Hb and heme-related products. Hb is incorporated into the kidney through the megalin/cubilin system, and after their oxidation and intracellular destabilization, heme is released and exerts its cytotoxic effect on the renal cells (particularly on the renal tubular epithelium) [66]. Heme consists of a tetrapyrrole ring with an iron atom bound in the center, coordinated to four pyrrole rings [67]. Heme released from the RBC generates oxidative stress, promoting the oxidation of proteins and lipids [68,69], altering the integrity of the cells, and damaging the DNA [70]. The structural instability of heme is essential for the induction of oxidative stress and inflammatory response [71]. Because of its structural properties, especially the hydrophobicity of the porphyrin ring, heme can be incorporated in the lipid bilayer that constitutes cell membranes, where it increases cellular susceptibility to oxidative damage [72]. Additionally, free iron is a potent oxidant and can generate free radicals through the Fenton reaction.

Heme has proinflammatory properties, including leukocyte activation and migration, increased expression of adhesion molecules, and the induction of acute-phase proteins. Thus, heme promotes endothelial activation and elicits the expression of adhesion molecules such as ICAM-1, VCAM-1, E-selectin, P-selectin, and von Willebrand factor [73–75], which facilitates the recruitment and migration of leukocytes [73,76].

Heme also promotes direct pro-inflammatory effects, for example, by activating the production of leukotriene B4 in tissue macrophages, which acts as a chemotactic agent of neutrophils [77]. Additionally, heme can act directly on neutrophils by delaying their apoptosis [78], enhancing their harmful effect on tissue [78]. Heme has been identified as a damage-associated molecular pattern (DAMP), a group of endogenous molecules derived from damaged cells capable of promoting and exacerbating the immune response. These DAMPs are recognized by pattern-recognition receptors (PRRs), within the family of TLRs. Specifically, heme is a ligand of a member of this family—the TLR4 receptor [79]. The activation of TLR4 by heme induces an inflammatory response through the activation of the transcription factor NF-kB [75,80]. As a ligand of TLR4, heme promotes the activation of several downstream signaling pathways, such as c-Jun kinases, p38, and MAPK [81], thus inducing an inflammatory response throughout MCP-1 production [82]. The TLR4 antagonist TAK-242 reduced these heme side effects, suggesting a direct relationship between inflammation and heme through TLR4 in renal tubular cells. Another pathway involved in the inflammation induced by heme is the activation of the NLRP3 (nitrogen permease regulator-like 3) inflammasome, leading to the release of different cytokines and chemokines involved in the recruitment of monocytes/macrophages [83].

6. Can We Envision a Therapeutic Approach for Hematuria-Associated Diseases?

There are no specific therapies to decrease adverse effects associated with hematuria in glomerular diseases. However, the more plausible therapeutic option would be oriented towards the prevention of hematuria bouts and treatment of the nephrotoxic effect of hematuria on renal cells.

6.1. *Treatment for the Prevention of Gross Hematuria Bouts*

Since hematuria was considered as just a benign symptom for decades, no significant effort has been made to treat macrohematuria. Indeed, the Kidney Disease: Improving Global Outcomes (KDIGO) guidelines only recommend supportive treatment for IgAN patients in this context, although this population is at high risk of developing acute or chronic kidney failure [21]. Immunosuppressor therapy, and most specifically corticosteroids, seems a logical option to treat macrohematuria episodes because inflammation is implicated in this phenomenon and because patients with IgAN, ANCA-vasculitis, or lupus nephritis that respond to this therapy usually experience hematuria disappearance. However, to date, there is no evidence to support this hypothesis.

The introduction of budesonide—a new oral corticosteroid with fewer systemic adverse events—provides opportunities to further explore therapeutic approaches for patients with persistent episodes of macroscopic hematuria [84]. Interestingly, budesonide treatment reduced hematuria in IgAN patients from the NEFIGAN clinical trial [85]. Since macrohematuria bouts are usually preceded by upper respiratory infection, tonsillectomy may be considered as another approach in IgAN patients with recurrent tonsillitis, though the results are contradictory [86].

6.2. *Treatment of the Nephrotoxic Effect of Hematuria*

No drug therapy has yet been tested in the management of nephrotoxicity induced by glomerular hematuria. However, based on the actual knowledge of pathogenesis of the damage, some therapeutic options could be effective: (1) alkalinization of the urine to reduce the dissociation of iron from the Hb, (2) diuretics to tubular obstruction by RBC casts, (3) iron chelators (deferiprone or deferoxamine) to decrease iron-nephrotoxicity, and (4) anti-oxidant and anti-inflammatory drugs, such as N-acetylcysteine or Nrf2 inducers. Although there are no current studies reporting beneficial effects on hematuria, a recent paper showed that the administration of N-acetylcysteine prevented Scr increase in 5/6 nephrectomized rats with warfarin-induced AKI [87].

7. Conclusions

Hematuria is a common urinary finding present in several glomerular diseases and patients with bad control of coagulation, among other conditions. Recent studies indicate a pathological role of hematuria in renal damage by promoting AKI and progression to CKD. The renal damage mediated by hematuria is related to nephrotoxic actions of Hb and heme on tubular cells, although data from our studies may suggest that the podocyte may be another cellular target of these molecules. Inflammation and oxidative stress are key processes involved in hematuria-related diseases, and may be plausible targets to develop novel therapeutic approaches.

References

1. Woolhandler, S.; Pels, R.J.; Bor, D.H.; Himmelstein, D.U.; Lawrence, R.S. Dipstick urinalysis screening of asymptomatic adults for urinary tract disorders. I. Hematuria and proteinuria. *JAMA* **1989**, *262*, 1214–1219. [CrossRef] [PubMed]
2. Hiatt, R.A.; Ordoñez, J.D. Dipstick urinalysis screening, asymptomatic microhematuria, and subsequent urological cancers in a population-based sample. *Cancer Epidemiol. Biomarkers Prev.* **1994**, *3*, 439–443.
3. Ramirez, S.P.B.; Kapke, A.; Port, F.K.; Wolfe, R.A.; Saran, R.; Pearson, J.; Hirth, R.A.; Messana, J.M.; Daugirdas, J.T. Dialysis Dose Scaled to Body Surface Area and Size-Adjusted, Sex-Specific Patient Mortality. *Clin. J. Am. Soc. Nephrol.* **2012**, *7*, 1977–1987. [CrossRef] [PubMed]
4. Chadban, S.J.; Briganti, E.M.; Kerr, P.G.; Dunstan, D.W.; Welborn, T.A.; Zimmet, P.Z.; Atkins, R.C. Prevalence of kidney damage in Australian adults: The AusDiab kidney study. *J. Am. Soc. Nephrol.* **2003**, *14*, S131–S138. [CrossRef] [PubMed]

5. Ong, L.M.; Punithavathi, N.; Thurairatnam, D.; Zainal, H.; Beh, M.L.; Morad, Z.; Lee, S.Y.; Bavanandan, S.; Kok, L.S. Prevalence and risk factors for proteinuria: The National Kidney Foundation of Malaysia Lifecheck Health Screening programme. *Nephrology* **2013**, *18*, 569–575. [CrossRef]
6. Vivante, A.; Afek, A.; Frenkel-Nir, Y.; Tzur, D.; Farfel, A.; Golan, E.; Chaiter, Y.; Shohat, T.; Skorecki, K.; Calderon-Margalit, R. Persistent asymptomatic isolated microscopic hematuria in Israeli adolescents and young adults and risk for end-stage renal disease. *JAMA* **2011**, *306*, 729–736. [CrossRef] [PubMed]
7. Hajar, F.; Taleb, M.; Aoun, B.; Shatila, A. Dipstick urine analysis screening among asymptomatic school children. *N. Am. J. Med. Sci.* **2011**, 179–184. [CrossRef] [PubMed]
8. Chen, W.; Liu, Q.; Wang, H.; Chen, W.; Johnson, R.J.; Dong, X.; Li, H.; Ba, S.; Tan, J.; Luo, N.; et al. Prevalence and risk factors of chronic kidney disease: A population study in the Tibetan population. *Nephrol. Dial. Trans.* **2011**, *26*, 1592–1599. [CrossRef] [PubMed]
9. Murakami, M.; Hayakawa, M.; Yanagihara, T.; Hukunaga, Y. Proteinuria screening for children. *Kidney Int. Suppl.* **2005**, S23–S27. [CrossRef]
10. Cohen, R.A.; Brown, R.S. Clinical practice. Microscopic hematuria. *N. Engl. J. Med.* **2003**, *348*, 2330–2338. [CrossRef] [PubMed]
11. Moreno, J.A.; Martin-Cleary, C.; Gutierrez, E.; Rubio-Navarro, A.; Ortiz, A.; Praga, M.; Egido, J. Haematuria: The forgotten CKD factor? *Nephrol. Dial. Trans.* **2012**, *27*, 28–34. [CrossRef] [PubMed]
12. Rychlik, I.; Jancova, E.; Tesar, V.; Kolsky, A.; Lacha, J.; Stejskal, J.; Stejskalova, A.; Dusek, J.; Herout, V. The Czech registry of renal biopsies. Occurrence of renal diseases in the years 1994-2000. *Nephrol. Dial. Trans.* **2004**, *19*, 3040–3049. [CrossRef]
13. Maixnerova, D.; Jancova, E.; Skibova, J.; Rysava, R.; Rychlik, I.; Viklicky, O.; Merta, M.; Kolsky, A.; Reiterova, J.; Neprasova, M.; et al. Nationwide biopsy survey of renal diseases in the Czech Republic during the years 1994–2011. *J. Nephrol.* **2015**, *28*, 39–49. [CrossRef]
14. Schena, F.P. Survey of the Italian Registry of Renal Biopsies. Frequency of the renal diseases for 7 consecutive years. The Italian Group of Renal Immunopathology. *Nephrol. Dial. Trans.* **1997**, *12*, 418–426. [CrossRef]
15. Paripović, D.; Kostić, M.; Kruščić, D.; Spasojević, B.; Lomić, G.; Marković-Lipkovski, J.; Basta-Jovanović, G.; Smoljanić, Ž.; Peco-Antić, A. Indications and results of renal biopsy in children: A 10-year review from a single center in Serbia. *J. Nephrol.* **2012**, *25*, 1054–1059. [CrossRef] [PubMed]
16. Polito, M.G.; de Moura, L.A.R.; Kirsztajn, G.M. An overview on frequency of renal biopsy diagnosis in Brazil: Clinical and pathological patterns based on 9617 native kidney biopsies. *Nephrol. Dial. Trans.* **2010**, *25*, 490–496. [CrossRef] [PubMed]
17. Yuste, C.; Rivera, F.; Moreno, J.A.; López-Gómez, J.M. Haematuria on the Spanish Registry of Glomerulonephritis. *Sci. Rep.* **2016**, *6*, 19732. [CrossRef] [PubMed]
18. Haas, M.; Racusen, L.C.; Bagnasco, S.M. IgA-dominant postinfectious glomerulonephritis: A report of 13 cases with common ultrastructural features. *Hum. Pathol.* **2008**, *39*, 1309–1316. [CrossRef] [PubMed]
19. Ding, J.Y.C.; Ibañez, D.; Gladman, D.D.; Urowitz, M.B. Isolated Hematuria and Sterile Pyuria May Indicate Systemic Lupus Erythematosus Activity. *J. Rheumatol.* **2015**, *42*, 437–440. [CrossRef] [PubMed]
20. Rhee, R.L.; Davis, J.C.; Ding, L.; Fervenza, F.C.; Hoffman, G.S.; Kallenberg, C.G.M.; Langford, C.A.; McCune, W.J.; Monach, P.A.; Seo, P.; et al. The Utility of Urinalysis in Determining the Risk of Renal Relapse in ANCA-Associated Vasculitis. *Clin. J. Am. Soc. Nephrol.* **2018**, *13*, 251–257. [CrossRef]
21. Gutiérrez, E.; González, E.; Hernández, E.; Morales, E.; Martínez, M.A.; Usera, G.; Praga, M. Factors that determine an incomplete recovery of renal function in macrohematuria-induced acute renal failure of IgA nephropathy. *Clin. J. Am. Soc. Nephrol.* **2007**, *2*, 51–57. [CrossRef] [PubMed]
22. Sevillano, A.M.; Gutiérrez, E.; Yuste, C.; Cavero, T.; Mérida, E.; Rodríguez, P.; García, A.; Morales, E.; Fernández, C.; Martínez, M.A.; et al. Remission of Hematuria Improves Renal Survival in IgA Nephropathy. *J. Am. Soc. Nephrol.* **2017**, *28*, 3089–3099. [CrossRef]
23. Moroni, G.; Pozzi, C.; Quaglini, S.; Segagni, S.; Banfi, G.; Baroli, A.; Picardi, L.; Colzani, S.; Simonini, P.; Mihatsch, M.J.; et al. Long-term prognosis of diffuse proliferative glomerulonephritis associated with infection in adults. *Nephrol. Dial. Trans.* **2002**, *17*, 1204–1211. [CrossRef]
24. Sethi, S.; Fervenza, F.C. Membranoproliferative Glomerulonephritis—A New Look at an Old Entity. *N. Engl. J. Med.* **2012**, *366*, 1119–1131. [CrossRef]
25. Wyatt, R.J.; Julian, B.A. IgA Nephropathy. *N. Engl. J. Med.* **2013**, *368*, 2402–2414. [CrossRef]
26. D'Agati, V.D.; Kaskel, F.J.; Falk, R.J. Focal Segmental Glomerulosclerosis. *N. Engl. J. Med.* **2011**, *365*, 2398–2411.[CrossRef]

27. Sethi, S.; Zand, L.; Nasr, S.H.; Glassock, R.J.; Fervenza, F.C. Focal and segmental glomerulosclerosis: Clinical and kidney biopsy correlations. *Clin. Kidney J.* **2014**, *7*, 531–537. [CrossRef]
28. Medjeral-Thomas, N.R.; O'Shaughnessy, M.M.; O'Regan, J.A.; Traynor, C.; Flanagan, M.; Wong, L.; Teoh, C.W.; Awan, A.; Waldron, M.; Cairns, T.; et al. C3 glomerulopathy: Clinicopathologic features and predictors of outcome. *Clin. J. Am. Soc. Nephrol.* **2014**, *9*, 46–53. [CrossRef]
29. Pickering, M.C.; D'Agati, V.D.; Nester, C.M.; Smith, R.J.; Haas, M.; Appel, G.B.; Alpers, C.E.; Bajema, I.M.; Bedrosian, C.; Braun, M.; et al. C3 glomerulopathy: Consensus report. *Kidney Int.* **2013**, *84*, 1079–1089. [CrossRef]
30. Kovačević, Z.; Jovanović, D.; Rabrenović, V.; Dimitrijević, J.; Djukanović, J. Asymptomatic microscopic haematuria in young males. *Int. J. Clin. Pract.* **2008**, *62*, 406–412. [CrossRef] [PubMed]
31. Deltas, C.; Pierides, A.; Voskarides, K. The role of molecular genetics in diagnosing familial hematuria(s). *Pediatr. Nephrol.* **2012**, *27*, 1221–1231. [CrossRef]
32. Deltas, C.; Pierides, A.; Voskarides, K. Molecular genetics of familial hematuric diseases. *Nephrol. Dial. Trans.* **2013**, *28*, 2946–2960. [CrossRef]
33. Kashtan, C.E. Familial hematuria. *Pediatr. Nephrol.* **2009**, *24*, 1951–1958. [CrossRef] [PubMed]
34. Brodsky, S.V.; Satoskar, A.; Chen, J.; Nadasdy, G.; Eagen, J.W.; Hamirani, M.; Hebert, L.; Calomeni, E.; Nadasdy, T. Acute Kidney Injury During Warfarin Therapy Associated With Obstructive Tubular Red Blood Cell Casts: A Report of 9 Cases. *Am. J. Kidney Dis.* **2009**, *54*, 1121–1126. [CrossRef] [PubMed]
35. Escoli, R.; Santos, P.; Andrade, S.; Carvalho, F. Dabigatran-Related Nephropathy in a Patient with Undiagnosed IgA Nephropathy. *Case Rep. Nephrol.* **2015**, *2015*, 298261. [CrossRef]
36. Brodsky, S.V.; Mhaskar, N.S.; Thiruveedi, S.; Dhingra, R.; Reuben, S.C.; Calomeni, E.; Ivanov, I.; Satoskar, A.; Hemminger, J.; Nadasdy, G.; et al. Acute kidney injury aggravated by treatment initiation with apixaban: Another twist of anticoagulant-related nephropathy. *Kidney Res. Clin. Pract.* **2017**, *36*, 387–392. [CrossRef]
37. Brodsky, S.; Eikelboom, J.; Hebert, L.A. Anticoagulant-Related Nephropathy. *J. Am. Soc. Nephrol.* **2018**, *29*, 2787–2793. [CrossRef] [PubMed]
38. Shin, J.-I.; Luo, S.; Alexander, G.C.; Inker, L.A.; Coresh, J.; Chang, A.R.; Grams, M.E. Direct Oral Anticoagulants and Risk of Acute Kidney Injury in Patients With Atrial Fibrillation. *J. Am. Coll. Cardiol.* **2018**, *71*, 251–252. [CrossRef]
39. Chan, Y.-H.; Yeh, Y.-H.; See, L.-C.; Wang, C.-L.; Chang, S.-H.; Lee, H.-F.; Wu, L.-S.; Tu, H.-T.; Kuo, C.-T. Acute Kidney Injury in Asians With Atrial Fibrillation Treated With Dabigatran or Warfarin. *J. Am. Coll. Cardiol.* **2016**, *68*, 2272–2283. [CrossRef]
40. Yao, X.; Tangri, N.; Gersh, B.J.; Sangaralingham, L.R.; Shah, N.D.; Nath, K.A.; Noseworthy, P.A. Renal Outcomes in Anticoagulated Patients With Atrial Fibrillation. *J. Am. Coll. Cardiol.* **2017**, *70*, 2621–2632. [CrossRef] [PubMed]
41. Brodsky, S.V.; Nadasdy, T.; Rovin, B.H.; Satoskar, A.A.; Nadasdy, G.M.; Wu, H.M.; Bhatt, U.Y.; Hebert, L.A. Warfarin-related nephropathy occurs in patients with and without chronic kidney disease and is associated with an increased mortality rate. *Kidney Int.* **2011**, *80*, 181–189. [CrossRef]
42. Lechner, S.M.; Abbad, L.; Boedec, E.; Papista, C.; Le Stang, M.-B.; Moal, C.; Maillard, J.; Jamin, A.; Bex-Coudrat, J.; Wang, Y.; et al. IgA1 Protease Treatment Reverses Mesangial Deposits and Hematuria in a Model of IgA Nephropathy. *J. Am. Soc. Nephrol.* **2016**, *27*, 2622–2629. [CrossRef]
43. Robert, T.; Berthelot, L.; Cambier, A.; Rondeau, E.; Monteiro, R.C. Molecular Insights into the Pathogenesis of IgA Nephropathy. *Trends Mol. Med.* **2015**, *21*, 762–775. [CrossRef]
44. Suzuki, Y.; Suzuki, H.; Nakata, J.; Sato, D.; Kajiyama, T.; Watanabe, T.; Tomino, Y. Pathological role of tonsillar B cells in IgA nephropathy. *Clin. Dev. Immunol.* **2011**, *2011*, 639074. [CrossRef]
45. Meng, T.; Li, X.; Ao, X.; Zhong, Y.; Tang, R.; Peng, W.; Yang, J.; Zou, M.; Zhou, Q. Hemolytic Streptococcus may exacerbate kidney damage in IgA nephropathy through CCL20 response to the effect of Th17 cells. *PLoS ONE* **2014**, *9*, e108723. [CrossRef]
46. Nishikawa, Y.; Shibata, R.; Ozono, Y.; Ichinose, H.; Miyazaki, M.; Harada, T.; Kohno, S. Streptococcal M protein enhances TGF-beta production and increases surface IgA-positive B cells in vitro in IgA nephropathy. *Nephrol. Dial. Trans.* **2000**, *15*, 772–777. [CrossRef]
47. Barratt, J.; Smith, A.C.; Feehally, J. The pathogenic role of IgA1 O-linked glycosylation in the pathogenesis of IgA nephropathy. *Nephrology (Carlton)* **2007**, *12*, 275–284. [CrossRef]

48. Cox, S.N.; Sallustio, F.; Serino, G.; Loverre, A.; Pesce, F.; Gigante, M.; Zaza, G.; Stifanelli, P.F.; Ancona, N.; Schena, F.P. Activated innate immunity and the involvement of CX3CR1-fractalkine in promoting hematuria in patients with IgA nephropathy. *Kidney Int.* **2012**, *82*, 548–560. [CrossRef]
49. Nakatani, K.; Yoshimoto, S.; Iwano, M.; Asai, O.; Samejima, K.; Sakan, H.; Terada, M.; Hasegawa, H.; Nose, M.; Saito, Y. Fractalkine expression and CD16+ monocyte accumulation in glomerular lesions: Association with their severity and diversity in lupus models. *Am. J. Physiol. Renal Physiol.* **2010**, *299*, F207–16. [CrossRef]
50. Ayoub, I.; Birmingham, D.; Rovin, B.; Hebert, L. Commentary on the Current Guidelines for the Diagnosis of Lupus Nephritis Flare. *Curr. Rheumatol. Rep.* **2019**, *21*, 12. [CrossRef]
51. Moreno, J.A.; Martin-Cleary, C.; Gutierrez, E.; Toldos, O.; Blanco-Colio, L.M.; Praga, M.; Ortiz, A.; Egido, J. AKI Associated with Macroscopic Glomerular Hematuria: Clinical and Pathophysiologic Consequences. *Clin. J. Am. Soc. Nephrol.* **2012**, *7*, 175–184. [CrossRef] [PubMed]
52. Gutiérrez, E.; Egido, J.; Rubio-Navarro, A.; Buendía, I.; Blanco Colio, L.M.; Toldos, O.; Manzarbeitia, F.; de Lorenzo, A.; Sanchez, R.; Ortiz, A.; et al. Oxidative stress, macrophage infiltration and CD163 expression are determinants of long-term renal outcome in macrohematuria-induced acute kidney injury of IgA nephropathy. *Nephron. Clin. Pract.* **2012**, *121*, c42–53. [CrossRef]
53. Rubio-Navarro, A.; Sanchez-Niño, M.D.; Guerrero-Hue, M.; García-Caballero, C.; Gutiérrez, E.; Yuste, C.; Sevillano, Á.; Praga, M.; Egea, J.; Román, E.; et al. Podocytes are new cellular targets of haemoglobin-mediated renal damage. *J. Pathol.* **2018**, *244*. [CrossRef]
54. Duan, Z.-Y.; Cai, G.-Y.; Bu, R.; Lu, Y.; Hou, K.; Chen, X.-M. Selection of urinary sediment miRNAs as specific biomarkers of IgA nephropathy. *Sci. Rep.* **2016**, *6*, 23498. [CrossRef] [PubMed]
55. Duan, Z.-Y.; Cai, G.-Y.; Li, J.-J.; Bu, R.; Chen, X.-M. Urinary Erythrocyte-Derived miRNAs: Emerging Role in IgA Nephropathy. *Kidney Blood Press. Res.* **2017**, *42*, 738–748. [CrossRef]
56. Tan, K.; Chen, J.; Li, W.; Chen, Y.; Sui, W.; Zhang, Y.; Dai, Y. Genome-wide analysis of microRNAs expression profiling in patients with primary IgA nephropathy. *Genome* **2013**, *56*, 161–169. [CrossRef]
57. Goto, M.; Wakai, K.; Kawamura, T.; Ando, M.; Endoh, M.; Tomino, Y. A scoring system to predict renal outcome in IgA nephropathy: A nationwide 10-year prospective cohort study. *Nephrol. Dial. Trans.* **2009**, *24*, 3068–3074. [CrossRef]
58. Barraca, D.; Moreno, J.A.; Aragoncillo, I.; Praga, M.; Gutiérrez, E.; Vega, A.; Egido, J.; Rubio-Navarro, A.; Mahillo, I.; Santos, A.; et al. Haematuria Increases Progression of Advanced Proteinuric Kidney Disease. *PLoS ONE* **2015**, *10*, e0128575.
59. Orlandi, P.F.; Fujii, N.; Roy, J.; Chen, H.Y.; Lee Hamm, L.; Sondheimer, J.H.; He, J.; Fischer, M.J.; Rincon-Choles, H.; Krishnan, G.; et al. Hematuria as a risk factor for progression of chronic kidney disease and death: Findings from the Chronic Renal Insufficiency Cohort (CRIC) Study. *BMC Nephrol.* **2018**, *19*, 1–11. [CrossRef] [PubMed]
60. Schulman, G.; Berl, T.; Beck, G.J.; Remuzzi, G.; Ritz, E.; Shimizu, M.; Kikuchi, M.; Shobu, Y. Risk factors for progression of chronic kidney disease in the EPPIC trials and the effect of AST-120. *Clin. Exp. Nephrol.* **2018**, *22*, 299–308. [CrossRef] [PubMed]
61. Lin, H.Y.H.; Niu, S.W.; Kuo, I.C.; Lim, L.M.; Hwang, D.Y.; Lee, J.J.; Hwang, S.J.; Chen, H.C.; Hung, C.C. Hematuria and Renal Outcomes in Patients With Diabetic Chronic Kidney Disease. *Am. J. Med. Sci.* **2018**, *356*, 268–276. [CrossRef]
62. Levey, A.S.; Cattran, D.; Friedman, A.; Miller, W.G.; Sedor, J.; Tuttle, K.; Kasiske, B.; Hostetter, T. Proteinuria as a surrogate outcome in CKD: report of a scientific workshop sponsored by the National Kidney Foundation and the US Food and Drug Administration. *Am. J. Kidney Dis.* **2009**, *54*, 205–226. [CrossRef] [PubMed]
63. Berthoux, F.; Mohey, H.; Laurent, B.; Mariat, C.; Afiani, A.; Thibaudin, L. Predicting the Risk for Dialysis or Death in IgA Nephropathy. *J. Am. Soc. Nephrol.* **2011**, *22*, 752–761. [CrossRef]
64. Le, W.; Liang, S.; Hu, Y.; Deng, K.; Bao, H.; Zeng, C.; Liu, Z. Long-term renal survival and related risk factors in patients with IgA nephropathy: Results from a cohort of 1155 cases in a Chinese adult population. *Nephrol. Dial. Trans.* **2012**, *27*, 1479–1485. [CrossRef] [PubMed]
65. Coppo, R.; Fervenza, F.C. Persistent Microscopic Hematuria as a Risk Factor for Progression of IgA Nephropathy: New Floodlight on a Nearly Forgotten Biomarker. *J. Am. Soc. Nephrol.* **2017**, *28*, 2831–2834. [CrossRef] [PubMed]

66. Tracz, M.J.; Alam, J.; Nath, K.A. Physiology and Pathophysiology of Heme: Implications for Kidney Disease. *J. Am. Soc. Nephrol.* **2007**, *18*, 414–420. [CrossRef]
67. Kumar, S.; Bandyopadhyay, U. Free heme toxicity and its detoxification systems in human. *Toxicol. Lett.* **2005**, *157*, 175–188. [CrossRef]
68. Vincent, S.H. Oxidative effects of heme and porphyrins on proteins and lipids. *Semin. Hematol.* **1989**, *26*, 105–113. [PubMed]
69. TAPPEL, A.L. The mechanism of the oxidation of unsaturated fatty acids catalyzed by hematin compounds. *Arch. Biochem. Biophys.* **1953**, *44*, 378–395. [CrossRef]
70. Aft, R.L.; Mueller, G.C. Hemin-mediated DNA strand scission. *J. Biol. Chem.* **1983**, *258*, 12069–12072.
71. Dutra, F.F.; Bozza, M.T. Heme on innate immunity and inflammation. *Front. Pharmacol.* **2014**, *5*, 115. [CrossRef]
72. Balla, G.; Jacob, H.S.; Eaton, J.W.; Belcher, J.D.; Vercellotti, G.M. Hemin: A possible physiological mediator of low density lipoprotein oxidation and endothelial injury. *Arterioscler. Thromb. J. Vasc. Biol.* **1991**, *11*, 1700–1711. [CrossRef]
73. Wagener, F.A.; Feldman, E.; de Witte, T.; Abraham, N.G. Heme induces the expression of adhesion molecules ICAM-1, VCAM-1, and E selectin in vascular endothelial cells. *Proc. Soc. Exp. Biol. Med.* **1997**, *216*, 456–463. [CrossRef]
74. Immenschuh, S.; Vijayan, V.; Janciauskiene, S.; Gueler, F. Heme as a Target for Therapeutic Interventions. *Front. Pharmacol.* **2017**, *8*, 146. [CrossRef]
75. Belcher, J.D.; Chen, C.; Nguyen, J.; Milbauer, L.; Abdulla, F.; Alayash, A.I.; Smith, A.; Nath, K.A.; Hebbel, R.P.; Vercellotti, G.M. Heme triggers TLR4 signaling leading to endothelial cell activation and vaso-occlusion in murine sickle cell disease. *Blood* **2014**, *123*, 377–390. [CrossRef]
76. Graça-Souza, A.V.; Arruda, M.A.B.; de Freitas, M.S.; Barja-Fidalgo, C.; Oliveira, P.L. Neutrophil activation by heme: Implications for inflammatory processes. *Blood* **2002**, *99*, 4160–4165. [CrossRef] [PubMed]
77. Monteiro, A.P.T.; Pinheiro, C.S.; Luna-Gomes, T.; Alves, L.R.; Maya-Monteiro, C.M.; Porto, B.N.; Barja-Fidalgo, C.; Benjamim, C.F.; Peters-Golden, M.; Bandeira-Melo, C.; et al. Leukotriene B4 mediates neutrophil migration induced by heme. *J. Immunol.* **2011**, *186*, 6562–6567. [CrossRef]
78. Arruda, M.A.; Rossi, A.G.; de Freitas, M.S.; Barja-Fidalgo, C.; Graça-Souza, A. V Heme inhibits human neutrophil apoptosis: Involvement of phosphoinositide 3-kinase, MAPK, and NF-kappaB. *J. Immunol.* **2004**, *173*, 2023–2030. [CrossRef]
79. Figueiredo, R.T.; Fernandez, P.L.; Mourao-Sa, D.S.; Porto, B.N.; Dutra, F.F.; Alves, L.S.; Oliveira, M.F.; Oliveira, P.L.; Graça-Souza, A.V.; Bozza, M.T. Characterization of heme as activator of Toll-like receptor 4. *J. Biol. Chem.* **2007**, *282*, 20221–20229. [CrossRef]
80. Lin, T.; Sammy, F.; Yang, H.; Thundivalappil, S.; Hellman, J.; Tracey, K.J.; Warren, H.S. Identification of hemopexin as an anti-inflammatory factor that inhibits synergy of hemoglobin with HMGB1 in sterile and infectious inflammation. *J. Immunol.* **2012**, *189*, 2017–2022. [CrossRef] [PubMed]
81. Medzhitov, R. Origin and physiological roles of inflammation. *Nature* **2008**, *454*, 428–435. [CrossRef]
82. Nath, K.A.; Belcher, J.D.; Nath, M.C.; Grande, J.P.; Croatt, A.J.; Ackerman, A.W.; Katusic, Z.S.; Vercellotti, G.M. Role of TLR4 signaling in the nephrotoxicity of heme and heme proteins. *Am. J. Physiol. Renal Physiol.* **2018**, *314*, F906–F914. [CrossRef]
83. Komada, T.; Usui, F.; Kawashima, A.; Kimura, H.; Karasawa, T.; Inoue, Y.; Kobayashi, M.; Mizushina, Y.; Kasahara, T.; Taniguchi, S.; et al. Role of NLRP3 Inflammasomes for Rhabdomyolysis-induced Acute Kidney Injury. *Sci. Rep.* **2015**, *5*, 10901. [CrossRef]
84. Lee, C.M.; Hardy, C.M. Cocoa feeding and human lactose intolerance. *Am. J. Clin. Nutr.* **1989**, *49*, 840–844. [CrossRef]
85. Fellström, B.C.; Barratt, J.; Cook, H.; Coppo, R.; Feehally, J.; de Fijter, J.W.; Floege, J.; Hetzel, G.; Jardine, A.G.; Locatelli, F.; et al. Targeted-release budesonide versus placebo in patients with IgA nephropathy (NEFIGAN): A double-blind, randomised, placebo-controlled phase 2b trial. *Lancet* **2017**, *389*, 2117–2127. [CrossRef]
86. Floege, J.; Barbour, S.J.; Cattran, D.C.; Hogan, J.J.; Nachman, P.H.; Tang, S.C.W.; Wetzels, J.F.M.; Cheung, M.; Wheeler, D.C.; Winkelmayer, W.C.; et al. Management and treatment of glomerular diseases (part 1):

Conclusions from a Kidney Disease: Improving Global Outcomes (KDIGO) Controversies Conference. *Kidney Int.* **2019**, *95*, 268–280. [CrossRef]

87. Ware, K.; Qamri, Z.; Ozcan, A.; Satoskar, A.A.; Nadasdy, G.; Rovin, B.H.; Hebert, L.A.; Nadasdy, T.; Brodsky, S. V N-acetylcysteine ameliorates acute kidney injury but not glomerular hemorrhage in an animal model of warfarin-related nephropathy. *Am. J. Physiol. Renal Physiol.* **2013**, *304*, F1421–F1427. [CrossRef] [PubMed]

12

Salt Inducible Kinase Signaling Networks: Implications for Acute Kidney Injury and Therapeutic Potential

Mary Taub

Biochemistry Dept, Jacobs School of Medicine and Biomedical Sciences, University at Buffalo, 955 Main Street Suite 4102, Buffalo, NY 14203, USA; biochtau@buffalo.edu

Abstract: A number of signal transduction pathways are activated during Acute Kidney Injury (AKI). Of particular interest is the Salt Inducible Kinase (SIK) signaling network, and its effects on the Renal Proximal Tubule (RPT), one of the primary targets of injury in AKI. The SIK1 network is activated in the RPT following an increase in intracellular Na^+ ($Na^+{}_{in}$), resulting in an increase in Na,K-ATPase activity, in addition to the phosphorylation of Class IIa Histone Deacetylases (HDACs). In addition, activated SIKs repress transcriptional regulation mediated by the interaction between cAMP Regulatory Element Binding Protein (CREB) and CREB Regulated Transcriptional Coactivators (CRTCs). Through their transcriptional effects, members of the SIK family regulate a number of metabolic processes, including such cellular processes regulated during AKI as fatty acid metabolism and mitochondrial biogenesis. SIKs are involved in regulating a number of other cellular events which occur during AKI, including apoptosis, the Epithelial to Mesenchymal Transition (EMT), and cell division. Recently, the different SIK kinase isoforms have emerged as promising drug targets, more than 20 new SIK2 inhibitors and activators having been identified by MALDI-TOF screening assays. Their implementation in the future should prove to be important in such renal disease states as AKI.

Keywords: kidney proximal tubule; acute kidney failure; signal transduction; transcription; CREB Regulated Transcriptional Coactivators (CRTC); cAMP Regulatory Element Binding Protein (CREB); Salt Inducible Kinase (SIK); Class IIa Histone Deacetylases (HDAC)

---

1. Introduction

Salt Inducible Kinase (SIK) was first discovered in the adrenal gland of rats on a high salt diet, where it plays a regulatory role in steroidogenesis [1]. Subsequently, a SIK network was identified that plays an important role in regulating Na^+ reabsorption in the Renal Proximal Tubule (RPT) [2]. SIK plays a number of additional roles, ranging from its roles in gene regulation, and the regulation of metabolism, to the roles played by SIK in cell survival, growth, the Epithelial to Mesenchymal Transition (EMT) as well as apoptosis. This report is concerned with the involvement of SIK in Acute Kidney Injury (AKI).

AKI is a heterogeneous group of conditions characterized by an abrupt decrease in the Glomerular Filtration Rate (GFR), followed by an increase in serum creatinine [3–5]. AKI arises as a consequence of ischemic and toxic insults, as well as radiation and ureteral obstruction [6,7]. Following the initiation and extension phases caused by the insults, the kidney goes through maintenance and recovery phases, during which repair occurs in cells that are sub-lethally damaged, in addition to the generation of new cells. There is a need to understand the underlying molecular changes that occur in the tubule epithelial cells during AKI, and the recovery period, so as to develop effective therapies. There is considerable evidence suggesting that signal transduction pathways that are activated during AKI involve different aspects of the SIK Networks, which opens up the possibility of new avenues for therapy.

2. Role of the Salt Inducible Kinase 1 (SIK1) Network in the Response of the Renal Proximal Tubule (RPT) to Injury

2.1. Initial Response of the Renal Proximal Tubule to Injury

Of particular interest in these regards, is the renal proximal tubule (RPT), one of the primary targets of injury in AKI [5]. The RPT primarily depends upon mitochondrial oxidative phosphorylation, rather than glycolysis [8]. Thus, ATP levels decline dramatically during hypoxia, resulting in a decrease in Na,K-ATPase activity, as well as an increase in intracellular Na^+ ($Na^+{}_{in}$). As a consequence, the capacity of the RPT to reabsorb Na^+ and other solutes is impaired. Impaired Na^+ reabsorption can present problems, because in order to survive, the body must retain Na^+ within an appropriate range (between 135 and 145 mEq/L). This level of Na^+ is necessary to maintain a normal blood pressure, support the function of muscles and nerves, and to preserve our body's fluid balance. One defense mechanism in the kidney, is Tubuloglomerular Feedback (TGF), which causes the Glomerular Filtration Rate (GFR) to decline when distal Na^+ levels increase, and in this manner acts so as to preserve Na^+ within a range compatible with renal tubular function (which may decline as a result of injury) [9]. In addition, tubule epithelial cells themselves possess defense mechanisms, including mechanisms that result in a response to changes in ionic balance. Although renal tubules are often viewed as being a central target in AKI, surprisingly little is known regarding these functional responses, which act to preserve renal tubule transport functions during AKI, including those in the RPT. Thus, it is important to gain an understanding of pertinent regulatory mechanisms involved in this nephron segment, and likely responses during AKI. Of particular interest in these regards is the SIK1 network, and its ability to regulate Na,K-ATPase, so as to maintain Na^+ homeostasis in the body.

2.2. Importance of Na,K-ATPase in Na^+ Reabsorption

As stated above, Na^+ plays a critical role in maintaining the homeostasis of bodily fluids, indirectly affecting the distribution of water in intravascular compartments, and ultimately, blood pressure [10]. Fluid as well as electrolyte disorders often develop during AKI, and fluid therapy (with its own inherent problems) is common [11]. Indeed, clinically employed saline solutions (154 mM) contain higher Na^+ levels than plasma (140 mM).

At the cellular level, the Na,K-ATPase is crucial in maintaining an appropriate Na^+/K^+ gradient across the plasma membrane (a requirement of all living cells). Presumably, the need for such a Na^+/K^+ gradient originated in primitive organisms, which were in an environment in which Na^+ was inhibitory, or even toxic, while K^+ was required for the activity of primitive enzymes (due to the preponderance of K^+ in the primitive environment) [12]. Thus, cells had to develop mechanisms to prevent the toxicity of intracellular Na^+. Indeed, if intracellular Na^+ levels are allowed to rise in mammalian cells, the intracellular environment risks intracellular "flooding" caused by a Donan equilibrium (i.e., intracellular swelling caused by an increase in the intracellular concentration of free cations over and above the extracellular level, due to the net negative charge of intracellular proteins). For this reason, mammalian cells have a Na,K-ATPase which ejects three intracellular Na^+ molecules in exchange for two extracellular K^+, at the expense of ATP [13]. Very importantly, the Na^+ gradient established by Na,K-ATPase provides the driving force for the cotransport of a number of solutes into the cell (amino acids, glucose, phosphate) with Na^+. In the case of the RPT, this is the first step in the transepithelial transport of these solutes.

Teleologically, it makes sense that cells are fortified to survive the continual changes in the ions in the extracellular milieu, including those that occur during exposure to a "toxic" environment. Protection from such external changes is provided by signaling systems that control the activity of membrane transporters, including Na,K-ATPase, and thereby permit renal cells to respond appropriately to changes not only in the external ionic environment, but also to metabolic challenges such as a decline in ATP levels, as well as oxidative stress and other toxic challenges. Of particular interest in these regards is the SIK Signaling Network and its role in the RPT during AKI.

2.3. SIK Structure and Function

SIKs are central components of a number of signaling pathways which are responsible for regulating a wide range of cellular processes in different organs. In subsequent studies, SIK1 was found to be homologous to AMP Kinase (AMPK), and for this reason, is included within the Sucrose Non-Fermenting 1 (SNF1)/AMPK family [14]. Three isoforms of SIK have been identified (SIK1, SIK2 and SIK3) which share common structural features, including a highly conserved, amino terminal kinase domain, a Sucrose Nonfermenting-1 Homology (SNH) domain, as well as a carboxy terminal phosphorylation domain (Figure 1). All three SIK isoforms are broadly expressed in a large number of tissues. Tissues which express amongst the highest levels of SIK1 include adipose tissue, as well as B and T cells. While heart and adipose tissue are amongst those with the highest level of SIK2 expression, other tissues, including the cerebral cortex and testes are amongst those with the highest levels of SIK3. However, the relative SIK expression level is not a necessary indicator of the importance of an individual SIK isoform in any particular tissue. When considering the kidney, SIK1 has been studied most extensively, although the kidney expresses moderate levels of all three SIK isoforms.

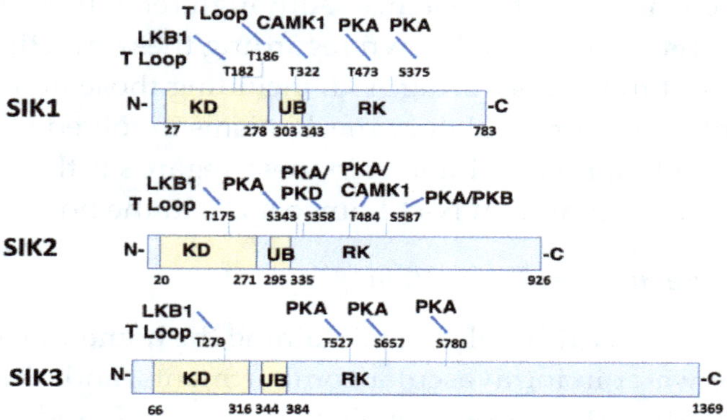

Figure 1. Domain Structure and Phosphorylation Sites of Salt Inducible Kinase (SIK) Isoforms. The domain structure of SIK1 (Uniprot P507059), SIK2 (Uniprot Q9Y2K2), and SIK3 (Uniprot Q9Y2K2) is shown including conserved Kinase Domain (KD), Ubiquitin Associated Domain (UB), and RK-rich region (RK). Identified phosphorylation sites are also illustrated, as well as the corresponding kinase (LKB1 (T182 SIK1, T175 SIK2, T221 SIK3), CaMK1 (T322 SIK1, T484 SIK2), PKA (T473 and S575 SIK1; S343, S358, T484 and S587 SIK2; T469, S551, S647 SIK3), and PKB (S587 SIK2)). T Loop indicates that the phosphorylation site is within the T activation loop. The amino and carboxy terminus of each SIK isoform are indicated by N- and C-, respectively. CaMK1, Calmodulin Activated Protein Kinase 1; PKA, Protein Kinase A; PKB, Protein Kinase B.

SIKs possess an activation loop within the kinase domain. Autophosphorylation occurs within the activation loop (Thr186 in SIK1), an event that is essential for kinase activity [15]. The catalytic activity of all SIK isoforms depends upon the phosphorylation of yet another residue within the activation loop (Thr182 in SIK1) by LKB1 [16]. LKB1 similarly phosphorylates all other members of the AMPK family. The activation loop of SIK1 and SIK2 is also phosphorylated by GSK-3β, although this phosphorylation event is not sufficient to activate SIK kinase activity [15]. Other domains of the SIKs also undergo phosphorylation by a number of protein kinases. For example, Calmodulin Activated Protein Kinase 1 (CaMK1) phosphorylates SIK1 within the UB domain, so as to increase SIK1 kinase activity. In contrast, CaMK1 phosphorylates SIK2 within the carboxy terminal domain, and in this manner similarly activates SIK kinase activity. Protein Kinase A (PKA) phosphorylates all three SIK isoforms in the carboxy terminal domain, depending upon the physiological condition [17].

A consequence of SIK phosphorylation by PKA is that SIKs become associated with cytoplasmic 14-3-3 proteins, which results in the sequestration of SIKs in the cytoplasm [17]. Thus, SIKs that have been phosphorylated by PKA can no longer phosphorylate nuclear proteins, including CRTCs, and class IIa HDACs.

2.4. SIK1 Signaling Network and Na,K-ATPase

2.4.1. Role of SIK1 in Na^+ Sensing: Acute Response

Of particular interest to this report, is the role of SIK1 in Na^+ sensing. In RPT cells, SIK1 is associated with a complex associated with the basolateral membrane, containing the Na, K-ATPase [12]. A number of proteins are associated with the SIK1/Na,K-ATPase complex, including Protein Phosphatase 2A (PP2A), and Protein Methylesterase-1 (PME-1), which constantly demethylates (and thus inactivates) PP2A. As illustrated in Figure 2, the increase in intracellular Na^+ ($Na^+{}_{in}$), which occurs following an increase in luminal Na^+, is followed by the activation of Na^+/Ca^{2+} exchange activity, and, as a consequence, an increase in intracellular Ca^{2+} ($Ca^{2+}{}_{in}$).

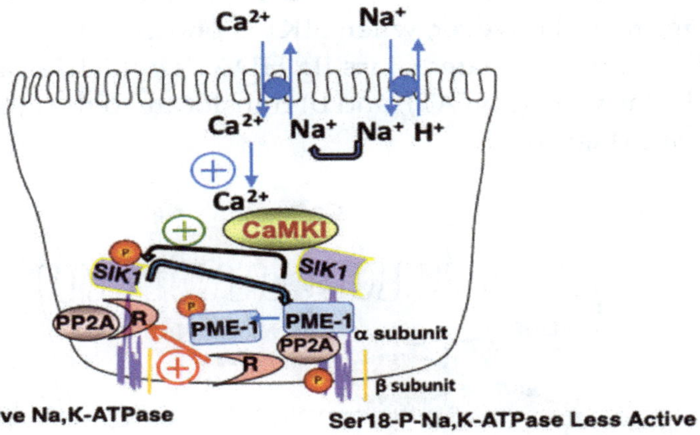

Figure 2. Model of the Basolateral SIK1 Network. An increase in luminal Na^+ results in an increase in $Na^+{}_{in}$, the activation of Na^+/Ca^{2+} exchange, and an increase in $Ca^{2+}{}_{in}$, which activates CaMK1. Activated CaMK1 phosphorylates SIK1 at Thr322 and activates basolateral SIK1, which as a consequence, phosphorylates PME-1, which dissociates from the Na,K-ATPase complex. PP2A remains demethylated, associates with its regulatory subunit (R), and in this activated state, dephosphorylates Ser18 of the catalytic subunit of Na,K-ATPase (i.e., the α subunit), activating the transporter. If the indicated reaction has a positive effect upon activity, it is indicated by a plus contained within a circle.

Ultimately, the increase in $Ca^{2+}{}_{in}$ results in CaMK1 activation, which in turn phosphorylates and activates SIK1. SIK1 then activates basolateral Na,K-ATPase, albeit indirectly [12]. Towards these ends, activated SIK1 phosphorylates PME1, which dissociates from the SIK1/Na,K-ATPase/PP2A complex. As a consequence, the PP2A catalytic subunit is no longer demethylated by PME1, and thus the activity of PP2A remains low. This is because PP2A only achieves its full catalytic activity following its demethylation, which allows the PP2A catalytic subunit to interact with the PP2A regulatory subunit, and dephosphorylate the catalytic subunit (i.e., the α subunit) of the Na,K-ATPase. The retention of the Na,K-ATPase in the basolateral membrane increases under these conditions, resulting in increased transport activity.

2.4.2. Relevance of the SIK1 Signaling Network and Na,K-ATPase to AKI

The SIK1 signaling network described above is responsible for eliciting the initial responses of the RPT to insults that result in AKI. An increase in luminal Na^+ ($Na^+{}_{in}$) occurs in response to a number of these insults, particularly when the GFR decreases (during the initiation phase of AKI), and luminal Na^+ increases. Intracellular ATP levels often decline during the initiation phase of AKI (often in response to hypoxia). A consequence of such a decline in intracellular ATP is reduced Na,K-ATPase activity, and, as a result, an increase in $Na^{+}{}_{in}$ (which decreases the driving force for transepithelial transport). From our knowledge of the SIK1 network [12], such acute increases in $Na^{+}{}_{in}$ rapidly activate the basolateral SIK1s, which are part of the Na,K-ATPase complex, and thereby initiate the events in the SIK1 network which counteract the tendency for Na^{+} reabsorption to decline during AKI (by increasing the quantity of basolateral Na,K-ATPases).

In addition to these immediate effects of an increase in $Na^{+}{}_{in}$ (which occurs during the initiation phase of AKI), during subsequent phases of AKI changes in gene expression occur which result in increased renal reabsorption, as well as other repair processes, due to changes occurring in other aspects of SIK networking.

2.5. *Transcriptional Effects of SIK1 Involving Its HDAC Kinase Activity and Relevance to AKI*

During the initiation phase of AKI, $Na^{+}{}_{in}$ increases, resulting in SIK1 activation, which in turn results in a transcriptional response due to the Class IIa Histone Deacetylase (HDAC) kinase activity of SIK1 [18,19]. Class IIa HDACs associate with such transcription factors as Myocyte Enhancer Factor 2C (MEF2C) and Nuclear Factor of Activated T cells (NFAT) on chromosomal DNA, so as to repress transcription (Figure 3). However, when SIK1 is phosphorylated at Thr322 by CAMK1 (and activated), activated SIK1 phosphorylates Class IIa HDACs, which, as a consequence, a) dissociate from chromosomal MEF2 (as well as NFAT), and b) translocate to the cytoplasm, where they bind to cytoplasmic 14-3-3 proteins (Figure 3).

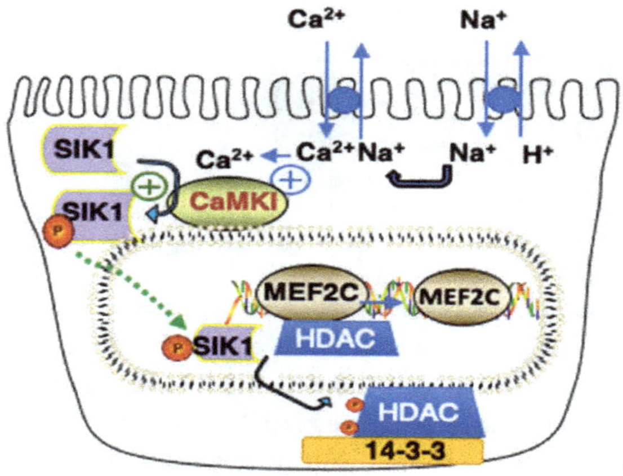

Figure 3. Model of Class IIa HDAC Kinase Phosphorylation by SIK1. An increase in $Na^{+}{}_{in}$ results in an increase in $Ca^{2+}{}_{in}$ due to activation of Na^{+}/Ca^{2+} exchange activity. SIK1 is phosphorylated at Thr322 by CAMK1 and activated, resulting in the phosphorylation of Class IIa HDACs associated with MEF2 transcriptions (as well as NFAT, not shown) on chromosomal DNA. As a consequence of their phosphorylation at two sites (Ser259 and Ser498 in the case of Human HDAC5), Class IIa HDACS translocate to the cytoplasm where they interact with 14-3-3 proteins. If the indicated reaction has a positive effect upon activity, it is indicated by a plus contained within a circle.

Following the dissociation of Class IIa HDACs from chromosomal DNA, transcription via MEF2 and NFAT is upregulated, increasing the expression of MEF2- (and NFAT-) regulated genes. Included amongst the genes upregulated following an increase in $Na^{+}{}_{in}$ are those encoding for Atrial Natriuretic Peptide (ANP) as well as α and β Myosin Heavy Chains (MHCs) [18]. Of particular interest in these regards, is the increased expression of ANP A and B, as well as α and β MHCs which has been reported during AKI [20–22]. Such an increase in the expression of ANP, may very well promote recovery during AKI. Indeed, ANP has been used in the management of AKI [23–25].

2.6. Involvement of SIK1 in Transcriptional Events Mediated by cAMP and Ca^{2+}

SIKs are also involved in regulating transcriptional events mediated by the cAMP Regulatory Element Binding Protein (CREB) and CREB Regulated Transcriptional Coactivators (CRTCs) [26]. Prostaglandin E_2 (PGE_2) is an example of an effector that acts via such a mechanism [27,28]. In the kidney, PGs are synthesized from Arachidonic acid by Cyclooxygenases (COXs), including constitutive COX1 and inducible COX2. Of particular interest in these regards, COX-2 inhibitors are a major cause of drug-induced AKI, and exacerbate reductions in the GFR caused by other agents such as Lipopolysaccharides (LPS) [29]. In addition, chemokines and cytokines including PGE_2 are produced during AKI (as early as the initiation phase) [9,29]. While they may have beneficial effects on the GFR, chemokines and cytokines also contribute to the inflammatory response [29].

PGE_2 in particular is known to regulate renal Na^+ handling, in a manner which depends upon the nephron segment [9]. PGE_2 interacts with its specific G Protein Coupled Receptors (GPCRs) (i.e., Prostaglandin E (EP) receptors) which are differentially expressed in tubule epithelial cells. Included amongst the GPCRs for PGE_2 are EP2 and EP4 receptors (which are coupled to Gs, which activates adenylate cyclase (AC)), as well as EP1 receptors (which is coupled to Gq, which activates Phospholipase C (PLC)) [30]. Following the interaction of PGE_2 with Gs coupled EP2 and EP4 receptors, intracellular cAMP increases, resulting in the phosphorylation SIK1 at Thr475 (by PKA), and SIK1 inactivation [27,31,32], unlike increases in $Na^+{}_{in}$ which result in SIK1 phosphorylation at Thr322 (by CAMK1), and SIK activation.

The PGE_2-mediated increase in Na,K-ATPase activity in primary rabbit RPT cell cultures is an example of transcriptional regulation which involves inhibitory effects of cAMP on SIK1 [33]. The Na,K-ATPase is a heterodimer, consisting of an α subunit, responsible for the catalytic activity, as well as a β subunit, a chaperone which facilitates the insertion of the Na,K-ATPase into the basolateral membrane. Although both subunits are present in Na,K-ATPase, an increase in the level of the β subunit alone can cause an overall increase in the level the heterodimer [34]. This occurs when the level of the β subunit is limiting to heterodimer formation (excess α subunit being degraded). In this case, transcriptional regulation of the Na,K-ATPase β subunit gene *atp1b1* becomes a critical determinant of the overall Na,K-ATPase level, and activity. The observed increase in the overall level of the Na,K-ATPase in the RPT cells following a prolonged incubation with PGE_2, can be explained by this type of regulation by the *atp1b1* gene [35].

Transcriptional regulation of the *atp1b1* gene by PGE_2 involves CREB, which binds to Prostaglandin Regulatory Elements, PGREs, located in the *atp1b1* promoter [36,37]. CREB binds constitutively to PGREs, even in the absence of the binding of effectors such as PGE_2 to their receptors (i.e., EP receptors in the case of PGE_2) (Figure 4A). Under these conditions, CREB Regulated Transcriptional Coactivators (CRTCs) are localized in the cytoplasm. Transcriptional regulation by CREB on the *atp1b1* promoter involves increases in cAMP as well as $Ca^{2+}{}_{in}$. PGE_2 interacts with both EP2, as well as EP1 receptors in primary RPT cells. When PGE_2 interacts with EP2 receptors, AC is activated, and subsequently, PKA. Activated PKA phosphorylates CREB (localized on the PGRE1 and PGRE3 sites on the *atp1b1* promoter), resulting in the recruitment of CREB Binding Protein (CBP) to phospho-CREB (pCREB) [36]. In order to obtain a maximal transcriptional response, CREB Regulated Transcriptional Coactivators (CRTCs) also associate with CREB on the *atp1b1* promoter [27] (Figure 4B). However, a second signaling event (an increase in Ca^{2+}) must occur if CRTCs are to interact with CREB [27,38]. This second signaling event is initiated by the interaction of PGE_2 with EP1 receptors, the activation of Phospholipase C (PLC), and an increase in $Ca^{2+}{}_{in}$ [31].

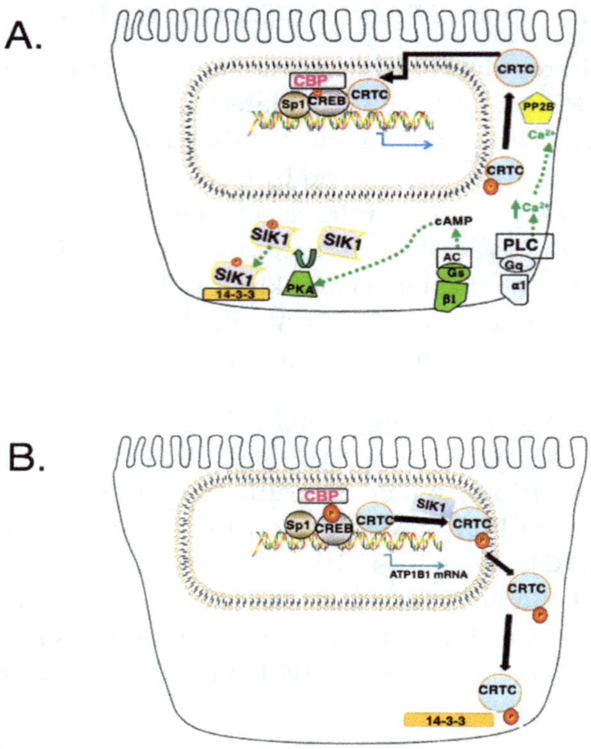

Figure 4. Establishment of a CREB/CRTC Interaction and its Disruption by SIK1. (**A**) Following a simultaneous increase in cAMP and $Ca^{2+}{}_{in}$, SIK1 is phosphorylated at Thr473 by PKA, which results in an interaction between PKA phosphorylated SIK1 and 14-3-3 proteins (which results in the sequestration of SIK1 in the cytoplasm, and which prevents the further phosphorylation of CRTCs by SIK1). CRTCs, which are phosphorylated (at Ser151 in the case of human CRTC1), are dephosphorylated by Calcineurin (i.e., Protein Phosphatase 2B (PP2B)). As a consequence, CRTCs translocate to the nucleus and interact with CREB, causing an increase in transcription, beyond that obtained with the Ser-133-pCREB/CBP interaction. (**B**) Following SIK1 activation (and its dephosphorylation at the PKA phosphorylation site), SIK1 no longer interacts with 14-3-3 proteins, which permits the nuclear translocation of SIK1. Once in the nucleus, SIK1 phosphorylates CRTCs, which translocate to the cytoplasm.

Notably, the binding of CRTCs to CREB on the *atp1b1* promoter is limited by SIK1 [27]. In order for CRTCs to interact with CREB, CRTCs must be in the nucleus (Figure 4A). However, activated SIK1 phosphorylates CRTCs, which causes CRTCs to translocate to the cytoplasm where they interact with 14-3-3 proteins (Figure 4B) [27].

Two simultaneous signaling events must occur in order for cytoplasmic CRTCs to reenter the nucleus (Figure 4A) [39]. First, intracellular cAMP must increase (due to the activation of AC, by Gs coupled EP2 in the case of PGE_2), and second, $Ca^{2+}{}_{in}$ must increase (due to the activation of PLC, by Gq coupled EP1 in the case of PGE_2). Following an AC-mediated increase in cAMP, PKA (which is activated) phosphorylates SIK1 at Thr475, inactivating SIK1, which no longer phosphorylates CRTCs. CRTCs must in addition be dephosphorylated in order to enter the nucleus. The dephosphorylation of CRTCs depends upon the activation of Calcineurin, which occurs when $Ca^{2+}{}_{in}$ increases. Calcineurin (i.e., Protein Phosphatase 2B (PP2B)), is a calcium- and calmodulin-dependent serine/threonine protein phosphatase.

2.7. Summary of the Three Major SIK1 Networks and Their Relevance to Acute Kidney Injury (AKI)

Thus, to summarize, the regulation of the transport and reabsorptive functions of the RPT depends upon three different signaling pathways involving SIK1. Two of these pathways are activated when $Na^{+}{}_{in}$ increases (which occurs following increases in luminal Na^{+}), and involve on one hand, the direct phosphorylation of PME1 by activated SIK1 basolateral SIK1 (in the first pathway), and on the other hand the direct phosphorylation of class IIA HDACs by activated nuclear SIK1 (in the second pathway). As a consequence, 1) pre-existing Na,K-ATPases are retained in the basolateral membrane in the first pathway, and 2) transcriptional regulation by MEF2 and NFAT transcription factors increases in the second pathway. A third component of the SIK1 network, transcriptional regulation by CRTCs (and CREB), is inhibited when SIK1 is activated, due to the phosphorylation of CRTCs by SIK1. This latter event may occur in the absence of an increase in $Na^+{}_{in}$ (i.e., when SIK1 is activated by LKB1 or CAMK).

The two SIK1 signal transduction pathways, which are activated following an increase in $Na^+{}_{in}$, both play a role during the initial phase of AKI. During this phase, a) luminal Na^+ increases due to TGF, and b) intracellular ATP levels may decline due to ischemia and/or a toxic insult. In this latter case, Na^+ extrusion by Na,K-ATPase declines, as this transporter depends upon cellular energy levels. As a consequence, $Na^+{}_{in}$ increases further, resulting in a) a further activation of SIK1, and increase in Na,K-ATPase activity (via PP2A), as well as b) protective effects elicited as a consequence of the expression of NFAT-regulated genes (a result of the class IIa HDAC Kinase activity of SIK1). During these responses, activated SIK1 can also restrict chronic, transcriptional regulation of Na,K-ATPase by CREB (through the phosphorylation of CRTCs).

The restrictive effect of SIK1 on transcriptional regulation of Na,K-ATPase by CREB and CRTCs is alleviated, however, when SIK1 is phosphorylated, and inhibited by PKA. This occurs in response to cytokines (such as PGE_2) which are produced during the maintenance and recovery phases of AKI. During this time, the necessary increases in intracellular cAMP and $Ca^{2+}{}_{in}$ required for the interaction of CRTCs with CREB on the *atp1b1* promoter must occur if RPT transport activity is to increase over the long term.

The SIK1 signaling networks described above are evolutionarily highly conserved, including the SIK1 signaling events responsible for maintaining cellular Na^+ homeostasis [40]. SIK1 orthologues have been reported in a diverse range of animal cells ranging from mouse, zebrafish, and drosophila, to Caenorhabditis elegans [12]. Even plants express the orthologous SOS2 and SOS3, which permit adaptions to drought, as well as increases in the salinity of the soil [41].

3. Other Roles of SIKs

3.1. Roles of SIK2 and SIK3 in Gluconeogenesis and Lipogenesis

SIKs are regulators of a diverse range of cellular functions which are much broader than those activated by ionic imbalances. Indeed, each of the three different SIK isoforms plays a variety of roles, in different tissues [26]. Examples discussed below include the role of SIK3 in hepatic gluconeogenesis [42], as well as the role of SIK2 in lipogenesis in adipocytes [43].

3.1.1. Role of SIK2 and SIK3 in Gluconeogenesis in the Liver

When blood glucose levels are high, insulin, which is produced, stimulates the phosphorylation and activation of Akt in the liver [38]. Akt in turn phosphorylates hepatic FOXO transcription factors, which become sequestered in the cytoplasm. Under these conditions, SIK3, which is activated by LKB1, phosphorylates CRTC2 and CRTC3 (as well as Class IIa HDACs), resulting in the sequestration of these proteins in the cytoplasm. As a consequence, gluconeogenic gene expression is repressed.

In contrast, during fasting, glucagon is produced, with a resultant increase in hepatocyte cAMP, the activation of AC, which as a consequence, phosphorylates (and inactivates) SIK3 [38]. Subsequently, CRTC2 and CRTC3 are dephosphorylated by calcineurin, and translocate to the nucleus, where they interact with pCREB (and CBP) on the promoters of gluconeogenic genes, including genes encoding for Phosphoenol Pyruvate Carboxykinase (PEPCK) and Glucose 6 Phosphatase (G6Pase).

At the same time (i.e., during fasting), hepatic class IIa HDACs and FOXO1 become dephosphorylated (due to the inhibition of SIK3), and translocate to the nucleus [44]. HDAC4 and HDAC5 (Class IIa HDACs) interact with FOXO1 on IRE sites in the PEPCK and G6Pase promoters, where they recruit HDAC3 (a Class I HDAC), which deacetylates FOXO1, thereby stimulating transcription. Thus, both CRTCs and Class IIa HDACs act so as to stimulate the expression of these hepatic gluconeogenic genes.

3.1.2. Role of SIK2 and Activating Transcription Factor 3 (ATF3) in Lipid Metabolism in Adipocytes

SIKs, HDACs and CRTCs similarly play a role in transcriptional regulation in other insulin-sensitive tissues, including adipocytes [38]. In white adipocytes, catecholamines (which are produced by the hypothalamus during fasting) stimulate lipolysis by activating β adrenergic receptors (and thus PKA) resulting in the phosphorylation of hormone-sensitive lipase [45]. Activated PKA also phosphorylates, and inactivates SIK2, which results in an increase in the transcription of ATF3 (ATF3 being a CREB, and CRTC dependent gene). ATF3 acts as a transcriptional repressor of the insulin responsive GLUT4 gene, as well as the adiponectin gene. In contrast, in the fed state SIK2 becomes dephosphorylated and activated, which results in the phosphorylation of CRTC2 (as well as HDAC4), and reduced expression of ATF3. The ultimate result is increased expression of GLUT4 and glucose uptake, promoting lipogenesis.

3.1.3. Relevance to the Kidney

Although the kidney is not generally noted as being an insulin-sensitive tissue, the RPT nevertheless does have gluconeogenic capacity, that is reportedly inhibited by insulin as well as glucose, by a mechanism which involves the inactivation of FOXO1 [46]. Very likely this mechanism involves SIK3, which very likely phosphorylates class IIa HDACs in the kidney (as in the liver), thereby preventing the interaction of class IIa HDACs (and HDAC3, a Class I HDAC) with FOXO1 on IREs in the PEPCK and G6Pase promoters (an interaction which is very likely just as necessary for the activation of FOXO1 in the kidney, in addition to the liver). Little is known about the effects of catecholamines on ATF3 expression in the kidney. However, ATF3 is rapidly induced during ischemia/reperfusion injury, and suppresses the expression of inflammatory cytokines (including IL-6 and IL-12b) during AKI (as indicated by studies with AFT3 deficient mice) [47]. Catecholamines (or other renal effectors that activate PKA) may be responsible for the induction of ATF3 in the kidney during AKI by stimulating the phosphorylation and inactivation of SIK2 by PKA (as observed in white adipocytes), thereby resulting in increased transcription of AFT3 (due to a CREB/CRTC1 interaction in the kidney as occurs in white adipocytes).

3.2. *Role of SIK2 in Mitochondrial Biogenesis and Its Relevance to AKI*

During AKI, the ability of the RPT to carry out is reabsorptive functions is impaired in part due to a reduced capacity to generate sufficient levels of ATP. In addition, Reactive Oxygen Species (ROS) are generated due to injuries affecting the mitochondria. These problems can be alleviated by means of mitochondrial biogenesis, which depends upon the expression of the Peroxisome Proliferator-Activated Receptor γ Co-activator-1α (PGC-1α) gene, which in turn depends upon SIKs.

3.2.1. Role of SIK2 in Regulating PGC-1α Adipocytes

In adipocytes, the PKA mediated activation of CREB, and its interaction with CRTC2 (which occurs following the inhibition of SIK2), results in increased expression of PGC-1α [48]. PGC-1α functions to induce Uncoupling protein 1 (UCP-1), as well as other mitochondrial genes and transcription factors. The ultimate result is mitochondrial biogenesis, and an increased oxidative capacity. In white adipocytes, inducers of PGC-1α include β adrenergic agonists, thyroid hormone, and in brown adipocytes, insulin. Insulin acts as an inducer in brown adipocytes by activating Phosphoinositol 3-Kinase (PI3K) as well as Akt, and ultimately phosphorylating SIK2 (at Ser587). In contrast, SIK1 has been implicated in regulating the expression of PGC-1α in skeletal muscle [49]. In skeletal muscle, important promoter elements for the PGC-1α gene include a regulatory element for CREB (i.e., a CRE), as well as MEF2. Thus, SIK1 regulates PGC-1α gene expression via its ability to phosphorylate CRTCs [50], as well as class IIA HDACs [19].

3.2.2. Regulation of Mitochondrial Biogenesis during AKI

In the RPT, mitochondrial biogenesis is particularly important in maintaining the energy demands of the RPT after injury, including injuries that result in AKI [51]. This is because the RPT primarily depends upon mitochondrial oxidative metabolism to produce the ATP necessary to carry out its reabsorptive functions, having a very limited capacity for glycolysis [29]. Thus, following injuries to the RPT, the remaining viable, transporting RPT cells may very well require additional mitochondria in order to meet their energy requirements.

Several small molecules such as resveratrol and isoflavone-derived compounds, induce mitochondrial biogenesis in the RPT, and have been used to alleviate deleterious effects of injuries to the RPT [52]. While resveratrol has been observed to increase mitochondrial biogenesis through the activation of AMPK in fibroblasts, a similar AMPK activation has not been observed in RPT cells [52]. Thus, the SIK network may be involved. Indeed, a recent report indicates that the mitochondrial biogenesis that occurs after the formoterol-induced recovery from ischemia-reperfusion injury is mediated by β adrenergic receptors [53]. Similarly, mitochondrial biogenesis occurs in brown adipocytes in response to catecholamines and occurs via a mechanism which involves the phosphorylation and inhibition of SIK2 [48].

The induction of mitochondrial biogenesis following injury to the RPT is also an important means of overcoming damage caused by Reactive Oxygen Species (ROS). ROS production occurs more often when the mitochondrial electron transport chain becomes more reduced as a consequence of cellular injuries [4,54,55]. This problem is alleviated when mitochondrial biogenesis occurs, which causes oxidative substrates to be distributed to more mitochondria. As a consequence, the degree to which the electron transport chain becomes reduced in individual mitochondria (and hence the degree that ROS production occurs) decreases.

As stated above, mitochondrial biogenesis is mediated by PGC-1α, whose expression depends upon the interaction of CRTCs with CREB, which in turn depends upon SIK. Following its induction, PGC-1α interacts with FOXO3 so as to increase the expression of the antioxidant genes CAT, SOD2, and GPX1 (which encode for catalase, superoxide dismutase and glutathione peroxidase, respectively) [55,56]. Indeed, these same antioxidant enzymes are induced in the kidney response to AKI [57,58]. Therefore, an understanding of the role of the SIK network in this process is important.

3.3. *Yet Other Roles Known to Be Played by SIKs in Events Which Occur during AKI*

A number of other metabolic events and cellular processes that occur during AKI are also known to involve SIKs. Included amongst the metabolic events is the decline in Fatty Acid (FA) oxidation in the RPT, which results in the Epithelial to Mesenchymal Transition (EMT). In addition, lethal damage during AKI results in apoptosis, and sublethal damage in repair processes, and ultimately cell division. The decline in FA oxidation, and apoptosis, as well as the progression of cells through the cell cycle, and ultimately, cell division involve SIKs.

3.3.1. Fatty Acid Oxidation

ATP Production in the RPT Is Generated by FA Oxidation, Which Declines in AKI

As stated above, RPT cells are included amongst the most energy demanding cells in the body, expending extensive quantities of ATP in order to meet their reabsorptive requirements. However, following a hypoxic or toxic insult, there is a major decline in cellular ATP and metabolism. ATP production by the RPT is primarily generated by the oxidation of FAs in mitochondria as well as peroxisomes. This process is largely shut down during AKI and for a lengthy period thereafter [54]. The FAs utilized by RPT cells are generated by their uptake by FA transporters such as CD36, the deacylation of phospholipids, and other metabolic events. Free FAs are first metabolized by Carnitine Palmitoyl-Transferase 1 (CPT-1), so as to form acyl carnitine derivatives, which enter mitochondria and peroxisomes [54]. After entering mitochondria and peroxisomes, the metabolism of FAs then depends upon enzymes including mitochondrial medium chain acyl COA dehydrogenase (MCAD) and peroxisomal acyl-CoA oxidase (ACOX1). However, both CPT-1 and ACOX1 enzymatic activity declines following ischemia/reperfusion injury, and MCAD activity declines as a consequence of cisplatin-induced AKI [54]. RPT cells have only a limited capacity to metabolize glucose in lieu of FAs. Thus, the decline in ATP levels that occurs in the RPT during AKI can be prolonged, with severe consequences.

SIK2 Regulates FA Oxidation in Other Tissues

Of particular interest in these regards, are the studies indicating that SIK2 regulates FA oxidation, in the liver, skeletal muscle, as well as in adipocytes [45]. Indeed, the levels of ACOX1, CPT1 and MCAD all decline in SIK2 KO mice. Thus, inactivation of SIK2 is an explanation for the decline in FA oxidation in RPT cells during AKI. Presumably then, interventions which specifically result in SIK2 activation would be expected to counteract the decline in FA oxidation (and resulting reductions in ATP levels).

Decreased FA Oxidation Results in EMT in the RPT

A number of studies indicate that the decrease in FA Oxidation that occurs during AKI results in EMT [54]. For example, studies with HK2 cells indicate that such a decrease in FA oxidation, and lipid accumulation precedes a glucose-induced morphological change typical of the EMT. Similarly, RPT cell cultures treated with the CPT-1 inhibitor Etoxmoxir undergo EMT. However, an alternative explanation for the EMT observed in the RPT during AKI (as well as during a decline in FA oxidation) is that it is a result of a TGFβ-mediated downregulation of cell–cell junctional constituents including E-cadherin.

Involvement of SIK1 in EMT

The studies of Vanlandewijck et al. [59] indicate that TGFβ downregulates E-cadherin through the activation of SIK1, which phosphorylates the polarity complex protein Par3 (a regulator of tight junction assembly), resulting in the degradation of Par3 by the proteasomes and lysosomes, an event which ultimately results in EMT. In addition, other kinases such as LKB1 maintain epithelial cell polarity, by activating SIKs, causing transcriptional repressors such as Snail1 to be downregulated (thereby preventing repression of E-Cadherin) [60].

TGFβ is a key profibrotic factor that is activated during AKI, and promotes EMT in the RPT [61]. Following repeated injury, RPT cells which have undergone EMT may fail to either re-differentiate, or to regain normal mitochondrial and metabolic function. Instead, these damaged RPT cells produce large quantities of TGFβ, which perpetuates the EMT, and prevents the proliferation necessary for repair. As a consequence, events can be initiated which result in Chronic Kidney Disease (CKD) [61]. Presumably, TGFβ production is responsible for perpetuating these problems. Conceivably, this cycle of events may be prevented by the use of SIK1 inhibitors to prevent signal transduction events which have been initiated via TGFβ receptors.

3.3.2. Role of SIKs in Apoptosis

Transient ischemia which occurs as a result of hypovolemia, hypotension and/or heart failure is a common cause of AKI. As stated above, the RPT is particularly susceptible to ischemic damage, which results in their detachment from their substratum, and death (either by apoptosis or necrosis) [62]. The apoptosis which occurs in the RPT during ischemia is a means of removing damaged, dysfunctional cells from the kidney. A number of studies indicate that p53 plays an important role in the apoptosis, cell cycle arrest and autophagy that occurs in the RPT when AKI is induced by ischemia, cisplatin and even folic acid [62]. Of particular interest in these regards are recent studies indicating that p53-dependent anoikis (a subtype of apoptosis resulting from a lack of cell adhesion) is mediated by SIK1 [63].

3.3.3. Pro-Survival Roles of SIKs and Epigenetics

Prosurvival Role of SIK1 in Myocytes Involves SIK1's HDAC Kinase Activity

A number of studies indicate that in addition, SIK1 has a pro-survival role (pertinent to cells which have been damaged, but are not destined to undergo apoptosis). Studies with transgenic mice with the targeted expression of a dominant negative CREB (ACREB), indicated that the survival of the differentiated cells in the targeted tissues decreased in the absence of functional CREB protein [19,64–66]. Initially, investigators thought that CREB was directly responsible for increasing cell survival and differentiation in the targeted tissues. However, subsequent studies indicated that CREB promoted cell survival (and differentiation) indirectly, by inducing the expression of the Snf1lk gene (encoding SIK1), resulting in an elevated level of activated SIK1 [19]. The activated SIK1 was observed to phosphorylate Class IIa HDACs, an event which was lost in vitro when the SIK1 phosphorylation site was removed by mutation [67]. The ultimate result of SIK1 phosphorylation in vivo was increased cell survival.

The initial studies indicating that SIK1 promoted cell survival were conducted with mice in which ACREB was targeted to skeletal muscle [67]. In skeletal muscle, previous studies indicated that the myogenic program depends upon MEF2 transcriptional activity. The binding of Class IIa HDACs to MEF2 transcription factors on chromosomal DNA inhibits MEF2-mediated transcription, and thus myogenesis. However, CREB activation was observed to induce SIK1 expression (which no longer occurred in ACREB skeletal muscle). Normally, the phosphorylation of Class IIa HDACs by SIK1 (and their translocation to the cytoplasm), results in increased MEF2 transcriptional activity and myogenesis (events which are impaired in ACREB mice). The discovery of that SIK1 is a pro-survival factor that promotes myogenesis, resulting in a reassessment of many previous studies.

Involvement of Epigenetics and Class IIa HDACs in Regeneration of Damaged Kidneys

A number of recent studies indicate that a number of epigenetic events, including histone acetylation, are important in the regeneration of damaged kidneys [68]. Indeed, a decrease in histone acetylation has been reported in RPTs subjected to energy depletion, while during the subsequent recovery period HDAC5 (a class IIa HDAC) was downregulated, and histone acetylation increased [69]. SIK1 may very well play a role in this process.

3.3.4. Role of SIKs in Cell Growth and Hypertrophy

Cell Division and Hypertrophy during AKI

In the normal kidney, RPT cells divide very slowly [70]. Cell division only occurs as a means to replace tubule epithelial cells, which are lost very slowly into the urine. However, following an ischemic or toxic insult, many RPT cells, which were previously quiescent, enter the cell cycle (even when there is massive necrosis and apoptosis). Many of the tubule epithelial cells which enter the cell cycle immediately after an ischemic or toxic insult spend a lengthy period in G2/M, secreting factors such as TGFβ, which result in fibrosis [71]. A large proportion of the epithelial cells which enter the cell cycle immediately after an ischemic or toxic insult have extensive DNA damage, leading to a mitotic catastrophe [70].

Subsequently, during the recovery period of AKI, additional RPT cells, including those which are sub-lethally injured, enter the cell cycle, and may divide [29]. The newly generated RPT cells migrate to regions which have been denuded as a consequence of injury, where they assume the polarized morphology required for transepithelial transport.

In recent studies, Lazzeri et al. [72] tracked the fate of individual tubular cells in conditional Pax8/Confetti mice during AKI. The results indicate that regeneration of new tubule epithelial cells during AKI is not as extensive as previously thought, even though kidney function recovers. Renal functional recovery could be attributed to some of the original tubule epithelial cells, in addition to limited progenitor driven regeneration. A number of the original tubule epithelial cells (or remnant cells) which were in the cell cycle, actually, went through endocycles (i.e., alternative cell cycles without cell division). Tubule epithelial cells which had undergone endoreplication cycles were often polyploid, and had undergone hypertrophy. Notably, endocycling cells and hypertrophy was also observed in the kidneys of patients after AKI.

Role of SIKs in Hypertrophy and Cell Division

As discussed above, the hypertrophy of atrial myocytes has been attributed to the activation of SIK1, in particular following an increase in intracellular Na^+ [18]. Recent studies by Popov et al. [73] indicate that SIK2 activation also causes hypertrophy in cardiac myocytes. In rats expressing a hypertensive variant of the α-adducin gene, the expression of SIK2 is elevated, as well as genes associated with left ventricle hypertrophy (LVH). Similarly, in mice on a high salt diet, LVH can be prevented by the ablation of sik2. Although not reported in the case of cardiac tissue, the SIK3 isoform is essential for chondrocyte hypertrophy during skeletal development [74]. However, the SIK Isoform(s) involved in renal hypertrophy have not been identified.

A number of recent studies indicate that SIKs regulate cell proliferation, particularly under conditions of stress. SIK2 promotes G1/S progression presumably due to its ability to phosphorylate the p85 α subunit of Phosphoinositide 3 Kinase (PI3K) [75], which mediates signaling in response to a number of growth factors. In addition, SIK2 is localized in centrosomes, where it acts as a "centrosome kinase" required for mitotic spindle formation [76]. The SIK3 isoform similarly is a mitotic regulator [77,78]. Indeed, mitosis is extended following a SIK3 knockdown. The increased duration of mitosis following a SIK3 knockdown has been attributed to a SIK3 requirement for mitotic exit. Although the metaphase plate forms normally when SIK3 is depleted, the onset of anaphase is delayed.

4. Summary and Therapeutic Potential

All three SIK isoforms are expressed in the RPT, and most likely play distinct roles in the preservation and reacquisition of renal function during AKI. Presently, the role played by each of the SIK isoforms during AKI can be surmised from investigations conducted with the renal SIK1 network, as well as with the SIK2 and SIK3 isoforms in other tissues, as summarized below.

During the initiation and extension phases of AKI, renal reabsorptive function declines and cytokines are produced. Activation of the SIK1 network during this time period results in an acute increase in the number of basolateral Na,K-ATPases (due to a SIK1 mediated decrease in basolateral PME activity, and an increase in dephosphorylated Na,K-ATPase (by activated PP2A)). The SIK1 activation caused by an increase in $Ca^{2+}{}_{in}$, also results in an increase in the phosphorylation of Class IIa HDACs by SIK1, transcriptional activation of NFAT2, which positively regulates the expression of the ANP and MHC genes. Thus, the development of SIK1 activators is needed so as to promote the expression of the SIK1 network during the early stages of AKI. The use of physiologic activators such as norepinephrine may have similar effects.

Needless to say, SIK1 activation may not always be beneficial. TGFβ (whose production starts during the early stages AKI) activates SIK1, and in this manner induces EMT. TGFβ production has the potential to continue for prolonged periods during AKI [61]. Thus, SIK1 inhibitors can presumably be employed to alleviate the long-term deleterious effects of TGFβ, including EMT and fibrosis.

PGE_2 is also produced during AKI. PGE_2 is a known mediator of inflammatory responses. Nevertheless, AKI was aggravated when microsomal Prostaglandin Synthase 2 (i.e., mPGES-2, which is responsible for renal PGE_2 production) was down-regulated, and this was associated with increased apoptosis [79]. These latter results suggest that PGE_2 promotes recovery from AKI. This can presumably be explained by a) the PKA-mediated inhibition of SIK1 which occurs as a consequence of the interaction of PGE_2 with either EP2 or EP4 receptors, as well as b) the Ca^{2+}-mediated activation of calcineurin, which results in the dephosphorylation of CRTC1, and its interaction with pCREB in RPT cells. As a consequence, not only does the expression of the *atp1b1* gene increase, as well as the level of the Na,K-ATPase in RPT cells, but in addition, ATF3 expression increases. Such an increase in the expression of ATF3 (observed in vivo when ATF3 is overexpressed in mice by adenoviral mediated gene transfer) has been observed to result in a reduction of ischemia-reperfusion injury [80]. Thus, SIK1 inhibition at least during the latter stages of AKI presumably promotes recovery.

An increase in mitochondrial biogenesis during the initial phases of AKI is expected to cause an increase in reabsorption, as well as a decrease in the level of ROS. As summarized above, the SIK2 isoform has been observed to restrict mitochondrial biogenesis, due to its ability to phosphorylate CRTCs, thereby preventing the interaction of CRTCs with CREB, and reducing transcription of the PGC1-α gene. This limitation can be overcome, presumably by the inhibition of the SIK2 isoform per se during the initiation phase of AKI.

However, the cell cycle progression which occurs during subsequent phases of AKI depends upon SIK2. Not only is the p85 α subunit of PI3 Kinase is a substrate of SIK2 (PI3K promoting cell cycle entry) [81], but, in addition, SIK2 is required for cell division itself, being a centrosome kinase [76]. Similarly, the SIK3 isoform is required for mitotic exit. These processes would be promoted by targeting either SIK2 or SIK3 via an activating drug.

Studies conducted both in vitro with cultured renal cells as well as in vivo with transgenic animals are needed in order to evaluate whether the different SIK isoforms participate as anticipated in the events occurring during the different phases of AKI. In addition to employing siRNA and CRISPR technology, a number of expression vectors can be employed, including kinase dead SIK K56M [16], as well as SIK phosphomutants which cannot be phosphorylated by either LKB1, CaMK1 or PKA, the mutants being T182A, T322A, or T577A, respectively in the case of SIK1 [12,16,67]. Similar SIK mutants have been employed in studies with the other SIK isoforms [82,83]. In addition to employing the in vitro approach, studies conducted in vivo with mice possessing targeted knockouts should also prove to be invaluable when studying the role of SIKs in AKI. For example, the use of a mouse strain which expresses CRE recombinase under the control of the SGLT2 promoter will permit targeting of specific SIK knockouts to the RPT [84].

5. Development of Clinical Kinase Drugs

Protein kinases have emerged as major drug targets, because their functions within signaling networks are deregulated in a number of disease states [85]. Currently, more than 37 kinase inhibitors have been approved for human use, and the number is expected to increase dramatically, because more than 250 kinase inhibitors are undergoing clinical trials [85]. A number of these drugs target the ATP binding site, which has led to concerns of selectivity. This has led to chemoproteomic target screens of a multitude of kinase inhibitors [85]. Although a number of clinical kinase inhibitors have been found to be nonselective, at the same time other inhibitors were found to be extremely selective, including drugs targeting Mitogen Activated Protein Kinase (MAPK) and the Epidermal Growth Factor Receptor (EGFR). In addition, chemoproteomics have found some unexpected, yet promising drug targets, including SIK2.

SIK2 became of interest as a drug target when a small-molecule screening found that a number of kinase inhibitors that enhanced IL-10 production (and inhibited TNFα production) by murine bone-marrow-derived dendritic cells (including the FDA approved drugs dasatinib and bosutinib) actually targeted SIK2 [86]. The SIK inhibitor HG-9-91-01 was observed to have similar effects. In order to identify additional SIK2 inhibitors, MALDI-TOF screening assays have been conducted. In such studies, Heap et al. [87] were able to screen for SIK2 inhibitors, while assaying the phosphorylation of CHKtide, a peptide derived from CHK1 protein kinase involved in DNA repair (CHKtide had been previously identified in a kinase screen as being a good SIK substrate). Not only did Heap et al. [87] successfully identify SIK2 inhibitors, but in addition obtained evidence of activators [87]. Using a similar chemoproteomic screening approach, 21 additional SIK2 inhibitors were identified by Klaeger et al. [85]. Further progress is needed in validating the newly identified SIK2 inhibitors and activators, in addition to identifying drugs specifically targeting the other SIK isoforms.

Acknowledgments: The author thanks Sudha Garimella, Dongwook Kim, Trivikram Rajkhowa, and Facundo Cutuli for their experimental work that inspired this review.

References

1. Okamoto, M.; Takemori, H.; Katoh, Y. Salt-inducible kinase in steroidogenesis and adipogenesis. *Trends Endocrinol. Metab.* **2004**, *15*, 21–26. [CrossRef] [PubMed]
2. Jaitovich, A.; Bertorello, A.M. Intracellular sodium sensing: SIK1 network, hormone action and high blood pressure. *Biochim. Et Biophys. Acta* **2010**, *1802*, 1140–1149. [CrossRef] [PubMed]
3. Makris, K.; Spanou, L. Acute Kidney Injury: Definition, Pathophysiology and Clinical Phenotypes. *Clin. Biochem. Rev.* **2016**, *37*, 85–98. [PubMed]
4. Pavlakou, P.; Liakopoulos, V.; Eleftheriadis, T.; Mitsis, M.; Dounousi, E. Oxidative Stress and Acute Kidney Injury in Critical Illness: Pathophysiologic Mechanisms-Biomarkers-Interventions, and Future Perspectives. *Oxid Med. Cell Longev.* **2017**, *2017*, 6193694. [CrossRef] [PubMed]
5. Zuk, A.; Bonventre, J.V. Acute Kidney Injury. *Annu. Rev. Med.* **2016**, *67*, 293–307. [CrossRef]
6. Moore, P.K.; Hsu, R.K.; Liu, K.D. Management of Acute Kidney Injury: Core Curriculum 2018. *Am. J. Kidney Dis.* **2018**, *72*, 136–148. [CrossRef] [PubMed]
7. Levey, A.S.; James, M.T. Acute Kidney Injury. *Ann. Intern. Med.* **2017**, *167*, ITC66–ITC80. [CrossRef]
8. Lan, R.; Geng, H.; Singha, P.K.; Saikumar, P.; Bottinger, E.P.; Weinberg, J.M.; Venkatachalam, M.A. Mitochondrial Pathology and Glycolytic Shift during Proximal Tubule Atrophy after Ischemic AKI. *J. Am. Soc. Nephrol.* **2016**, *27*, 3356–3367. [CrossRef]
9. Morrell, E.D.; Kellum, J.A.; Hallows, K.R.; Pastor-Soler, N.M. Epithelial transport during septic acute kidney injury. *Nephrol. Dial. Transpl.* **2014**, *29*, 1312–1319. [CrossRef]
10. Strazzullo, P.; Leclercq, C. Sodium. *Adv. Nutr.* **2014**, *5*, 188–190. [CrossRef]
11. Ding, X.; Cheng, Z.; Qian, Q. Intravenous Fluids and Acute Kidney Injury. *Blood Purif.* **2017**, *43*, 163–172. [CrossRef] [PubMed]
12. Sjostrom, M.; Stenstrom, K.; Eneling, K.; Zwiller, J.; Katz, A.I.; Takemori, H.; Bertorello, A.M. SIK1 is part of a cell sodium-sensing network that regulates active sodium transport through a calcium-dependent process. *Proc. Natl. Acad. Sci. USA.* **2007**, *104*, 16922–16927. [CrossRef] [PubMed]
13. Skou, J.C.; Esmann, M. The Na,K-ATPase. *J. Bioenerg. Biomembr.* **1992**, *24*, 249–261. [PubMed]
14. Sakamoto, K.; Bultot, L.; Goransson, O. The Salt-Inducible Kinases: Emerging Metabolic Regulators. *Trends Endocrinol Metab.* **2018**, *29*, 827–840. [CrossRef] [PubMed]
15. Hashimoto, Y.K.; Satoh, T.; Okamoto, M.; Takemori, H. Importance of autophosphorylation at Ser186 in the A-loop of salt inducible kinase 1 for its sustained kinase activity. *J. Cell Biochem.* **2008**, *104*, 1724–1739. [CrossRef] [PubMed]
16. Katoh, Y.; Takemori, H.; Lin, X.Z.; Tamura, M.; Muraoka, M.; Satoh, T.; Tsuchiya, Y.; Min, L.; Doi, J.; Miyauchi, A.; et al. Silencing the constitutive active transcription factor CREB by the LKB1-SIK signaling cascade. *Febs. J.* **2006**, *273*, 2730–2748. [CrossRef] [PubMed]
17. Sonntag, T.; Vaughan, J.M.; Montminy, M. 14-3-3 proteins mediate inhibitory effects of cAMP on salt-inducible kinases (SIKs). *Febs. J.* **2018**, *285*, 467–480. [CrossRef] [PubMed]
18. Popov, S.; Venetsanou, K.; Chedrese, P.J.; Pinto, V.; Takemori, H.; Franco-Cereceda, A.; Eriksson, P.; Mochizuki, N.; Soares-da-Silva, P.; Bertorello, A.M. Increases in intracellular sodium activate transcription and gene expression via the salt-inducible kinase 1 network in an atrial myocyte cell line, American journal of physiology. *Heart Circ. Physiol.* **2012**, *303*, H57–H65. [CrossRef]
19. Berdeaux, R.; Goebel, N.; Banaszynski, L.; Takemori, H.; Wandless, T.; Shelton, G.D.; Montminy, M. SIK1 is a class II HDAC kinase that promotes survival of skeletal myocytes. *Nat. Med.* **2007**, *13*, 597–603. [CrossRef]
20. Vesely, D.L. Natriuretic peptides and acute renal failure. *Am. J. Physiol. Ren. Physiol.* **2003**, *285*, F167–F177. [CrossRef]
21. Kim, S.W.; Lee, J.; Park, J.W.; Hong, J.H.; Kook, H.; Choi, C.; Choi, K.C. Increased expression of atrial natriuretic peptide in the kidney of rats with bilateral ureteral obstruction. *Kidney Int.* **2001**, *59*, 1274–1282. [CrossRef] [PubMed]
22. Takei, Y.; Sims, T.N.; Urmson, J.; Halloran, P.F. Central role for interferon-gamma receptor in the regulation of renal MHC expression. *J. Am. Soc. Nephrol.* **2000**, *11*, 250–261. [PubMed]
23. Arulkumaran, N.; Prowle, J.R. Natriuretic Peptides: A Role in Early Septic Acute Kidney Injury? *Anesthesiology* **2018**, *129*, 235–237. [CrossRef] [PubMed]

24. Ueda, K.; Hirahashi, J.; Seki, G.; Tanaka, M.; Kushida, N.; Takeshima, Y.; Nishikawa, Y.; Fujita, T.; Nangaku, M. Successful treatment of acute kidney injury in patients with idiopathic nephrotic syndrome using human atrial natriuretic Peptide. *Intern. Med.* **2014**, *53*, 865–869. [CrossRef] [PubMed]
25. Nigwekar, S.U.; Navaneethan, S.D.; Parikh, C.R.; Hix, J.K. Atrial natriuretic peptide for management of acute kidney injury: A systematic review and meta-analysis. *Clin. J. Am. Soc. Nephrol.* **2009**, *4*, 261–272. [CrossRef]
26. Wein, M.N.; Foretz, M.; Fisher, D.E.; Xavier, R.J.; Kronenberg, H.M. Salt-Inducible Kinases: Physiology, Regulation by cAMP, and Therapeutic Potential. *Trends Endocrinol Metab.* **2018**, *29*, 723–735. [CrossRef] [PubMed]
27. Taub, M.; Garamella, S.; Kim, D.; Rajkhowa, T.; Cutuli, F. Renal Proximal Tubule Na,K-ATPase is Controlled by CREB Regulated Transcriptional CoActivators as well as Salt Inducible Kinase 1. *Cell. Signal.* **2015**, *27*, 2568–2578. [CrossRef]
28. MacKenzie, K.F.; Clark, K.; Naqvi, S.; McGuire, V.A.; Noehren, G.; Kristariyanto, Y.; van den Bosch, M.; Mudaliar, M.; McCarthy, P.C.; Pattison, M.J.; et al. PGE(2) induces macrophage IL-10 production and a regulatory-like phenotype via a protein kinase A-SIK-CRTC3 pathway. *J. Immunol.* **2013**, *190*, 565–577. [CrossRef]
29. Basile, D.P.; Anderson, M.D.; Sutton, T.A. Pathophysiology of acute kidney injury. *Compr. Physiol.* **2012**, *2*, 1303–1353.
30. Breyer, M.D.; Breyer, R.M. Prostaglandin E receptors and the kidney. *Am. J. Physiol. Ren. Physiol.* **2000**, *279*, F12–F23. [CrossRef]
31. Matlhagela, K.; Taub, M. Involvement of EP1 and EP2 receptors in the regulation of the Na,K-ATPase by prostaglandins in MDCK cells. *Prostaglandins Other Lipid Mediat.* **2006**, *79*, 101–113. [CrossRef] [PubMed]
32. Herman, M.B.; Rajkhowa, T.; Cutuli, F.; Springate, J.E.; Taub, M. Regulation of renal proximal tubule Na-K-ATPase by prostaglandins. *Am. J. Physiol. Ren. Physiol.* **2010**, *298*, F1222–F1234. [CrossRef] [PubMed]
33. Taub, M.; Borsick, M.; Geisel, J.; Rajkhowa, T.; Allen, C. Regulation of the Na,K-ATPase in MDCK cells by prostaglandin E1: A role for calcium as well as cAMP. *Exp. Cell Res.* **2004**, *299*, 1–14. [CrossRef] [PubMed]
34. Geering, K. The functional role of the beta-subunit in the maturation and intracellular transport of sodium-potassium ATPase. *FEBS Lett.* **1991**, *285*, 189–193. [CrossRef]
35. Taub, M. Gene Level Regulation of Na,K-ATPase in the Renal Proximal Tubule Is Controlled by Two Independent but Interacting Regulatory Mechanisms Involving Salt Inducible Kinase 1 and CREB-Regulated Transcriptional Coactivators. *Int. J. Mol. Sci.* **2018**, *19*, 2086–2095. [CrossRef] [PubMed]
36. Matlhagela, K.; Borsick, M.; Rajkhowa, T.; Taub, M. Identification of a Prostaglandin-responsive Element in the Na,K-ATPase {beta}1 Promoter That Is Regulated by cAMP and Ca2+: Evidence for an interactive role of cAMP regulatory element-bindin protein and Sp1. *J. Biol. Chem.* **2005**, *280*, 334–346. [CrossRef]
37. Matlhagela, K.; Taub, M. Regulation of the Na-K-ATPase beta(1)-subunit promoter by multiple prostaglandin-responsive elements. *Am. J. Physiol. - Ren. Physiol.* **2006**, *291*, F635–F646. [CrossRef]
38. Altarejos, J.Y.; Montminy, M. CREB and the CRTC co-activators: Sensors for hormonal and metabolic signals, Nature reviews. *Mol. Cell Biol.* **2011**, *12*, 141–151.
39. Nakajima, T.; Uchida, C.; Anderson, S.F.; Parvin, J.D.; Montminy, M. Analysis of a cAMP-responsive activator reveals a two-component mechanism for transcriptional induction via signal-dependent factors. *Genes Dev.* **1997**, *11*, 738–747. [CrossRef]
40. Bertorello, A.M.; Zhu, J.K. SIK1/SOS2 networks: Decoding sodium signals via calcium-responsive protein kinase pathways. *Pflug. Arch. - Eur. J. Physiol.* **2009**, *458*, 613–619. [CrossRef]
41. Ji, H.; Pardo, J.M.; Batelli, G.; Van Oosten, M.J.; Bressan, R.A.; Li, X. The Salt Overly Sensitive (SOS) pathway: Established and emerging roles. *Mol. Plant.* **2013**, *6*, 275–286. [CrossRef] [PubMed]
42. Itoh, Y.; Sanosaka, M.; Fuchino, H.; Yahara, Y.; Kumagai, A.; Takemoto, D.; Kagawa, M.; Doi, J.; Ohta, M.; Tsumaki, N.; et al. Salt-inducible Kinase 3 Signaling Is Important for the Gluconeogenic Programs in Mouse Hepatocytes. *J. Biol. Chem.* **2015**, *290*, 17879–17893. [CrossRef] [PubMed]
43. Du, J.; Chen, Q.; Takemori, H.; Xu, H. SIK2 can be activated by deprivation of nutrition and it inhibits expression of lipogenic genes in adipocytes. *Obes. (Silver Spring)* **2008**, *16*, 531–538. [CrossRef] [PubMed]
44. Liu, Y.; Dentin, R.; Chen, D.; Hedrick, S.; Ravnskjaer, K.; Schenk, S.; Milne, J.; Meyers, D.J.; Cole, P.; Yates III, J.; et al. A fasting inducible switch modulates gluconeogenesis via activator/coactivator exchange. *Nature* **2008**, *456*, 269–273. [CrossRef] [PubMed]
45. Park, J.; Yoon, Y.S.; Han, H.S.; Kim, Y.H.; Ogawa, Y.; Park, K.G.; Lee, C.H.; Kim, S.T.; Koo, S.H. SIK2 is critical in the regulation of lipid homeostasis and adipogenesis *in vivo*. *Diabetes* **2014**, *63*, 3659–3673. [CrossRef]

[PubMed]
46. Sasaki, M.; Sasako, T.; Kubota, N.; Sakurai, Y.; Takamoto, I.; Kubota, T.; Inagi, R.; Seki, G.; Goto, M.; Ueki, K.; et al. Dual Regulation of Gluconeogenesis by Insulin and Glucose in the Proximal Tubules of the Kidney. *Diabetes* **2017**, *66*, 2339–2350. [CrossRef] [PubMed]
47. Li, H.F.; Cheng, C.F.; Liao, W.J.; Lin, H.; Yang, R.B. ATF3-mediated epigenetic regulation protects against acute kidney injury. *J. Am. Soc. Nephrol.* **2010**, *21*, 1003–1013. [CrossRef] [PubMed]
48. Muraoka, M.; Fukushima, A.; Viengchareun, S.; Lombes, M.; Kishi, F.; Miyauchi, A.; Kanematsu, M.; Doi, J.; Kajimura, J.; Nakai, R.; et al. Involvement of SIK2/TORC2 signaling cascade in the regulation of insulin-induced PGC-1alpha and UCP-1 gene expression in brown adipocytes. *Am. J. Physiol. Endocrinol Metab.* **2009**, *296*, E1430–E1439. [CrossRef] [PubMed]
49. Nixon, M.; Stewart-Fitzgibbon, R.; Fu, J.; Akhmedov, D.; Rajendran, K.; Mendoza-Rodriguez, M.G.; Rivera-Molina, Y.A.; Gibson, M.; Berglund, E.D.; Justice, N.J.; et al. Skeletal muscle salt inducible kinase 1 promotes insulin resistance in obesity. *Mol. Metab.* **2016**, *5*, 34–46. [CrossRef]
50. Wu, Z.; Huang, X.; Feng, Y.; Handschin, C.; Feng, Y.; Gullicksen, P.S.; Bare, O.; Labow, M.; Spiegelman, B.; Stevenson, S.C. Transducer of regulated CREB-binding proteins (TORCs) induce PGC-1alpha transcription and mitochondrial biogenesis in muscle cells. *Proc. Natl. Acad. Sci. USA.* **2006**, *103*, 14379–14384. [CrossRef]
51. Rasbach, K.A.; Schnellmann, R.G. PGC-1alpha over-expression promotes recovery from mitochondrial dysfunction and cell injury. *Biochem. Biophys. Res. Commun.* **2007**, *355*, 734–739. [CrossRef] [PubMed]
52. Funk, J.A.; Odejinmi, S.; Schnellmann, R.G. SRT1720 induces mitochondrial biogenesis and rescues mitochondrial function after oxidant injury in renal proximal tubule cells. *J. Pharm. Exp.* **2010**, *333*, 593–601. [CrossRef] [PubMed]
53. Cameron, R.B.; Gibbs, W.S.; Miller, S.R.; Dupre, T.V.; Megyesi, J.; Beeson, C.C.; Schnellmann, R.G. Proximal Tubule beta 2-Adrenergic Receptor Mediates Formoterol-Induced Recovery of Mitochondrial and Renal Function after Ischemia-Reperfusion Injury. *J. Pharm. Exp.* **2019**, *369*, 173–180. [CrossRef] [PubMed]
54. Simon, N.; Hertig, A. Alteration of Fatty Acid Oxidation in Tubular Epithelial Cells: From Acute Kidney Injury to Renal Fibrogenesis. *Front. Med. (Lausanne)* **2015**, *2*, 52. [CrossRef] [PubMed]
55. Weinberg, J.M. Mitochondrial biogenesis in kidney disease. *J. Am. Soc. Nephrol.* **2011**, *22*, 431–436. [CrossRef]
56. Olmos, Y.; Valle, I.; Borniquel, S.; Tierrez, A.; Soria, E.; Lamas, S.; Monsalve, M. Mutual dependence of Foxo3a and PGC-1alpha in the induction of oxidative stress genes. *J. Biol. Chem.* **2009**, *284*, 14476–14484. [CrossRef] [PubMed]
57. Singh, I.; Gulati, S.; Orak, J.K.; Singh, A.K. Expression of antioxidant enzymes in rat kidney during ischemia-reperfusion injury. *Mol. Cell Biochem.* **1993**, *125*, 97–104. [CrossRef]
58. Tran, M.; Parikh, S.M. Mitochondrial biogenesis in the acutely injured kidney. *Nephron Clin. Pr.* **2014**, *127*, 42–45. [CrossRef]
59. Vanlandewijck, M.; Dadras, M.S.; Lomnytska, M.; Mahzabin, T.; Lee Miller, M.; Busch, C.; Brunak, S.; Heldin, C.H.; Moustakas, A. The protein kinase SIK downregulates the polarity protein Par3. *Oncotarget* **2018**, *9*, 5716–5735. [CrossRef]
60. Goodwin, J.M.; Svensson, R.U.; Lou, H.J.; Winslow, M.M.; Turk, B.E.; Shaw, R.J. An AMPK-independent signaling pathway downstream of the LKB1 tumor suppressor controls Snail1 and metastatic potential. *Mol Cell* **2014**, *55*, 436–450. [CrossRef]
61. Gewin, L.S. Transforming Growth Factor-beta in the Acute Kidney Injury to Chronic Kidney Disease Transition. *Nephron* **2019**, 1–4. [CrossRef] [PubMed]
62. Havasi, A.; Borkan, S.C. Apoptosis and acute kidney injury. *Kidney Int.* **2011**, *80*, 29–40. [CrossRef] [PubMed]
63. Cheng, H.; Liu, P.; Wang, Z.C.; Zou, L.; Santiago, S.; Garbitt, V.; Gjoerup, O.V.; Iglehart, J.D.; Miron, A.; Richardson, A.L.; et al. SIK1 couples LKB1 to p53-dependent anoikis and suppresses metastasis. *Sci. Signal.* **2009**, *2*, ra35. [CrossRef] [PubMed]
64. Watson, P.A.; Birdsey, N.; Huggins, G.S.; Svensson, E.; Heppe, D.; Knaub, L. Cardiac-specific overexpression of dominant-negative CREB leads to increased mortality and mitochondrial dysfunction in female mice. *Am. J. Physiol. Heart Circ. Physiol.* **2010**, *299*, H2056–H2068. [CrossRef]
65. Jhala, U.S.; Canettieri, G.; Screaton, R.A.; Kulkarni, R.N.; Krajewski, S.; Reed, J.; Walker, J.; Lin, X.; White, M.; Montminy, M. cAMP promotes pancreatic beta-cell survival via CREB-mediated induction of IRS2. *Genes Dev.* **2003**, *17*, 1575–1580. [CrossRef]
66. Sakamoto, K.; Karelina, K.; Obrietan, K. CREB: A multifaceted regulator of neuronal plasticity and protection. *J. Neurochem.* **2011** *116*, 1–9. [CrossRef] [PubMed]

67. Stewart, R.; Akhmedov, D.; Robb, C.; Leiter, C.; Berdeaux, R. Regulation of SIK1 abundance and stability is critical for myogenesis. *Proc. Natl. Acad. Sci. USA.* **2013**, *110*, 117–122. [CrossRef]

68. Dressler, G.R.; Patel, S.R. Epigenetics in kidney development and renal disease. *Transl. Res.* **2015**, *165*, 166–176. [CrossRef]

69. Marumo, T.; Hishikawa, K.; Yoshikawa, M.; Fujita, T. Epigenetic regulation of BMP7 in the regenerative response to ischemia. *J. Am. Soc. Nephrol.* **2008**, *19*, 1311–1320. [CrossRef]

70. Thomasova, D.; Anders, H.J. Cell cycle control in the kidney. *Nephrol. Dial. Transpl.* **2015**, *30*, 1622–1630. [CrossRef]

71. Wu, C.F.; Chiang, W.C.; Lai, C.F.; Chang, F.C.; Chen, Y.T.; Chou, Y.H.; Wu, T.H.; Linn, G.R.; Ling, H.; Wu, K.D.; et al. Transforming growth factor beta-1 stimulates profibrotic epithelial signaling to activate pericyte-myofibroblast transition in obstructive kidney fibrosis. *Am. J. Pathol.* **2013**, *182*, 118–131. [CrossRef] [PubMed]

72. Lazzeri, E.; Angelotti, M.L.; Peired, A.; Conte, C.; Marschner, J.A.; Maggi, L.; Mazzinghi, B.; Lombardi, D.; Melica, M.E.; Nardi, S.; et al. Endocycle-related tubular cell hypertrophy and progenitor proliferation recover renal function after acute kidney injury. *Nat. Commun.* **2018**, *9*, 1344. [CrossRef] [PubMed]

73. Popov, S.; Takemori, H.; Tokudome, T.; Mao, Y.; Otani, K.; Mochizuki, N.; Pires, N.; Pinho, M.J.; Franco-Cereceda, A.; Torielli, L.; et al. Lack of salt-inducible kinase 2 (SIK2) prevents the development of cardiac hypertrophy in response to chronic high-salt intake. *PLoS ONE* **2014**, *9*, e95771. [CrossRef] [PubMed]

74. Sasagawa, S.; Takemori, H.; Uebi, T.; Ikegami, D.; Hiramatsu, K.; Ikegawa, S.; Yoshikawa, H.; Tsumaki, N. SIK3 is essential for chondrocyte hypertrophy during skeletal development in mice. *Development* **2012**, *139*, 1153–1163. [CrossRef] [PubMed]

75. Miranda, F.; Mannion, D.; Liu, S.; Zheng, Y.; Mangala, L.S.; Redondo, C.; Herrero-Gonzalez, S.; Xu, R.; Taylor, C.; Chedom, D.F.; et al. Salt-Inducible Kinase 2 Couples Ovarian Cancer Cell Metabolism with Survival at the Adipocyte-Rich Metastatic Niche. *Cancer Cell* **2016**, *30*, 273–289. [CrossRef] [PubMed]

76. Ahmed, A.A.; Lu, Z.; Jennings, N.B.; Etemadmoghadam, D.; Capalbo, L.; Jacamo, R.O.; Barbosa-Morais, N.; Le, X.F.; Australian Ovarian Cancer Study Group; Vivas-Mejia, P.; et al. SIK2 is a centrosome kinase required for bipolar mitotic spindle formation that provides a potential target for therapy in ovarian cancer. *Cancer Cell* **2010**, *18*, 109–121. [CrossRef] [PubMed]

77. Wehr, M.C.; Holder, M.V.; Gailite, I.; Saunders, R.E.; Maile, T.M.; Ciirdaeva, E.; Instrell, R.; Jiang, M.; Howell, M.; Rossner, M.J.; et al. Salt-inducible kinases regulate growth through the Hippo signalling pathway in Drosophila. *Nat. Cell Biol.* **2013**, *15*, 61–71. [CrossRef]

78. Chen, H.; Huang, S.; Han, X.; Zhang, J.; Shan, C.; Tsang, Y.H.; Ma, H.T.; Poon, R.Y. Salt-inducible kinase 3 is a novel mitotic regulator and a target for enhancing antimitotic therapeutic-mediated cell death. *Cell Death Dis.* **2014**, *5*, e1177. [CrossRef]

79. Li, Y.; Xia, W.; Zhao, F.; Wen, Z.; Zhang, A.; Huang, S.; Jia, Z.; Zhang, Y. Prostaglandins in the pathogenesis of kidney diseases. *Oncotarget* **2018**, *9*, 26586–26602. [CrossRef]

80. Yoshida, T.; Sugiura, H.; Mitobe, M.; Tsuchiya, K.; Shirota, S.; Nishimura, S.; Shiohira, S.; Ito, H.; Nobori, K.; Gullans, S.R.; et al. ATF3 protects against renal ischemia-reperfusion injury. *J. Am. Soc. Nephrol.* **2008**, *19*, 217–224. [CrossRef]

81. Chen, F.; Chen, L.; Qin, Q.; Sun, X. Salt-Inducible Kinase 2: An Oncogenic Signal Transmitter and Potential Target for Cancer Therapy. *Front. Oncol.* **2019**, *9*, 18. [CrossRef] [PubMed]

82. Patel, K.; Foretz, M.; Marion, A.; Campbell, D.G.; Gourlay, R.; Boudaba, N.; Tournier, E.; Titchenell, P.; Peggie, M.; Deak, M.; et al. The LKB1-salt-inducible kinase pathway functions as a key gluconeogenic suppressor in the liver. *Nat. Commun.* **2014**, *5*, 4535. [CrossRef] [PubMed]

83. Honda, T.; Fujiyama, T.; Miyoshi, C.; Ikkyu, A.; Hotta-Hirashima, N.; Kanno, S.; Mizuno, S.; Sugiyama, F.; Takahashi, S.; Funato, H.; et al. A single phosphorylation site of SIK3 regulates daily sleep amounts and sleep need in mice. *Proc. Natl. Acad. Sci. USA.* **2018**, *115*, 10458–10463. [CrossRef] [PubMed]

84. Igarashi, P. Kidney-specific gene targeting. *J. Am. Soc. Nephrol.* **2004**, *15*, 2237–2239. [CrossRef] [PubMed]

85. Klaeger, S.; Heinzlmeir, S.; Wilhelm, M.; Polzer, H.; Vick, B.; Koenig, P.A.; Reinecke, M.; Ruprecht, B.; Petzoldt, S.; Meng, C.; et al. The target landscape of clinical kinase drugs. *Science* **2017**, *358*. [CrossRef] [PubMed]

86. Sundberg, T.B.; Choi, H.G.; Song, J.H.; Russell, C.N.; Hussain, M.M.; Graham, D.B.; Khor, B.; Gagnon, J.; O'Connell, D.J.; Narayan, K.; et al. Small-molecule screening identifies inhibition of salt-inducible kinases as

a therapeutic strategy to enhance immunoregulatory functions of dendritic cells. *Proc. Natl. Acad. Sci. USA.* **2014**, *111*, 12468–12473. [CrossRef]

87. Heap, R.E.; Hope, A.G.; Pearson, L.A.; Reyskens, K.; McElroy, S.P.; Hastie, C.J.; Porter, D.W.; Arthur, J.S.C.; Gray, D.W.; Trost, M. Identifying Inhibitors of Inflammation: A Novel High-Throughput MALDI-TOF Screening Assay for Salt-Inducible Kinases (SIKs). *Slas. Discov.* **2017**, *22*, 1193–1202. [CrossRef] [PubMed]

13

Renal Benefits of SGLT 2 Inhibitors and GLP-1 Receptor Agonists: Evidence Supporting a Paradigm Shift in the Medical Management of Type 2 Diabetes

Vjera Ninčević [1,2], Tea Omanović Kolarić [1,2], Hrvoje Roguljić [1,3], Tomislav Kizivat [4,5], Martina Smolić [1,2] and Ines Bilić Ćurčić [1,6,*]

1 Department of Pharmacology, Faculty of Medicine, Josip Juraj Strossmayer University of Osijek, J. Huttlera 4, 31000 Osijek, Croatia; vnincevic@mefos.hr (V.N.); tomanovic@mefos.hr (T.O.K.); hrvoje.roguljic@mefos.hr (H.R.); martina.smolic@mefos.hr (M.S.)

2 Department of Pharmacology and Biochemistry, Faculty of Dental Medicine and Health, Josip Juraj Strossmayer University of Osijek, Crkvena 21, 31000 Osijek, Croatia

3 Department for Cardiovascular Disease, University Hospital Osijek, 4, 31000 Osijek, Croatia

4 Clinical Institute of Nuclear Medicine and Radiation Protection, University Hospital Osijek, 31000 Osijek, Croatia; tkizivat@mefos.hr

5 Department for Nuclear Medicine and Oncology, Faculty of Medicine, Josip Juraj Strossmayer University of Osijek; J. Huttlera 4, 31000 Osijek, Croatia

6 Department of Diabetes, Endocrinology and Metabolism Disorders, University Hospital Osijek, 31000 Osijek, Croatia

* Correspondence: ibcurcic@mefos.hr

Abstract: Diabetic nephropathy (DN) is one of the most perilous side effects of diabetes mellitus type 1 and type 2 (T1DM and T2DM).). It is known that sodium/glucose cotransporter 2 inhibitors (SGLT 2i) and glucagone like peptide-1 receptor agonists (GLP-1 RAs) have renoprotective effects, but the molecular mechanisms are still unknown. In clinical trials GLP-1 analogs exerted important impact on renal composite outcomes, primarily on macroalbuminuria, possibly through suppression of inflammation-related pathways, however enhancement of natriuresis and diuresis is also one of possible mechanisms of nephroprotection. Dapagliflozin, canagliflozin, and empagliflozin are SGLT2i drugs, useful in reducing hyperglycemia and in their potential renoprotective mechanisms, which include blood pressure control, body weight loss, intraglomerular pressure reduction, and a decrease in urinary proximal tubular injury biomarkers. In this review we have discussed the potential synergistic and/or additive effects of GLP 1 RA and SGLT2 inhibitors on the primary onset and progression of kidney disease, and the potential implications on current guidelines of diabetes type 2 management.

Keywords: diabetic nephropathy; diabetes mellitus; GLP-1 receptor agonists; SGLT2 inhibitors; molecular mechanisms

1. Introduction

Diabetic nephropathy (DN) is a complication of diabetes mellitus, both type I and II, caused by changes in microvasculature [1], and which can lead to end-stage renal disease and cardiovascular disease [2,3]. Moreover, it is the leading cause of chronic kidney disease, affecting 30–40% of patients with diabetes mellitus type 1 and 25–40% of patients with diabetes type 2 [4–7].

In its classic definition DN is defined as increased protein excretion in urine [8]. Major representations of diabetes in renal disease include persistent albuminuria, loss of podocytes, glomerular hypertrophy, matrix expansion, and thickening of the glomerular basement membrane [9,10]. The first stages of DN are characterized by microalbuminuria, a small increase in albumin excretion in urine [11–13]. Later stages are defined by macroalbuminuria or proteinuria leading to a decreased glomerular filtration rate [8].

Pathogenesis and progression of diabetic kidney disease are most likely a result of interactions between metabolic and hemodynamic changes which are caused by onset of diabetes [14], but also other factors including genetic predisposition [15], generation of reactive oxygen species (ROS) caused by hyperglycemia [14–16], and inflammation [17].

Studies have shown that diabetic kidney disease can lead to end stage renal disease in 30–40% of diabetes mellitus (DM) patients [18], implying that genetic variations could have impact on the start and progression of DM and the end stage renal disease. Genome-wide studies have been conducted to identify potential candidate genes of importance to DM and diabetic kidney disease [19]. More than fourteen genes have been identified as important to the development of diabetic kidney disease, among which are genes controlling lipid metabolism (*ADIPOQ*), glucose metabolism (*GCKR*), angiogenesis (*EPO promotor* gene), genes related to renal structure and function (*SHROOM3*), inflammation and oxidative stress related genes (*TGF-β1*), renin-angiotensin-aldosterone system related genes (*AGTR1*), and others [15]. Still, the complete effects of these genes and their variants are not completely clear. Results from these studies cannot be replicated among different races indicating race-specific gene polymorphisms or still significant environmental impacts.

Inflammation and chronic high levels of circulating glucose and its end metabolites are main causes of tissue damage in DM by, among other, creating high levels of oxidative and nitrosative stress in kidneys [20,21]. The effects of oxidative stress in other renal diseases like urolithiasis have been described [22]. High production of ROS and nitrosative species (NS) can cause damage to nuclear and mitochondrial DNA, induce apoptosis, and cause endoplasmic reticulum stress, and with this playing a role in cell death pathways such as apoptosis and necrosis in key cell types such as podocytes [20].

Considering the structural changes in diabetic kidney disease, they are similar in both DM1 and DM2, but are more heterogeneous and less predictable in association with clinical presentation in DM2 [23], probably because DM2 has unreliable onset timing, longer exposure to hyperglycemia before diagnosis, older patients, and patients that are treated with renin-angiotensin inhibitors before the onset of diabetes [24].

These structural alterations encompass modifications of several kidney departments. One of the first changes is thickening of the glomerular basal membrane, becoming apparent at 1.5 to 2 years from the diagnosis of DM, and which is closely followed by thickening of the capillary and tubular basement membrane [25–28]. Glomerular changes later include mesangial matrix expansion, loss of endothelial fenestrations, and loss of podocytes with effacement of foot processes [25]. The first signs of mesangial volume expansion are seen after 5–7 years of DM1 onset [27–30]. As DM progresses, segmental mesangiolysis appears and is considered to be connected with the development of micoaneurysms and Kimmelstal–Wilson nodules [31,32]. Subendothelial deposits of proteins forming periodic acid-Schiff-positive and electron-dense deposits accumulate in small arterioles, glomerular capillaries and microaneurysms result in exudative lesions and can cause luminal compromise [25]. Subepithelial deposits similar to subendothelial can be seen in Bowman's capsule and renal tubules. In the later stages of DM, glomerulopathy and interstitial changes grow together to segmental and global sclerosis [25]. Glomerular filtration, albuminuria, and hypertension in DM1 are strongly correlated with mesangial expansion, but to a less degree with glomerular basement membrane width [25].

2. GLP-1 Agonists in Diabetic Nephropathy

2.1. Classes of GLP-1 RA and Mechanism of Action

Glucagon-like peptide-1 (GLP-1) receptor agonists (RAs), an antidiabetic class of drugs, are known for their proven efficacy and safety profile [33]. They can be divided into human originated GLP-1

RAs, synthesized by various modifications of human GLP-1 active fragments, and agents derived from reptile Gila monster venom (exendin-4) [33,34]. Another classification of GLP-1 RAs is based on their pharmacokinetic profile, which divides these drugs into two different groups: short-acting (exenatide twice daily and lixisenatide) and long-acting agonists (once-weekly injected; dulaglutide, liraglutide, semaglutide, albiglutide) [33,34]. The half-lives of GLP-RAs vary between 2–3 h for short-acting agonists and 13 h to 7 days for long-acting agonists [33]. Up-to-date, above-mentioned 6 GLP-1 RAs have been approved for the treatment of patients with type 2 diabetes mellitus (T2DM), and all these drugs are administered by subcutaneous injection [33]. In general, GLP-1 RAs exert various beneficial effects in T2DM: enhancement of glucose-dependent insulin secretion, acceleration of β-cells proliferation and inhibition of β-cells apoptosis, inhibition of motility and gastric emptying, and a stimulation of the sensations of satiety and fullness by direct action on the central nervous system, with reduction in body weight [34–37]. Many other effects are still being investigated, among them reduction in systolic and diastolic blood pressure and improvements in lipid profile [33,38–42]. The main difference between the two groups is the fact that short-acting GLP-1 RAs while delaying gastric emptying, mostly lower postprandial plasma glucose, whereas the long-acting agonists predominantly exhibit insulinotropic and glucagonostatic actions, consequently exerting a much greater effect on fasting glucose concentrations. Various meta-analysis showed that long-acting agonists were more successful in lowering HbA_{1C} compering to short-acting agonists [33,41,43–47]. More specifically, these studies demonstrated that the largest reduction in HbA_{1c} values was associated with dulaglutide and exenatide once weekly, whereas the smallest mean reduction was observed with albiglutide [48]. The same results were observed when comparing the effects on the reduction of body weight [33]. The advantages of liraglutide in comparison with exenatide were: less frequent nausea and vomiting (shorter duration of GI side effects at the beginning of the therapy), more efficacy in lowering glycemic parameters, fasting glucose, and improving the homeostatic model assessment of β cells [34]. Generally, the most often side effects of GLP-1 RA therapy are gastrointestinal events (nausea, vomiting, diarrhea; shorter duration in short-acting agonists because of their lack of substantial effects on gastric emptying), and injection-site reactions (notable for albiglutide and lixisenatide), immunogenicity (exendin-4 derivates are more likely to be associated with the development of antidrug antibodies compared to GLP-1 RAs modified from human GLP-1) [33,49,50]. Nevertheless, these adverse events are rarely serious or persistent, nor the cause of discontinuation of therapy, especially because of the high efficiency of these drugs.

2.2. Potential Nephroprotective Actions of GLP-1 Agonists

Among all the above-mentioned therapeutic effects (lowering glucose, reducing body-weight etc.), GLP-1 RAs exert possible nephroprotective effects in T2DM, which have been demonstrated in various studies. Yin W et al. showed that GLP-1 RAs reduced albuminuria and ameliorated kidney tubules and tubulointerstitial lesions in the diabetic nephropathy rats model [51]. GLP-1 RAs downregulated the expression of tubulointerstitial tumor necrosis factor alpha (TNFα), monocyte chemoattractant protein-1(MCP-1), collagen I, alpha-smooth muscle actin (α-SMA), and fibronectin (FN) which are all reported to play a role in the diabetic nephropathy [51]. Additionally, the level of C-peptide, which was found to inhibit tubulointerstitial fibrosis [52], was increased by GLP-1 RAs and this may be one of the ways of improving tubuluinterstitial and tubular injury in GK rats with diabetic nephropathy [51]. In the study of Kodera et al. various beneficial effects of exendin-4 were showed, with emphasis on the prevention of macrophage infiltration, decrease of protein levels of intercellular adhesion moleculi-1 (ICAM-1) and type IV collagen in glomeruli, as well as the decrease of oxidative stress (downregulation of *Nox4* gene expression) and nuclear factor-kB (known for contributing to cross-talk between inflammation and oxidative stress) activation in kidney tissue [53]. Furthermore, liraglutide is capable of inhibiting NAD(P)H oxidase through generation of cAMP, followed by activation of PKA or Epac2 [54–57]. Hendarto et al. confirmed the role of liraglutide in the normalization of oxidative stress markers and expression of renal NAD(P)H oxidase components (Nox4, gp91phox, p22phox, p47phox) in diabetic rats, but independently of lowering plasma glucose levels [58]. Similar results were demonstrated in the mouse model of diabetic nephrophathy with the crucial role of liraglutide in protection against renal oxidative stress and lowering of fibronectin accumulation in glomerular capillary walls [59]. Molecular mechanisms included in these actions are inhibition of NAD(P)H oxidase and activation of cAMP-PKA pathway as already explained [59]. The in vitro beneficial effects of liraglutide were also showed in various studies. Zhao et al. proved that liraglutide enhances cell viability in HK-2 cells (human proximal tubular cells) by downregulating caspase-3 expression [37]. Furthermore, mRNA and protein expression of GLP-1R was significantly enhanced by liraglutide, whereas the expression of the autophagic markers LC3-II and Beclin1 was ameliorated [37]. All these effects were blocked by the GLP-1R antagonist exendin-(9–39) [37]. Additionally, another study on HK2 cells treated with GLP1 RAs showed decrease in the expression of profibrotic factors like fibronectin, α-SMA, collagen I, and TNFα [51]. In the same study GLP-1RAs inhibited the activity of NF-κB and p38MAPK (two significant signaling pathways for kidney fibrosis) via GLP-1R [51]. Various studies confirmed the role of GLP-1RAs in water and electrolyte balance. One of the suggested mechanisms for this effect is inhibition of intestinal sodium–hydrogen exchanger isoform 3 (NHE3) activity [60]. This NHE3 exchanger is located on the renal proximal tubule, and GLP-1RA, by inhibiting its activity, enhance natriuresis and diuresis [61]. Accordingly, when adding GLP-1R blocker exendin-9, a decrease in renal excretion of sodium and water is observed [62]. Furthermore, exendin-9 has been connected with slight decrease in glomerular filtration rate (GFR), although it would be expected to increase GFR by increasing proximal tubular reabsorption, followed by inhibition of tubuloglomerular feedback signals and reduction in afferent arteriolar resistance [62]. However, this implicates another possible positive effect of GLP-1RA on nephroprotection and water/sodium balance [62]. Glomerular hyperfiltration enhanced by GLP-1RAs increases filtration and in the end excretion of electrolytes [61]. Finally, all these studies, which show the beneficial effects of GLP-1RAs in diabetic glomerular, tubulointerstitial, and tubular nephropathy, implicate the possible clinical use of these agents in treatment of diabetic nephropathy.

2.3. *Assessment of Nephroprotective Effect of GLP-1 Receptor Agonists in Clinical Trials*

Recent clinical trials demonstrate notable evidence of glucagon-like peptide-1 (GLP-1) agonists exerting renal benefits.

Between June 2012 and August 2013 the LIRA–RENAL trial examined the efficacy and safety profile of liraglutide in diabetic patients with moderate renal impairment (defined as eGFR 30–59 mL/min/1.73 m^2) [63]. This double blinded, randomized, placebo-controlled trial included 279 patients with type 2 DM who had HbA1c in the range of 7% to 10%. Addition of liraglutide to background glucose-lowering therapy reduced HbA1c more than placebo treatment (−1.05% vs. −0.38%). During the trial no deterioration of renal function was observed in patients treated with liraglutide in comparison with placebo. Furthermore, albuminuria assessed as the urinary albumin-to-creatinine ratio showed lower increase at week 26 in patients treated with liraglutide, although it was not significantly.

A more extensive and longer study of liraglutide treatment effect on renal outcomes in patients with diabetic nephropathy was the Liraglutide Effect and Action in Diabetes: Evaluation of Cardiovascular Outcome Results (LEADER) trial [64]. The LEADER trial included 9340 patients with type 2 diabetes and a high risk of cardiovascular disease with a median follow-up of 3.84 years. 23.1% of the trial population had mean estimated GFR less than 59 mL per minute per 1.73 m^2; and furthermore, microalbuminuria and macroalbuminuria were present at the baseline (26.3% and 10.5%, respectively). The renal outcome showed a lower rate of occurrence in the liraglutide group in comparison with placebo (5.7% vs. 7.2%). That was primarily the result of lower incidence of new-onset persistent macroalbuminuria in patients treated with liraglutide (3.4% vs. 4.6%). During the follow-up the urinary albumin-to-creatinine ratio growth was slower in liraglutide group while decline of estimated GFR and the rates of renal adverse effects were similar between the two groups. Interestingly, the effect of liraglutide on composite renal outcomes showed no difference in prespecified subgroups of patients with an elevated baseline renal risk, suggesting effectiveness of the liraglutide renal benefit to be an independent factor of stage of chronic kidney disease.

While the LEADER trial included patients with macroalbuminuria from the baseline to the onset of sustained albuminuria in the endpoint, the Evaluation of Lixisenatide in Acute Coronary Syndrome (ELIXA) trial assessed renal outcomes in patients only with normoalbuminuria or microalbuminuria [65]. This randomized, double blinded study primarily examined the effect on cardiovascular outcomes of short-acting GLP1 agonist lixisenatide in 6068 patients with type 2 diabetes and a recent acute coronary syndrome. Beside cardiovascular safety, the addition of lixisenatide to standard therapy showed beneficial impact on renal outcomes. The renoprotective effect manifested as lower rate of increase in urinary albumin-to-creatinine ratio, 34% in the placebo group vs. 24% in lixisenatide group. No significant difference was observed between the two groups in eGFR decline or doubling of serum creatinine, while overall incidence of renal adverse effects was low in both groups. Evidently the difference in pharmacokinetics of GLP-1 analogs, short-acting versus long-acting analogs, has no impact on renal composite outcomes. Somewhat different results were obtained in AWARD-7 study which examined the effect of long acting GLP-1 analog dulaglutide versus insulin glargine on renal outcomes in patients with diabetes type 2 and moderate-to-severe CKD [66]. 577 participants were randomized in three groups, dulaglutide 1.5 mg or 0.75 mg treated groups and insulin glargine group. The decline of eGFR after 52 weeks of treatment with dulaglutide was significantly smaller in dulaglutide treated patients compared to insulin group. The albuminuria decrease was similar between all treatment groups, with a slightly greater decrease of urinary albumin-to-creatinine ratio in dulaglutide treated patients. Although dulaglutide enhanced body loss, whether fat or muscle tissue, the study confirmed the beneficial renal effect of GLP-1 analog as an independent action. In the Trial to Evaluate Cardiovascular and other Long-term Outcomes with Semaglutide in Subjects with Type 2 Diabetes (SUSTAIN-6), the rate of persistent macroalbuminuria was lower in patients receiving semaglutide, than in those receiving placebo [67].

Taken together, GLP-1 analogs as antidiabetic medications show significant influence on renal composite outcomes, primarily on a new onset of macroalbuminuria as shown in Table 1. Numerous previous studies characterized development of albuminuria as an independent predictor of diabetic nephropathy progression with subsequent deterioration of estimated glomerular filtration and development of end stage renal disease [68–70]. Definitely, more intensive glycemic control achieved by addition of GLP-1 agonist to background antidiabetic therapy justifies a decrease of macroalbuminuria incidence in diabetic patients due to a well-known effect of serum high glucose concentration on increased filtration rate of proteins via glomerular capillary membrane and on impaired tubular reabsorption [71]. Another possible mechanism of GLP-1 beneficial renal effect could be suppression of inflammation-related pathways. Preclinical studies have unambiguously demonstrated anti-inflammatory and antioxidative effect of GLP-1 analogs [59,72]. This was also suggested during the LIRA-RENAL trial when lower concentration of inflammation marker hsCRP was obtained in liraglutid treated group in comparison with placebo [63]. Although the mechanism of beneficial renal effect of GLP-1 agonists still remains elusive, it is definitely achieved as a combined effect through glucose lowering treatment and extra-glycemic effects.

Table 1. The pharmacokinetic properties and renal outcomes of clinical trials with GLP-1 receptor agonists.

Drug.	Dose	Half Life (h)	Elimination	Clinical Study	Renal Benefit
Short-acting GLP-1 receptor agonists					
Exenatide	5–10 µg twice-daily s.c.	2.4	Mostly renal	/	/
Lixisenatide	10–20 µg once-daily s.c.	3.0	Mostly renal	ELIXA [65]	Lower rate of increase in urinary albumin-to-creatinine ratio
Long-acting GLP-1 receptor agonists					
Exenatide	2 mg QW s.c.	2.4	Mostly renal		
Liraglutide	0.6 mg, 1.2 mg or 1.8 mg once-daily s.c.	11.6–13.0	Peptidases and renal 6%; feces 5%	LEADER [64]	↓Nephropathy, ↓UACR, ↓RAS hormone, ↓Progression to macroalbuminuria, ↓Doubling of serum creatinine levels, ↓eGFR of ≤45 mL/min per 1.73 m^2, ↓The initiation of renal-replacement therapy, ↓Risk of end-stage renal disease or renal death, ↓Plasma renin concentration, renin activity, angiotensin II
Semaglutide	0.5–1.0 mg once-weekly s.c.	165.0–184.0	Peptidases and renal	SUSTAIN-6 [67]	↓Nephropathy >35%, ↓Progression to macroalbuminuria, ↓Doubling of serum creatinine levels, ↓eGFR of ≤45 mL/min per 1.73 m^2, ↓The initiation of renal-replacement therapy
Dulaglutide	0.75–1.5 mg once-weekly s.c.	~112.8	Peptidases and renal	AWARD VII [66]	Reduced albuminuria, slower decline in renal function
Albiglutide	30–50 mg once-weekly s.c.	~120.0	Peptidases and renal	/	/

Abbrevations: s.c., subcutaneous injection; eGFR, estimated glomerular filtration rate in mL/min/1.73m^2; UACR, urine albumin/creatinine ratio; RAS, renin-angiotensin system; CVR, cardiovascular risk, ↓ decline.

3. SGLT2 Inhibitors in Diabetic Nephropathy

3.1. Mechanism of Action

Sodium/glucose cotransporter 2 (SGLT2) inhibitors are orally administrated hypoglycemic drugs with a novel mechanism of action that is useful across a continuum of diabetes regardless of duration of diabetes, baseline Hba1c or concomitant antidiabetic therapy [73,74]. Glucose reabsorbtion takes place in the proximal tubule via the sodium dependent glucose transporters (SGLT), placed on the apical side of the proximal tubule cell through the basolateral Na, K-ATPase pump [75,76]. SGLT2 is expressed almost entirely in the renal proximal tubules, hence selective inhibition of this protein leads to renal glucose excretion and reduction of plasma glucose levels without influencing other metabolic processes [77]. Sodium glucose cotransporter 2 (SGLT2) is the main luminal glucose transporter placed in the S1 and S2 portions of the proximal tubule (PT) while sodium glucose cotransporter 1 (SGLT1) is placed in the S3 portion and supply fewer than 10% of entire luminal glucose transport [78]. SGLT2 on the apical membrane is connected with GLUT2 on the basolateral part and jointly they reabsorb up to 90% of filtered glucose beneath normoglycaemic conditions [79]. Increased renin angiotensin system (RAS) activity with SGLT2 inhibition is explained by the normal volume depletion with this kind of therapy [80], although a tendency for diminished GFR with SGLT2 inhibition is probably due to enlarged afferent tone over tubuloglomerular feedback [81]. Furthermore, maximal renoprotection from glomerular injury, renal fibrosis, and proteinuria was achieved when luseogliflozin (SGLT2 inhibitor) was combined with the ACE inhibitor, lisinopril [82]. At the early stage of kidney impairment, therapies that prevent the RAS activity are as well indicated, but these approaches are not completely beneficial [83]. One of the possible mechanisms of SGLT2 inhibitors is prevention of glucose influx to the kidney proximal tubular cell responsible for development of diabetic nephropathy [84–86]. Histological variation detected in the glomerulus is the traditional focal point in diabetic nephropathy, but it has become extensively recognized that the changes detected in tubulointerstitial fibrosis and in the tubulointerstitium correspond more firmly with impairment in renal function [79]. Dapagliflozin, canagliflozin, and empagliflozin are SGLT2i drugs, useful in reducing hyperglycemia and improvement of glycemic control. They are used in mild renal impairment and have combined beneficial effects such as the lowering of body weight and blood pressure (BP) [73]. The pharmacokinetic properties of SGLT2 inhibitors demonstrate an excellent oral bioavailability, a rather long elimination half-life permitting once daily administration, a short accumulation index, no active metabolites and restricted renal excretion [87]. Moreover, these drugs share an insignificant risk of drug–drug interactions [88]. The risk for hypoglycemia is low because inhibition of SGLT2 does not increase the excretion of insulin or impede with gluconeogenesis. Additionally, there are some indications that SGLT2 inhibition improves beta cell function, perhaps by reducing glucotoxicity [89,90]. Loss of excess calories mediated by glucose excretion in urine results in weight loss and can alleviate the weight gain induced by another classes of hypoglycemic agents. In patients with hypertension SGLT2 inhibitors lower blood pressure as well, probably due to glucosuria, subsequent natriuresis, and diuresis [91]. Absorption of dapagliflozin after oral administration is fast, reaching peak plasma concentrations in 1–2 h it. The main organs included in the metabolism of this drug are the liver and kidneys, where inactive metabolites are produced by enzyme uridine diphosphate-glucuronosyltransferase-1A9 (UGT1A9). Clearance of dapagliflozin by renal excretion is not significant, and there are no drug–drug interactions [88]. Dapagliflozin is capable of reducing body weight and fat mass, improving glycemic control and lowering blood pressure [92,93]. Following the treatment of T2DM with 5 or 10 mg dapagliflozin, a higher risk of mild to moderate urinary tract infections was observed, but without a final dose correlatin among UTI and glucosuria [94].Pharmacokinetic properties of canagliflozin include immediate absorption after oral administration, 65% oral bioavailability within a dose range of 50–300 mg, and in dose-dependent manner, high potential as 99% is bounded to plasma proteins, especially albumin, and finally it is metabolized generally to inactive metabolites [88,95]. As opposed to other SGLT2i, canagliflozin is also capable of minor inhibition of SGLT1. Canagliflozin postpones intestinal glucose absorption in addition to increasing UGE, followed by lowering of postprandial glucose and insulin levels [96]. Canagliflozin treatment is also associated with an UTI and symptomatic vulvovaginal adverse events in female patients with T2DM [97]. Empagliflozin is quickly absorbed in single oral doses achieving Cmax after 1.0–2.0 h. Drug-drug interactions among empagliflozin and other oral glucose lowering agents, cardiovascular medications or various other drugs with narrow therapeutic index were not observed [88,98]. In a fasting and postprandial state in T2DM patients, following administration of empagliflozin or dapagliflozin, paradoxical increase in endogenous glucose production was demonstrated [99]. Nevertheless, plasma glucose levels in these patients were reduced by empagliflozin [98]. Ferrannini et al. showed moderate association of a 10 and 25 mg empagliflozin dose and increased incidence of genital infections, but without increase in UTIs incidence [100]. The capacity of SGLT2i to decrease the plasma glucose levels is directly proportional to the glomerular filtration rate (GFR) and is reduced in chronic kidney disease (CKD). Nevertheless, research underway indicates that SGLT2i can contribute to nephroprotection in diabetes independently of glycemic control [73,101–103].

3.2. Evidence of Nephroprotection In Vitro and in Animal Models

Cultured human proximal renal tubular cells of patients with type 2 diabetes demonstrate noticeably enlarged levels of SGLT2 mRNA and protein and increased glucose transporter activity [104]. Several experiments using human proximal tubular cells (HK2) showed that SGLT2 inhibition reduced the output of inflammatory and fibrotic markers induced by high glucose levels [73]. The above-mentioned in vitro findings suggest that SGLT2 inhibitors can provide nephroprotection in diabetes by blocking glucose influx to proximal tubule cells [105]. In new preclinical trials, nephroprotection with SGLT2 inhibition has been observed after improvement of glycemic control [82,105–109].

Accordingly, the effect of SGLT2 inhibition on early kidney growth, inflammation, and fibrosis was proposed to result from blood glucose lowering [109]. Thus, blood glucose lowering effect could be responsible for SGLT2i inhibition of inflammation, fibrosis and early renal growth [105]. This hypothesis is supported by several recently published studies conducted in animal models. Inhibition of progression of albuminuria along with drop in plasma glucose by <15 mmol/L was observed in male db/db mice treated with dapagliflozin [107] and females treated with tofogliflozin [109]. Furthermore, Lin et al. showed decrease in albuminuria and glomerulosclerosis followed by improvement of hyperglycemia in male db/db mice treated with empagliflozin [108]. Vallon et al. demonstrated reduction of albuminuria, kidney hypertrophy, and markers of inflammation, proportional to glucose lowering effect in the T1DM model of male Akita mice treated with empagliflozin [105]. The effect of SGLT2 inhibition on diabetic nephropathy, autonomous of blood glucose decrease, was investigated in diabetic eNOS knockout mice [110], while further studies in fat Zucker rats have demonstrated that diabetes enhanced RNA expression of SGLT2 and SGLT1 within the kidney [111]. In addition, proximal tubular cells exposed to the urine of diabetic patients have shown an increase in SGLT2 expression [104]. Diversity of agents have been related to the modification in expression of SGLT1 and 2, including HNF1α and SGK1 [76]. Furthermore, exposure of proximal tubular cells to transforming growth factor β (TGFβ), a profibrotic cytokine, led to upregulation of SGLT2 expression [66].

Interleukin-6 (IL-6) and tumor necrosis factor-α (TNF-α) increased SGLT2 expression in cultured kidney cell lines after exposure for 96–120 h [112], while increase in SGLT2 expression has also been achieved through high glucose-induced pathway exceeding protein kinase A (PKA) and protein kinase C (PKC) reliant pathways [113,114]. Some studies have also shown interaction among the sodium glucose cotransporters and the renin–angiotensin–aldosterone model. For example, losartan decreased SGLT2 expression in diabetic rats in regular or high salt nutrition in animal models [115]. In diabetic rats, enhancement of GLUT2 expression and its translocation to the luminal surface of the proximal tubular cells was observed leading to an increase in glucose reabsorption [78]. One of the potential mechanisms involved in nephroprotection could be linked with a decrease in GLUT 9 expression, a major regulator of urate homeostasis [116–118]. The expression of certain profibrotic genes is diminished with empagliflozin, in line with the effects of first line anti-diabetic agent, metformin in diabetic rat model. Gallo at al. presented that a threshold of blood glucose lowering can be necessary to accomplished complete renoprotection in diabetes, since empagliflozin influenced some markers of fibrosis but had no effect on albuminuria and glomerular sclerosis. So, Gallo et al. suggested that adequate, and stable blood glucose lowering, perhaps with multiple medications, including higher- and/or multiple daily-dosing of SGLT2 inhibition in combination with a RAS blockade, can be necessary to accomplished maximal nephroprotection in diabetes [83].

3.3. Assessment of Nephroprotective Effect of SGLT 2 Inhibitors in Clinical Trials

Presently, short-term studies are available assuring of renal safety with SGLT2i drugs, however there are no long-term data confirming renal benefit [118] SGLT2i decreases albuminuria, the most important renal risk marker in DN [119]. The albuminuria-lowering effects of SGLT2i have been shown in various studies [120,121] but the precise mechanism is still not clear, and it seems to be independent of alterations in eGFR, systolic BP, body weight, or HbA1c [121]. A placebo-controlled study has demonstrated that canagliflozin 100 mg/day diminished albuminuria around 22% [120], likewise empagliflozin 25 mg/day decreased albuminuria roughly 35% relative to placebo in patients with chronic kidney disease and diabetes mellitus type 2 RAS-based drugs such as ACEi or ARBs, and SGLT2i could have complementary but different mechanisms of action, with diverse outcomes to the kidney system and a potential synergistic effect. In a recently published study, the combination of SGLT2i and RAS blockers was associated with additive nephroprotective effect in diabetic nephropathy compared to either medicament alone [106]. Heerspink et al. showed reduction of albuminuria with dapagliflozin 10 mg/day, compared to placebo in patients with hypertension and diabetes already treated with RAS blockers [121].

Decrease of uric acid in serum is another way where SGLT2i may achieve their nephroprotective effect. Elevated levels of uric acid or hyperuricemia, have been demonstrated to hugely correlate with the possibility of renal impairment in diabetes [122–124], and are responsible for microvascular complications in diabetes [125,126]. The beneficial effect of uric acid reduction in serum with SGLT2i can be clinically significant and has been shown in several studies [127–129]. The EMPA-REG outcome study has shown that empagliflozin therapy was associated with improvement in all renal function parameters in patients with estimated glomerular filtration rate of at least 30 mL per minute. Empagliflozin significantly decreased worsening or incident nephropathy, request for renal transplantation or dialysis and doubling of serum creatinine levels compared to placebo, while further analysis showed reduction in albuminuria [67].

In the DECLARE trial there was a 24% reduction with dapagliflozin in a composite renal outcome of a ≥40% decrease in estimated glomerular filtration rate (eGFR) (to <60 mL/min/1.73 m^2), end-stage renal disease (ESRD), or death from renal or CV causes compared with placebo [130]. Included patients had eGFR of at least 60 mL/min at baseline, emphasizing the potential role of dapagliflozin not only in treatment but in the prevention of diabetic nephropathy [131,132]. The CANVAS trial showed a 27% reduction in progression of albuminuria, with a 40% reduction in eGFR, need for renal-replacement therapy, or death from renal causes associated with the use of canagliflozin [131]. The CREDENCE study was the first large-scale outcome trial of an SGLT2 inhibitor canagliflozin with primary kidney outcome defined as doubling of serum creatinine, end-stage kidney disease, or death due to cardiovascular or kidney disease. Almost all patients included in the CREDENCE trial (99%) were treated with ACE inhibitors or ARBs compared to other trials (80%) [133], and had eGFR of 30 to <90 mL per minute as shown in Table 2. The trial was stopped early after a planned interim analysis based on positive results since the relative risk of the renal-specific composite outcome was lower by 34% and the relative risk of end-stage kidney disease was lower by 32%. These data demonstrate that renoprotection was accomplished via the whole spectrum of eGFR levels once again establishing nephroprotecitve effect irrispective of baseline kidney function. The nephroprotective effects of SGLT2i could also benefit cardiovascular outcomes by triggering neurohormonal activation and volume wasting [134,135]. Recent meta-analysis demonstrated that SGLT2 inhibitors reduced the risk of dialysis, transplantation, or death due to kidney disease in individuals with type 2 diabetes and provided protection against acute kidney injury, adding additional evidence endorsing SGLT2i therapy as a corner stone of nephroprotection in diabetics [133]. SGLT2i are not presently recommended in patients with an eGFR lower than 45 mL/min per 1.73 m^2, to a large degree because of deficient glycemic effectiveness [136,137]. Proof of renoprotection from the above mentioned trials, due to these limitations, is questionable [138].

Table 2. The pharmacokinetic properties and renal outcomes of clinical trials with SGLT2i.

Drug	Dose (mg)	Half Life (h)	Administration	Clinical Study/Outcome	Renal Benefit
Empagliflozin	10	11.9	Per os, once daily	EMPA-REG OUTCOME [67]/incident or worsening nephropathy and incident albuminuria	↓Nephropathy 39%, ↓Progression to macroalbuminuria, ↓Doubling of serum creatinine levels, ↓the initiation of renal-replacement therapy
Dapagliflozin	10	12.9	Per os, once daily	DECLARE [137]/beneficial effects defined by eGFR status and the attendance or absence of Atherosclerotic cardiovascular illness at baseline	↓eGFR of 40% or more to an eGFR of fewer than 60 mL/min per 1.73 m^2, ↓Combined risk of end-stage renal disease or renal death, ↓Early prevention and decrease in progression of chronic renal disease in patients with T2DM, 31% reduction in the risk of acute renal injury in the dapagliflozin group compared to placebo group
Canagliflozin	100	over 12	Per os, once daily	CANVAS [67,133]/incident albuminuria, incident of renal failure	↓acute ↓acute kidney injury ↓albuminuria ↓eGFR of 40% ↓the initiation of renal-replacementtherapy ↓death from renal causes kidney injury ↓albuminuria ↓eGFR of 40% ↓the initiation of renal-replacementtherapy ↓death from renal causes
				CREDENCE * [133]/patients with established CKD, incident albuminuria, composite of dialysis, transplantation or death due to renal disease	↓Acute kidney injury, Albuminuria, ↓eGFR of 40%, ↓The initiation of renal-replacement therapy, ↓Death from renal causes in acute kidney injury, ↓Doubling of serum creatinine levels ↓Risk of dialysis and transplantation, ↓Risk of end-stage renal, disease or renal death

Abbreviations: eGFR, estimated glomerular filtration rate in mL/min/1.73m^2, * fewer than 60 mL/min per 1.73m^2, * use of RASi was obligatory to entry into the CREDENCE trial; DKD, diabetic kidney disease, ↓ decline.

4. Implications of Potential Synergism of GLP 1 RA and SGLT2 Inhibitors on Prevention of Kidney Disease

Although glycemic control along with blood pressure control and blockade of renin–angiotensin–aldosterone system represents a cornerstone of the prevention of new-onset diabetic nephropathy, 30% of diabetic patients will develop significant renal insufficiency [102,139]. Therefore, novel therapeutic measures as well as diabetic polytherapy are a necessity in prevention and treatment of diabetes mellitus associated complications. Recent studies clearly demonstrate the renoprotective effects of GLP-1 receptor agonists primarily achieved through reduction of new onset microalbuminuria [140]. Although the molecular mechanisms of these beneficial effects are not fully clarified some of renal effects of these drugs have been emphasized. GLP1 receptors present in multiple renal cells are responsible for increased glomerular filtration rate, vasodilatation of the afferent arteriole, and enhanced natriuresis [62]. The state of hyperglycaemia causes enhanced reabsorption of Na+ in proximal tubule and reduced delivery of Na+ to the macula densa with consequent vasodilatation of afferent arteriole, glomerular hypertension, and hyperfiltration [4,141]. Both GLP 1 receptor agonists and SGLT2I promote natriuresis within the proximal tubule acting at different sites. Inhibition of SGLT2 co-transporter beside enhanced glucosuria results in increased natiuresis while GLP-1 receptor agonists promote natriuresis through inhibition of NHE3 (sodium hydrogen exchanger-3) transporter in proximale tubule. Increased delivery of Na+ to macula densa due to inhibition of SGLT2 triggers tubuloglomerlar feedback resulting in afferent vasoconstriction, reduced glomerular pressure and a 30–50% decrease in albuminuria [142]. Despite the natriuretic effect, mechanistic studies and clinical trials failed to exhibit renal hemodynamic vasoconstriction in response to GLP-1 RA treatment resulting in overall neutral GFR effect. However, GLP-1 RA treatment of diabetic patients undoubtedly reduces albuminuria probably due to suppression of inflammation-related pathways [139]. Combination of these antihyperglycemic agents characterizes complementary physiological effect on natriuresis while albuminuria reduction is achieved by different mechanisms. Taken together, potential synergistic and/or additive effects of SGLT2I and GLP-1 receptor agonists at renal function implicate direct beneficial impact on progression of diabetic kidney disease (Figure 1.). In addition, renal benefits could be achieved through common extrarenal effects such as weight reduction and lowering of blood pressure. However, to determine whether a synergistic or additive effect is in question, or perhaps a combination of the two, further studies in vitro and in vivo are needed comparing renal molecular mechanisms and clinical outcomes of combined therapy to each monocomponent separately.

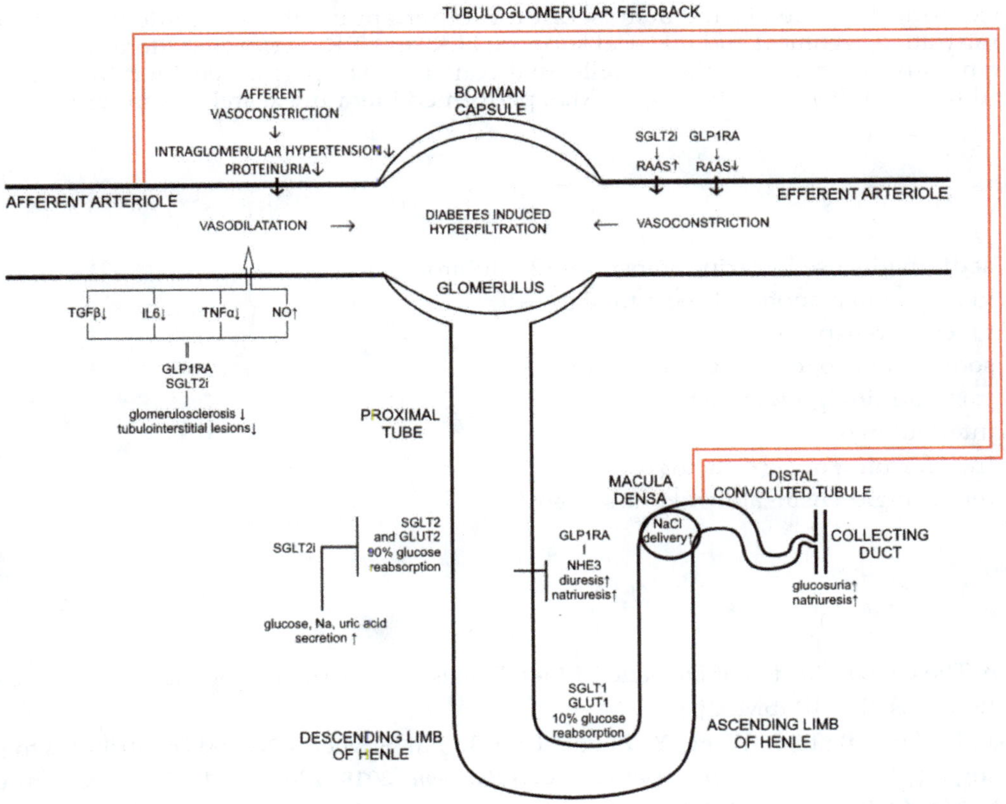

Figure 1. Mechanism of action of SGLT2i and GLP 1RA on kidney. SGLT2i inhibit glucose and sodium transport via SGLT2 and GLUT 2 transporters which are responsible for 90% of glucose reabsorption thus inducing glucosuria, diuresis, natriuresis, and uric acid excretion. At the same time GLP 1RA via NHE3 are also promoting diuresis and natriuresis. Influx of sodium to macula densa is increased thus affecting afferent vasoconstriction causing reduction in intraglomerular pressure and proteinuria through tubuloglomerular feedback. Both, GLP 1RA and SGLT2i induce suppression of inflammatory markers such as TGFβ, IL6, TNFα, decreasing glomerusclerosis and tubulointerstitial lesions and causing afferent vasoconstriction (induction of NO is also involved). GLP 1RA therapy leads to a decrease in RAAS activity causing efferent vasodilatation, while the effect of SGLT2i is quite the opposite, it increases RAAS activity due to natriuresis and volume depletion implying that positive effect on intraglomerular pressure is mediated completely through tubuloglomerular feedback; ↑ increase; ↓ decrease.

5. Conclusions

Both GLP 1 RA and SGLT2i may exhibit direct renoprotective effects through the suppression of inflammatory responses, inhibition of oxidative injury, and prevention of apoptosis as a result of the combined impact of glucose lowering treatment and extra-glycemic effects. Definitely, more intensive glycemic control achieved by addition of GLP-1 agonist and SGLT2i to background antidiabetic therapy justifies a potential benefit on renal function in diabetic patients, however it is obvious that other renoprotective mechanisms exist such as hemodynamic effects, blood pressure control, and body weight loss. Recently, based on the evidence from the trials mentioned above, new European Society of Cardiology (ESC) guidelines in association with European Association for the Study of Diabetes (EASD) position these drugs as the first therapy of choice in patients with diabetes and high cardiovascular risk overthrowing the long-standing paradigm of metformin as the first line therapy in DMT2 [143]. Given the importance of cardiovascular and renal risk reduction in diabetic patients achieved with those therapeutic options, it is only a matter of time before these two classes of drugs will become the gold standard in the treatment of type 2 diabetes.

Author Contributions: V.N. and T.O.K. conceived of and designed the article, and critically revised the manuscript; I.B.Ć. performed critical revision of the manuscript for important intellectual content, obtained funding, and provided administrative, technical and material support; H.R. and T.K. performed literature searches and critical revision of the manuscript for important intellectual content; M.S. performed literature searches, wrote the manuscript, and updated the text of the paper; M.S. performed literature searches and wrote the manuscript.

Abbreviations

SGLT2i	sodium glucose lowering transporter2 inhibitors
GLP1 RA	glucagon like peptide 1 receptor agonist
GLUT 2	glucose transporter 2
NHE3	sodium-hydrogen exchanger isoform 3
TGFβ	transforming growth factor β
IL6	interleukin 6
TNFα	transforming nuclear factor α
RAAS	renin–angiotensin–aldosterone system

References

1. Thomas, B. The Global Burden of Diabetic Kidney Disease: Time Trends and Gender Gaps. *Curr. Diabet. Rep.* **2019**, *19*, 18. [CrossRef] [PubMed]
2. Zha, F.; Bai, L.; Tang, B.; Li, J.; Wang, Y.; Zheng, P.; Ji, T.; Bai, S. MicroRNA-503 contributes to podocyte injury via targeting E2F3 in diabetic nephropathy. *J. Cell Biochem.* **2019**, *120*, 12574–12581. [CrossRef] [PubMed]
3. Murea, M.; Ma, L.; Freedman, B.I. Genetic and environmental factors associated with type 2 diabetes and diabetic vascular complications. *Rev. Diabet. Stud.* **2012**, *9*, 6–22. [CrossRef] [PubMed]
4. Abbiss, H.; Maker, G.L.; Trengove, R.D. Metabolomics Approaches for the Diagnosis and Understanding of Kidney Diseases. *Metabolites* **2019**, *9*, 34. [CrossRef] [PubMed]
5. Gross, J.L.; de Azevedo, M.J.; Silveiro, S.P.; Canani, L.H.; Caramori, M.L.; Zelmanovitz, T. Diabetic nephropathy: Diagnosis, prevention, and treatment. *Diabetes Care* **2005**, *28*, 164–176. [CrossRef] [PubMed]
6. Parving, H.H.; Lehnert, H.; Bröchner-Mortensen, J.; Gomis, R.; Andersen, S.; Arner, P. Irbesartan in Patients with Type 2 Diabetes and Microalbuminuria Study Group. The effect of irbesartan on the development of diabetic nephropathy in patients with type 2 diabetes. *N. Engl. J. Med.* **2001**, *345*, 870–878. [CrossRef]
7. Van der Kloet, F.M.; Tempels, F.W.; Ismail, N.; van der Heijden, R.; Kasper, P.T.; Rojas-Cherto, M.; van Doorn, R.; Spijksma, G.; Koek, M.; van der Greef, J.; et al. Discovery of early-stage biomarkers for diabetic kidney disease using ms-based metabolomics (FinnDiane study). *Metabolomics* **2012**, *8*, 109–119. [CrossRef]
8. Zelmanovitz, T.; Gerchman, F.; Balthazar, A.P.; Thomazelli, F.C.; Matos, J.D.; Canani, L.H. Diabetic nephropathy. *Diabet. Metab. Syndr.* **2009**, *1*, 10. [CrossRef]
9. Yoon, J.J.; Park, J.H.; Kim, H.J.; Jin, H.G.; Kim, H.Y.; Ahn, Y.M.; Kim, Y.C.; Lee, H.S.; Lee, Y.J.; Kang, D.G. Improves Glomerular Fibrosis and Renal Dysfunction in Diabetic Nephropathy Model. *Nutrients* **2019**, *11*, 553. [CrossRef]
10. Declèves, A.E.; Sharma, K. New pharmacological treatments for improving renal outcomes in diabetes. *Nat. Rev. Nephrol* **2010**, *6*, 371–380. [CrossRef]
11. Mogensen, C.E.; Christensen, C.K. Predicting diabetic nephropathy in insulin-dependent patients. *N. Engl. J. Med.* **1984**, *311*, 89–93. [CrossRef] [PubMed]
12. Parving, H.H.; Oxenbøll, B.; Svendsen, P.A.; Christiansen, J.S.; Andersen, A.R. Early detection of patients at risk of developing diabetic nephropathy. A longitudinal study of urinary albumin excretion. *Acta Endocrinol. (Copenh)* **1982**, *100*, 550–555. [CrossRef] [PubMed]
13. Viberti, G.C.; Hill, R.D.; Jarrett, R.J.; Argyropoulos, A.; Mahmud, U.; Keen, H. Microalbuminuria as a predictor of clinical nephropathy in insulin-dependent diabetes mellitus. *Lancet* **1982**, *1*, 1430–1432. [CrossRef]
14. Cao, Z.; Cooper, M.E. Pathogenesis of diabetic nephropathy. *J. Diabet. Investig.* **2011**, *2*, 243–247. [CrossRef] [PubMed]
15. Wei, L.; Xiao, Y.; Li, L.; Xiong, X.; Han, Y.; Zhu, X.; Sun, L. The Susceptibility Genes in Diabetic Nephropathy. *Kidney Dis. (Basel)* **2018** *4*, 226–237. [CrossRef] [PubMed]

16. Mahmoodnia, L.; Aghadavod, E.; Beigrezaei, S.; Rafieian-Kopaei, M. An update on diabetic kidney disease, oxidative stress and antioxidant agents. *J. Renal. Inj. Prev.* **2017**, *6*, 153–157. [CrossRef] [PubMed]
17. Pichler, R.; Afkarian, M.; Dieter, B.P.; Tuttle, K.R. Immunity and inflammation in diabetic kidney disease: Translating mechanisms to biomarkers and treatment targets. *Am. J. Physiol. Ren. Physiol.* **2017**, *312*, F716–F731. [CrossRef]
18. Hill, C.J.; Cardwell, C.R.; Patterson, C.C.; Maxwell, A.P.; Magee, G.M.; Young, R.J.; Matthews, B.; O'Donoghue, D.J.; Fogarty, D.G. Chronic kidney disease and diabetes in the national health service: A cross-sectional survey of the U.K. national diabetes audit. *Diabet. Med.* **2014**, *31*, 448–454. [CrossRef]
19. McDonough, C.W.; Palmer, N.D.; Hicks, P.J.; Roh, B.H.; An, S.S.; Cooke, J.N.; Hester, J.M.; Wing, M.R.; Bostrom, M.A.; Rudock, M.E.; et al. A genome-wide association study for diabetic nephropathy genes in African Americans. *Kidney Int.* **2011**, *79*, 563–572. [CrossRef]
20. Lindblom, R.; Higgins, G.; Coughlan, M.; de Haan, J.B. Targeting Mitochondria and Reactive Oxygen Species-Driven Pathogenesis in Diabetic Nephropathy. *Rev. Diabet. Stud.* **2015**, *12*, 134–156. [CrossRef]
21. Mittal, M.; Siddiqui, M.R.; Tran, K.; Reddy, S.P.; Malik, A.B. Reactive oxygen species in inflammation and tissue injury. *Antioxid. Redox Signal.* **2014**, *20*, 1126–1167. [CrossRef] [PubMed]
22. Kizivat, T.; Smolić, M.; Marić, I.; Tolušić Levak, M.; Smolić, R.; Bilić Čurčić, I.; Kuna, L.; Mihaljević, I.; Včev, A.; Tucak-Zorić, S. Antioxidant Pre-Treatment Reduces the Toxic Effects of Oxalate on Renal Epithelial Cells in a Cell Culture Model of Urolithiasis. *Int. J. Environ. Res. Public Health* **2017**, *14*, 109. [CrossRef] [PubMed]
23. Fioretto, P.; Caramori, M.L.; Mauer, M. The kidney in diabetes: Dynamic pathways of injury and repair. The Camillo Golgi Lecture 2007. *Diabetologia* **2008**, *51*, 1347–1355. [CrossRef] [PubMed]
24. Tervaert, T.W.; Mooyaart, A.L.; Amann, K.; Cohen, A.H.; Cook, H.T.; Drachenberg, C.B.; Ferrario, F.; Fogo, A.B.; Haas, M.; de Heer, E.; et al. Pathologic classification of diabetic nephropathy. *J. Am. Soc. Nephrol.* **2010**, *21*, 556–563. [CrossRef] [PubMed]
25. Alicic, R.Z.; Rooney, M.T.; Tuttle, K.R. Diabetic Kidney Disease: Challenges, Progress, and Possibilities. *Clin. J. Am. Soc. Nephrol.* **2017**, *12*, 2032–2045. [CrossRef] [PubMed]
26. Tyagi, I.; Agrawal, U.; Amitabh, V.; Jain, A.K.; Saxena, S. Thickness of glomerular and tubular basement membranes in preclinical and clinical stages of diabetic nephropathy. *Indian J. Nephrol.* **2008**, *18*, 64–69. [CrossRef]
27. Fioretto, P.; Mauer, M. Histopathology of diabetic nephropathy. *Semin. Nephrol.* **2007**, *27*, 195–207. [CrossRef]
28. Caramori, M.L.; Parks, A.; Mauer, M. Renal lesions predict progression of diabetic nephropathy in type 1 diabetes. *J. Am. Soc. Nephrol.* **2013**, *24*, 1175–1181. [CrossRef]
29. Drummond, K.; Mauer, M.; Group, I.D.N.S. The early natural history of nephropathy in type 1 diabetes: II. Early renal structural changes in type 1 diabetes. *Diabetes* **2002**, *51*, 1580–1587. [CrossRef]
30. Osterby, R.; Tapia, J.; Nyberg, G.; Tencer, J.; Willner, J.; Rippe, B.; Torffvit, O. Renal structures in type 2 diabetic patients with elevated albumin excretion rate. *APMIS* **2001**, *109*, 751–761. [CrossRef]
31. Saito, Y.; Kida, H.; Takeda, S.; Yoshimura, M.; Yokoyama, H.; Koshino, Y.; Hattori, N. Mesangiolysis in diabetic glomeruli: Its role in the formation of nodular lesions. *Kidney Int.* **1988**, *34*, 389–396. [CrossRef] [PubMed]
32. Stout, L.C.; Kumar, S.; Whorton, E.B. Focal mesangiolysis and the pathogenesis of the Kimmelstiel-Wilson nodule. *Hum. Pathol.* **1993**, *24*, 77–89. [CrossRef]
33. Gentilella, R.; Pechtner, V.; Corcos, A.; Consoli, A. Glucagon-like peptide-1 receptor agonists in type 2 diabetes treatment: Are they all the same? *Diabetes Metab Res. Rev.* **2019**, *35*, e3070. [CrossRef] [PubMed]
34. Gallwitz, B. Glucagon-like peptide-1 receptor agonists. In *Handbook of Incretin-Based Therapies in Type 2 Diabetes*; Gough, S., Ed.; Springer International Publishing Switzerland: Cham, Switzerland, 2016; pp. 31–43.
35. Baggio, L.L.; Drucker, D.J. Biology of incretins: GLP-1 and GIP. *Gastroenterology* **2007**, *132*, 2131–2157. [CrossRef]
36. Turton, M.D.; O'Shea, D.; Gunn, I.; Beak, S.A.; Edwards, C.M.; Meeran, K.; Choi, S.J.; Taylor, G.M.; Heath, M.M.; Lambert, P.D.; et al. A role for glucagon-like peptide-1 in the central regulation of feeding. *Nature* **1996**, *379*, 69–72. [CrossRef]
37. Zhao, X.; Liu, G.; Shen, H.; Gao, B.; Li, X.; Fu, J.; Zhou, J.; Ji, Q. Liraglutide inhibits autophagy and apoptosis induced by high glucose through GLP-1R in renal tubular epithelial cells. *Int. J. Mol. Med.* **2015**, *35*, 684–692. [CrossRef]
38. Nauck, M.A.; Duran, S.; Kim, D.; Johns, D.; Northrup, J.; Festa, A.; Brodows, R.; Trautmann, M. A comparison of twice-daily exenatide and biphasic insulin aspart in patients with type 2 diabetes who were suboptimally

controlled with sulfonylurea and metformin: A non-inferiority study. *Diabetologia* **2007**, *50*, 259–267. [CrossRef]

39. Buse, J.B.; Bergenstal, R.M.; Glass, L.C.; Heilmann, C.R.; Lewis, M.S.; Kwan, A.Y.; Hoogwerf, B.J.; Rosenstock, J. Use of twice-daily exenatide in Basal insulin-treated patients with type 2 diabetes: A randomized, controlled trial. *Ann. Intern. Med.* **2011**, *154*, 103–112. [CrossRef]
40. Weissman, P.N.; Carr, M.C.; Ye, J.; Cirkel, D.T.; Stewart, M.; Perry, C.; Pratley, R. HARMONY 4: Randomised clinical trial comparing once-weekly albiglutide and insulin glargine in patients with type 2 diabetes inadequately controlled with metformin with or without sulfonylurea. *Diabetologia* **2014**, *57*, 2475–2484. [CrossRef]
41. Wysham, C.; Blevins, T.; Arakaki, R.; Colon, G.; Garcia, P.; Atisso, C.; Kuhstoss, D.; Lakshmanan, M. Efficacy and safety of dulaglutide added onto pioglitazone and metformin versus exenatide in type 2 diabetes in a randomized controlled trial (AWARD-1). *Diabetes Care* **2014**, *37*, 2159–2167. [CrossRef]
42. Nauck, M.; Weinstock, R.S.; Umpierrez, G.E.; Guerci, B.; Skrivanek, Z.; Milicevic, Z. Efficacy and safety of dulaglutide versus sitagliptin after 52 weeks in type 2 diabetes in a randomized controlled trial (AWARD-5). *Diabetes Care* **2014**, *37*, 2149–2158. [CrossRef]
43. Drucker, D.J.; Buse, J.B.; Taylor, K.; Kendall, D.M.; Trautmann, M.; Zhuang, D.; Porter, L.; Group, D.-S. Exenatide once weekly versus twice daily for the treatment of type 2 diabetes: A randomised, open-label, non-inferiority study. *Lancet* **2008**, *372*, 1240–1250. [CrossRef]
44. Blevins, T.; Pullman, J.; Malloy, J.; Yan, P.; Taylor, K.; Schulteis, C.; Trautmann, M.; Porter, L. DURATION-5: Exenatide once weekly resulted in greater improvements in glycemic control compared with exenatide twice daily in patients with type 2 diabetes. *J. Clin. Endocrinol. Metab.* **2011**, *96*, 1301–1310. [CrossRef]
45. Buse, J.B.; Drucker, D.J.; Taylor, K.L.; Kim, T.; Walsh, B.; Hu, H.; Wilhelm, K.; Trautmann, M.; Shen, L.Z.; Porter, L.E.; et al. DURATION-1: Exenatide once weekly produces sustained glycemic control and weight loss over 52 weeks. *Diabetes Care* **2010**, *33*, 1255–1261. [CrossRef]
46. Buse, J.B.; Rosenstock, J.; Sesti, G.; Schmidt, W.E.; Montanya, E.; Brett, J.H.; Zychma, M.; Blonde, L.; Group, L.-S. Liraglutide once a day versus exenatide twice a day for type 2 diabetes: A 26-week randomised, parallel-group, multinational, open-label trial (LEAD-6). *Lancet* **2009**, *374*, 39–47. [CrossRef]
47. Abd El Aziz, M.S.; Kahle, M.; Meier, J.J.; Nauck, M.A. A meta-analysis comparing clinical effects of short- or long-acting GLP-1 receptor agonists versus insulin treatment from head-to-head studies in type 2 diabetic patients. *Diabetes Obes. Metab.* **2017**, *19*, 216–227. [CrossRef]
48. Zaccardi, F.; Htike, Z.Z.; Webb, D.R.; Khunti, K.; Davies, M.J. Benefits and Harms of Once-Weekly Glucagon-like Peptide-1 Receptor Agonist Treatments: A Systematic Review and Network Meta-analysis. *Ann. Intern. Med.* **2016**, *164*, 102–113. [CrossRef]
49. DeFronzo, R.A.; Ratner, R.E.; Han, J.; Kim, D.D.; Fineman, M.S.; Baron, A.D. Effects of exenatide (exendin-4) on glycemic control and weight over 30 weeks in metformin-treated patients with type 2 diabetes. *Diabetes Care* **2005**, *28*, 1092–1100. [CrossRef]
50. Lorenz, M.; Evers, A.; Wagner, M. Recent progress and future options in the development of GLP-1 receptor agonists for the treatment of diabesity. *Bioorg Med. Chem. Lett.* **2013**, *23*, 4011–4018. [CrossRef]
51. Yin, W.; Xu, S.; Wang, Z.; Liu, H.; Peng, L.; Fang, Q.; Deng, T.; Zhang, W.; Lou, J. Recombinant human GLP-1(rhGLP-1) alleviating renal tubulointestitial injury in diabetic STZ-induced rats. *Biochem. Biophys. Res. Commun.* **2018**, *495*, 793–800. [CrossRef]
52. Hills, C.E.; Al-Rasheed, N.; Willars, G.B.; Brunskill, N.J. C-peptide reverses TGF-beta1-induced changes in renal proximal tubular cells: Implications for treatment of diabetic nephropathy. *Am. J. Physiol. Ren. Physiol.* **2009**, *296*, F614–F621. [CrossRef] [PubMed]
53. Kodera, R.; Shikata, K.; Kataoka, H.U.; Takatsuka, T.; Miyamoto, S.; Sasaki, M.; Kajitani, N.; Nishishita, S.; Sarai, K.; Hirota, D.; et al. Glucagon-like peptide-1 receptor agonist ameliorates renal injury through its anti-inflammatory action without lowering blood glucose level in a rat model of type 1 diabetes. *Diabetologia* **2011**, *54*, 965–978. [CrossRef] [PubMed]
54. Leech, C.A.; Holz, G.G.; Habener, J.F. Signal transduction of PACAP and GLP-1 in pancreatic beta cells. *Ann. N. Y. Acad. Sci.* **1996**, *805*, 81–92. [CrossRef]
55. Holz, G.G. Epac: A new cAMP-binding protein in support of glucagon-like peptide-1 receptor-mediated signal transduction in the pancreatic beta-cell. *Diabetes* **2004**, *53*, 5–13. [CrossRef]
56. Bengis-Garber, C.; Gruener, N. Protein kinase A downregulates the phosphorylation of p47 phox in human

neutrophils: A possible pathway for inhibition of the respiratory burst. *Cell Signal.* **1996**, *8*, 291–296. [CrossRef]

57. Savitha, G.; Salimath, B.P. Cross-talk between protein kinase C and protein kinase A down-regulates the respiratory burst in polymorphonuclear leukocytes. *Cell Signal.* **1993**, *5*, 107–117. [CrossRef]
58. Hendarto, H.; Inoguchi, T.; Maeda, Y.; Ikeda, N.; Zheng, J.; Takei, R.; Yokomizo, H.; Hirata, E.; Sonoda, N.; Takayanagi, R. GLP-1 analog liraglutide protects against oxidative stress and albuminuria in streptozotocin-induced diabetic rats via protein kinase A-mediated inhibition of renal NAD(P)H oxidases. *Metabolism* **2012**, *61*, 1422–1434. [CrossRef]
59. Fujita, H.; Morii, T.; Fujishima, H.; Sato, T.; Shimizu, T.; Hosoba, M.; Tsukiyama, K.; Narita, T.; Takahashi, T.; Drucker, D.J.; et al. The protective roles of GLP-1R signaling in diabetic nephropathy: Possible mechanism and therapeutic potential. *Kidney Int.* **2014**, *85*, 579–589. [CrossRef]
60. Gutzwiller, J.P.; Hruz, P.; Huber, A.R.; Hamel, C.; Zehnder, C.; Drewe, J.; Gutmann, H.; Stanga, Z.; Vogel, D.; Beglinger, C. Glucagon-like peptide-1 is involved in sodium and water homeostasis in humans. *Digestion* **2006**, *73*, 142–150. [CrossRef]
61. Rieg, T.; Gerasimova, M.; Murray, F.; Masuda, T.; Tang, T.; Rose, M.; Drucker, D.J.; Vallon, V. Natriuretic effect by exendin-4, but not the DPP-4 inhibitor alogliptin, is mediated via the GLP-1 receptor and preserved in obese type 2 diabetic mice. *Am. J. Physiol. Renal. Physiol.* **2012**, *303*, F963–F971. [CrossRef]
62. Muskiet, M.H.A.; Tonneijck, L.; Smits, M.M.; van Baar, M.J.B.; Kramer, M.H.H.; Hoorn, E.J.; Joles, J.A.; van Raalte, D.H. GLP-1 and the kidney: From physiology to pharmacology and outcomes in diabetes. *Nat. Rev. Nephrol.* **2017**, *13*, 605–628. [CrossRef]
63. Davies, M.J.; Bain, S.C.; Atkin, S.L.; Rossing, P.; Scott, D.; Shamkhalova, M.S.; Bosch-Traberg, H.; Syrén, A.; Umpierrez, G.E. Efficacy and Safety of Liraglutide Versus Placebo as Add-on to Glucose-Lowering Therapy in Patients with Type 2 Diabetes and Moderate Renal Impairment (LIRA-RENAL): A Randomized Clinical Trial. *Diabetes Care* **2016**, *39*, 222–230. [CrossRef]
64. Mann, J.F.E.; Ørsted, D.D.; Buse, J.B. Liraglutide and Renal Outcomes in Type 2 Diabetes. *N. Engl. J. Med.* **2017**, *377*, 2197–2198. [CrossRef]
65. Muskiet, M.H.A.; Tonneijck, L.; Huang, Y.; Liu, M.; Saremi, A.; Heerspink, H.J.L.; van Raalte, D.H. Lixisenatide and renal outcomes in patients with type 2 diabetes and acute coronary syndrome: An exploratory analysis of the ELIXA randomised, placebo-controlled trial. *Lancet Diabetes Endocrinol.* **2018**, *6*, 859–869. [CrossRef]
66. Tuttle, K.R.; Lakshmanan, M.C.; Rayner, B.; Busch, R.S.; Zimmermann, A.G.; Woodward, D.B.; Botros, F.T. Dulaglutide versus insulin glargine in patients with type 2 diabetes and moderate-to-severe chronic kidney disease (AWARD-7): A multicentre, open-label, randomised trial. *Lancet Diabetes Endocrinol.* **2018**, *6*, 605–617. [CrossRef]
67. De Vos, L.C.; Hettige, T.S.; Cooper, M.E. New Glucose-Lowering Agents for Diabetic Kidney Disease. *Adv. Chronic Kidney Dis.* **2018**, *25*, 149–157. [CrossRef] [PubMed]
68. Fuhrman, D.Y.; Schneider, M.F.; Dell, K.M.; Blydt-Hansen, T.D.; Mak, R.; Saland, J.M.; Furth, S.L.; Warady, B.A.; Moxey-Mims, M.M.; Schwartz, G.J. Albuminuria, Proteinuria, and Renal Disease Progression in Children with CKD. *Clin. J. Am. Soc. Nephrol.* **2017**, *12*, 912–920. [CrossRef]
69. Fox, C.S.; Matsushita, K.; Woodward, M.; Bilo, H.J.; Chalmers, J.; Heerspink, H.J.; Lee, B.J.; Perkins, R.M.; Rossing, P.; Sairenchi, T.; et al. Associations of kidney disease measures with mortality and end-stage renal disease in individuals with and without diabetes: A meta-analysis. *Lancet* **2012**, *380*, 1662–1673. [CrossRef]
70. Lorenzo, V.; Saracho, R.; Zamora, J.; Rufino, M.; Torres, A. Similar renal decline in diabetic and non-diabetic patients with comparable levels of albuminuria. *Nephrol. Dial. Transplant.* **2010**, *25*, 835–841. [CrossRef]
71. Marso, S.P.; Bain, S.C.; Consoli, A.; Eliaschewitz, F.G.; Jódar, E.; Leiter, L.A.; Lingvay, I.; Rosenstock, J.; Seufert, J.; Warren, M.L.; et al. Semaglutide and Cardiovascular Outcomes in Patients with Type 2 Diabetes. *N. Engl. J. Med.* **2016**, *375*, 1834–1844. [CrossRef]
72. Muskiet, M.H.; Smits, M.M.; Morsink, L.M.; Diamant, M. The gut-renal axis: Do incretin-based agents confer renoprotection in diabetes? *Nat. Rev. Nephrol.* **2014**, *10*, 88–103. [CrossRef]
73. Panchapakesan, U.; Pegg, K.; Gross, S.; Komala, M.G.; Mudaliar, H.; Forbes, J.; Pollock, C.; Mather, A. Effects of SGLT2 inhibition in human kidney proximal tubular cells—Renoprotection in diabetic nephropathy? *PLoS ONE* **2013**, *8*, e54442. [CrossRef]
74. Katz, P.M.; Leiter, L.A. The Role of the Kidney and SGLT2 Inhibitors in Type 2 Diabetes. *Can. J. Diabetes* **2015**, *39* (Suppl. S5), S167–S175. [CrossRef]

75. Mather, A.; Pollock, C. Glucose handling by the kidney. *Kidney Int. Suppl.* **2011**, *79*, S1–S6. [CrossRef]
76. Mather, A.; Pollock, C. Renal glucose transporters: Novel targets for hyperglycemia management. *Nat. Rev. Nephrol.* **2010**, *6*, 307–311. [CrossRef]
77. Abdul-Ghani, M.A.; DeFronzo, R.A.; Norton, L. Novel hypothesis to explain why SGLT2 inhibitors inhibit only 30-50% of filtered glucose load in humans. *Diabetes* **2013**, *62*, 3324–3328. [CrossRef]
78. Marks, J.; Carvou, N.J.; Debnam, E.S.; Srai, S.K.; Unwin, R.J. Diabetes increases facilitative glucose uptake and GLUT2 expression at the rat proximal tubule brush border membrane. *J. Physiol.* **2003**, *553*, 137–145. [CrossRef]
79. Gilbert, R.E.; Cooper, M.E. The tubulointerstitium in progressive diabetic kidney disease: More than an aftermath of glomerular injury? *Kidney Int.* **1999**, *56*, 1627–1637. [CrossRef]
80. Cherney, D.Z.; Perkins, B.A.; Soleymanlou, N.; Xiao, F.; Zimpelmann, J.; Woerle, H.J.; Johansen, O.E.; Broedl, U.C.; von Eynatten, M.; Burns, K.D. Sodium glucose cotransport-2 inhibition and intrarenal RAS activity in people with type 1 diabetes. *Kidney Int.* **2014**, *86*, 1057–1058. [CrossRef]
81. Vallon, V.; Richter, K.; Blantz, R.C.; Thomson, S.; Osswald, H. Glomerular hyperfiltration in experimental diabetes mellitus: Potential role of tubular reabsorption. *J. Am. Soc. Nephrol.* **1999**, *10*, 2569–2576.
82. Kojima, N.; Williams, J.M.; Slaughter, T.N.; Kato, S.; Takahashi, T.; Miyata, N.; Roman, R.J. Renoprotective effects of combined SGLT2 and ACE inhibitor therapy in diabetic Dahl S rats. *Physiol. Rep.* **2015**, *3*, e12436. [CrossRef]
83. Gallo, L.A.; Ward, M.S.; Fotheringham, A.K.; Zhuang, A.; Borg, D.J.; Flemming, N.B.; Harvie, B.M.; Kinneally, T.L.; Yeh, S.M.; McCarthy, D.A.; et al. Erratum: Once daily administration of the SGLT2 inhibitor, empagliflozin, attenuates markers of renal fibrosis without improving albuminuria in diabetic db/db mice. *Sci. Rep.* **2016**, *6*, 28124. [CrossRef]
84. Johnson, D.W.; Saunders, H.J.; Brew, B.K.; Poronnik, P.; Cook, D.I.; Field, M.J.; Pollock, C.A. TGF-beta 1 dissociates human proximal tubule cell growth and Na(+)-H+ exchange activity. *Kidney Int.* **1998**, *53*, 1601–1607. [CrossRef]
85. Panchapakesan, U.; Pollock, C.A.; Chen, X.M. The effect of high glucose and PPAR-gamma agonists on PPAR-gamma expression and function in HK-2 cells. *Am. J. Physiol Renal Physiol.* **2004**, *287*, F528–F534. [CrossRef]
86. Qi, W.; Chen, X.; Holian, J.; Mreich, E.; Twigg, S.; Gilbert, R.E.; Pollock, C.A. Transforming growth factor-beta1 differentially mediates fibronectin and inflammatory cytokine expression in kidney tubular cells. *Am. J. Physiol. Renal Physiol.* **2006**, *291*, F1070–F1077. [CrossRef]
87. Scheen, A.J. Evaluating SGLT2 inhibitors for type 2 diabetes: Pharmacokinetic and toxicological considerations. *Expert Opin. Drug Metab. Toxicol.* **2014**, *10*, 647–663. [CrossRef]
88. Scheen, A.J. Drug-drug interactions with sodium-glucose cotransporters type 2 (SGLT2) inhibitors, new oral glucose-lowering agents for the management of type 2 diabetes mellitus. *Clin. Pharmacokinet.* **2014**, *53*, 295–304. [CrossRef]
89. Merovci, A.; Mari, A.; Solis-Herrera, C.; Xiong, J.; Daniele, G.; Chavez-Velazquez, A.; Tripathy, D.; Urban McCarthy, S.; Abdul-Ghani, M.; DeFronzo, R.A. Dapagliflozin lowers plasma glucose concentration and improves β-cell function. *J. Clin. Endocrinol. Metab.* **2015**, *100*, 1927–1932. [CrossRef]
90. Del Prato, S. Role of glucotoxicity and lipotoxicity in the pathophysiology of Type 2 diabetes mellitus and emerging treatment strategies. *Diabet. Med.* **2009**, *26*, 1185–1192. [CrossRef]
91. Wilding, J.P.; Blonde, L.; Leiter, L.A.; Cerdas, S.; Tong, C.; Yee, J.; Meininger, G. Efficacy and safety of canagliflozin by baseline HbA1c and known duration of type 2 diabetes mellitus. *J. Diabetes Complic.* **2015**, *29*, 438–444. [CrossRef]
92. Bolinder, J.; Ljunggren, Ö.; Johansson, L.; Wilding, J.; Langkilde, A.M.; Sjöström, C.D.; Sugg, J.; Parikh, S. Dapagliflozin maintains glycaemic control while reducing weight and body fat mass over 2 years in patients with type 2 diabetes mellitus inadequately controlled on metformin. *Diabetes Obes. Metab.* **2014**, *16*, 159–169. [CrossRef]
93. Engeli, S.; Jordan, J. Novel metabolic drugs and blood pressure: Implications for the treatment of obese hypertensive patients? *Curr. Hypertens Rep.* **2013**, *15*, 470–474. [CrossRef]
94. Johnsson, K.M.; Ptaszynska, A.; Schmitz, B.; Sugg, J.; Parikh, S.J.; List, J.F. Urinary tract infections in patients with diabetes treated with dapagliflozin. *J. Diabetes Complic.* **2013**, *27*, 473–478. [CrossRef]
95. Elkinson, S.; Scott, L.J. Canagliflozin: First global approval. *Drugs* **2013**, *73*, 979–988. [CrossRef]
96. Polidori, D.; Sha, S.; Mudaliar, S.; Ciaraldi, T.P.; Ghosh, A.; Vaccaro, N.; Farrell, K.; Rothenberg, P.; Henry, R.R.

Canagliflozin lowers postprandial glucose and insulin by delaying intestinal glucose absorption in addition to increasing urinary glucose excretion: Results of a randomized, placebo-controlled study. *Diabetes Care* **2013**, *36*, 2154–2161. [CrossRef]

97. Nyirjesy, P.; Zhao, Y.; Ways, K.; Usiskin, K. Evaluation of vulvovaginal symptoms and Candida colonization in women with type 2 diabetes mellitus treated with canagliflozin, a sodium glucose co-transporter 2 inhibitor. *Curr. Med. Res. Opin.* **2012**, *28*, 1173–1178. [CrossRef]
98. Scheen, A.J. Pharmacokinetic and pharmacodynamic profile of empagliflozin, a sodium glucose co-transporter 2 inhibitor. *Clin. Pharmacokinet.* **2014**, *53*, 213–225. [CrossRef]
99. Ferrannini, E.; Muscelli, E.; Frascerra, S.; Baldi, S.; Mari, A.; Heise, T.; Broedl, U.C.; Woerle, H.J. Metabolic response to sodium-glucose cotransporter 2 inhibition in type 2 diabetic patients. *J. Clin. Invest.* **2014**, *124*, 499–508. [CrossRef]
100. Ferrannini, E.; Berk, A.; Hantel, S.; Pinnetti, S.; Hach, T.; Woerle, H.J.; Broedl, U.C. Long-term safety and efficacy of empagliflozin, sitagliptin, and metformin: An active-controlled, parallel-group, randomized, 78-week open-label extension study in patients with type 2 diabetes. *Diabetes Care* **2013**, *36*, 4015–4021. [CrossRef]
101. Gerich, J.E. Role of the kidney in normal glucose homeostasis and in the hyperglycaemia of diabetes mellitus: Therapeutic implications. *Diabet. Med.* **2010**, *27*, 136–142. [CrossRef]
102. Cherney, D.Z.; Scholey, J.W.; Jiang, S.; Har, R.; Lai, V.; Sochett, E.B.; Reich, H.N. The effect of direct renin inhibition alone and in combination with ACE inhibition on endothelial function, arterial stiffness, and renal function in type 1 diabetes. *Diabetes Care* **2012**, *35*, 2324–2330. [CrossRef] [PubMed]
103. De Nicola, L.; Gabbai, F.B.; Liberti, M.E.; Sagliocca, A.; Conte, G.; Minutolo, R. Sodium/glucose cotransporter 2 inhibitors and prevention of diabetic nephropathy: Targeting the renal tubule in diabetes. *Am. J. Kidney Dis.* **2014**, *64*, 16–24. [CrossRef] [PubMed]
104. Rahmoune, H.; Thompson, P.W.; Ward, J.M.; Smith, C.D.; Hong, G.; Brown, J. Glucose transporters in human renal proximal tubular cells isolated from the urine of patients with non-insulin-dependent diabetes. *Diabetes* **2005**, *54*, 3427–3434. [CrossRef] [PubMed]
105. Vallon, V.; Gerasimova, M.; Rose, M.A.; Masuda, T.; Satriano, J.; Mayoux, E.; Koepsell, H.; Thomson, S.C.; Rieg, T. SGLT2 inhibitor empagliflozin reduces renal growth and albuminuria in proportion to hyperglycemia and prevents glomerular hyperfiltration in diabetic Akita mice. *Am. J. Physiol. Renal Physiol.* **2014**, *306*, F194–F204. [CrossRef] [PubMed]
106. Kojima, N.; Williams, J.M.; Takahashi, T.; Miyata, N.; Roman, R.J. Effects of a new SGLT2 inhibitor, luseogliflozin, on diabetic nephropathy in T2DN rats. *J. Pharmacol. Exp. Ther.* **2013**, *345*, 464–472. [CrossRef] [PubMed]
107. Terami, N.; Ogawa, D.; Tachibana, H.; Hatanaka, T.; Wada, J.; Nakatsuka, A.; Eguchi, J.; Horiguchi, C.S.; Nishii, N.; Yamada, H.; et al. Long-term treatment with the sodium glucose cotransporter 2 inhibitor, dapagliflozin, ameliorates glucose homeostasis and diabetic nephropathy in db/db mice. *PLoS ONE* **2014**, *9*, e100777. [CrossRef] [PubMed]
108. Lin, B.; Koibuchi, N.; Hasegawa, Y.; Sueta, D.; Toyama, K.; Uekawa, K.; Ma, M.; Nakagawa, T.; Kusaka, H.; Kim-Mitsuyama, S. Glycemic control with empagliflozin, a novel selective SGLT2 inhibitor, ameliorates cardiovascular injury and cognitive dysfunction in obese and type 2 diabetic mice. *Cardiovasc. Diabetol.* **2014**, *13*, 148. [CrossRef]
109. Nagata, T.; Fukuzawa, T.; Takeda, M.; Fukazawa, M.; Mori, T.; Nihei, T.; Honda, K.; Suzuki, Y.; Kawabe, Y. Tofogliflozin, a novel sodium-glucose co-transporter 2 inhibitor, improves renal and pancreatic function in db/db mice. *Br. J. Pharmacol.* **2013**, *170*, 519–531. [CrossRef] [PubMed]
110. Gangadharan Komala, M.; Gross, S.; Mudaliar, H.; Huang, C.; Pegg, K.; Mather, A.; Shen, S.; Pollock, C.A.; Panchapakesan, U. Inhibition of kidney proximal tubular glucose reabsorption does not prevent against diabetic nephropathy in type 1 diabetic eNOS knockout mice. *PLoS ONE* **2014**, *9*, e108994. [CrossRef]
111. Tabatabai, N.M.; Sharma, M.; Blumenthal, S.S.; Petering, D.H. Enhanced expressions of sodium-glucose cotransporters in the kidneys of diabetic Zucker rats. *Diabetes Res. Clin. Pract.* **2009**, *83*, e27–e30. [CrossRef]
112. Maldonado-Cervantes, M.I.; Galicia, O.G.; Moreno-Jaime, B.; Zapata-Morales, J.R.; Montoya-Contreras, A.; Bautista-Perez, R.; Martinez-Morales, F. Autocrine modulation of glucose transporter SGLT2 by IL-6 and TNF-α in LLC-PK(1) cells. *J. Physiol. Biochem.* **2012**, *68*, 411–420. [CrossRef] [PubMed]
113. Beloto-Silva, O.; Machado, U.F.; Oliveira-Souza, M. Glucose-induced regulation of NHEs activity and SGLTs expression involves the PKA signaling pathway. *J. Membr. Biol.* **2011**, *239*, 157–165. [CrossRef] [PubMed]

114. Ghezzi, C.; Wright, E.M. Regulation of the human Na+-dependent glucose cotransporter hSGLT2. *Am. J. Physiol. Cell Physiol.* **2012**, *303*, C348–C354. [CrossRef] [PubMed]
115. Osorio, H.; Bautista, R.; Rios, A.; Franco, M.; Santamaría, J.; Escalante, B. Effect of treatment with losartan on salt sensitivity and SGLT2 expression in hypertensive diabetic rats. *Diabetes Res. Clin. Pract.* **2009**, *86*, e46–e49. [CrossRef] [PubMed]
116. Doblado, M.; Moley, K.H. Facilitative glucose transporter 9, a unique hexose and urate transporter. *Am. J. Physiol. Endocrinol. Metab.* **2009**, *297*, E831–E835. [CrossRef] [PubMed]
117. Cain, L.; Shankar, A.; Ducatman, A.M.; Steenland, K. The relationship between serum uric acid and chronic kidney disease among Appalachian adults. *Nephrol. Dial. Transplant.* **2010**, *25*, 3593–3599. [CrossRef]
118. Komala, M.G.; Panchapakesan, U.; Pollock, C.; Mather, A. Sodium glucose cotransporter 2 and the diabetic kidney. *Curr. Opin. Nephrol. Hypertens* **2013**, *22*, 113–119. [CrossRef]
119. De Zeeuw, D.; Remuzzi, G.; Parving, H.H.; Keane, W.F.; Zhang, Z.; Shahinfar, S.; Snapinn, S.; Cooper, M.E.; Mitch, W.E.; Brenner, B.M. Proteinuria, a target for renoprotection in patients with type 2 diabetic nephropathy: Lessons from RENAAL. *Kidney Int.* **2004**, *65*, 2309–2320. [CrossRef]
120. Yale, J.F.; Bakris, G.; Cariou, B.; Yue, D.; David-Neto, E.; Xi, L.; Figueroa, K.; Wajs, E.; Usiskin, K.; Meininger, G. Efficacy and safety of canagliflozin in subjects with type 2 diabetes and chronic kidney disease. *Diabetes Obes. Metab.* **2013**, *15*, 463–473. [CrossRef]
121. Heerspink, H.J.; Johnsson, E.; Gause-Nilsson, I.; Cain, V.A.; Sjöström, C.D. Dapagliflozin reduces albuminuria in patients with diabetes and hypertension receiving renin-angiotensin blockers. *Diabetes Obes. Metab.* **2016**, *18*, 590–597. [CrossRef]
122. Chonchol, M.; Shlipak, M.G.; Katz, R.; Sarnak, M.J.; Newman, A.B.; Siscovick, D.S.; Kestenbaum, B.; Carney, J.K.; Fried, L.F. Relationship of uric acid with progression of kidney disease. *Am. J. Kidney Dis.* **2007**, *50*, 239–247. [CrossRef] [PubMed]
123. Goicoechea, M.; de Vinuesa, S.G.; Verdalles, U.; Ruiz-Caro, C.; Ampuero, J.; Rincón, A.; Arroyo, D.; Luño, J. Effect of allopurinol in chronic kidney disease progression and cardiovascular risk. *Clin. J. Am. Soc. Nephrol.* **2010**, *5*, 1388–1393. [CrossRef] [PubMed]
124. Iseki, K.; Oshiro, S.; Tozawa, M.; Iseki, C.; Ikemiya, Y.; Takishita, S. Significance of hyperuricemia on the early detection of renal failure in a cohort of screened subjects. *Hypertens Res.* **2001**, *24*, 691–697. [CrossRef] [PubMed]
125. Hovind, P.; Rossing, P.; Johnson, R.J.; Parving, H.H. Serum uric acid as a new player in the development of diabetic nephropathy. *J. Ren. Nutr.* **2011**, *21*, 124–127. [CrossRef]
126. Kang, D.H.; Nakagawa, T.; Feng, L.; Watanabe, S.; Han, L.; Mazzali, M.; Truong, L.; Harris, R.; Johnson, R.J. A role for uric acid in the progression of renal disease. *J. Am. Soc. Nephrol.* **2002**, *13*, 2888–2897. [CrossRef]
127. Cefalu, W.T.; Leiter, L.A.; Yoon, K.H.; Arias, P.; Niskanen, L.; Xie, J.; Balis, D.A.; Canovatchel, W.; Meininger, G. Efficacy and safety of canagliflozin versus glimepiride in patients with type 2 diabetes inadequately controlled with metformin (CANTATA-SU): 52 week results from a randomised, double-blind, phase 3 non-inferiority trial. *Lancet* **2013**, *382*, 941–950. [CrossRef]
128. Bailey, C.J.; Gross, J.L.; Pieters, A.; Bastien, A.; List, J.F. Effect of dapagliflozin in patients with type 2 diabetes who have inadequate glycaemic control with metformin: A randomised, double-blind, placebo-controlled trial. *Lancet* **2010**, *375*, 2223–2233. [CrossRef]
129. Wilding, J.P.; Ferrannini, E.; Fonseca, V.A.; Wilpshaar, W.; Dhanjal, P.; Houzer, A. Efficacy and safety of ipragliflozin in patients with type 2 diabetes inadequately controlled on metformin: A dose-finding study. *Diabetes Obes. Metab.* **2013**, *15*, 403–409. [CrossRef]
130. Home, P. Cardiovascular outcome trials of glucose-lowering medications: An update. *Diabetologia* **2019**, *62*, 357–369. [CrossRef]
131. Neal, B.; Perkovic, V.; Matthews, D.R. Canagliflozin and Cardiovascular and Renal Events in Type 2 Diabetes. *N. Engl. J. Med.* **2017**, *377*, 2099. [CrossRef]
132. Mosenzon, O.; Wiviott, S.D.; Cahn, A.; Rozenberg, A.; Yanuv, I.; Goodrich, E.L.; Murphy, S.A.; Heerspink, H.J.L.; Zelniker, T.A.; Dwyer, J.P.; et al. Effects of dapagliflozin on development and progression of kidney disease in patients with type 2 diabetes: An analysis from the DECLARE-TIMI 58 randomised trial. *Lancet Diabetes Endocrinol.* **2019**, *7*, 606–617. [CrossRef]
133. Neuen, B.L.; Young, T.; Heerspink, H.J.L.; Neal, B.; Perkovic, V.; Billot, L.; Mahaffey, K.W.; Charytan, D.M.; Wheeler, D.C.; Arnott, C.; et al. SGLT2 inhibitors for the prevention of kidney failure in patients with type 2 diabetes: A systematic review and meta-analysis. *Lancet Diabetes Endocrinol.* **2019**, *7*, 845–854. [CrossRef]

134. Zinman, B.; Wanner, C.; Lachin, J.M.; Fitchett, D.; Bluhmki, E.; Hantel, S.; Mattheus, M.; Devins, T.; Johansen, O.E.; Woerle, H.J.; et al. Empagliflozin, Cardiovascular Outcomes, and Mortality in Type 2 Diabetes. *N. Engl. J. Med.* **2015**, *373*, 2117–2128. [CrossRef] [PubMed]
135. Schernthaner, G.; Schernthaner-Reiter, M.H.; Schernthaner, G.H. EMPA-REG and Other Cardiovascular Outcome Trials of Glucose-lowering Agents: Implications for Future Treatment Strategies in Type 2 Diabetes Mellitus. *Clin. Ther.* **2016**, *38*, 1288–1298. [CrossRef] [PubMed]
136. Kalra, S.; Singh, V.; Nagrale, D. Sodium-Glucose Cotransporter-2 Inhibition and the Glomerulus: A Review. *Adv. Ther.* **2016**, *33*, 1502–1518. [CrossRef] [PubMed]
137. Heerspink, H.J.L.; Kosiborod, M.; Inzucchi, S.E.; Cherney, D.Z.I. Renoprotective effects of sodium-glucose cotransporter-2 inhibitors. *Kidney Int.* **2018**, *94*, 26–39. [CrossRef]
138. Molitch, M.E.; Adler, A.I.; Flyvbjerg, A.; Nelson, R.G.; So, W.Y.; Wanner, C.; Kasiske, B.L.; Wheeler, D.C.; de Zeeuw, D.; Mogensen, C.E. Diabetic kidney disease: A clinical update from Kidney Disease: Improving Global Outcomes. *Kidney Int.* **2015**, *87*, 20–30. [CrossRef]
139. Cherney, D.Z.I.; Bakris, G.L. Novel therapies for diabetic kidney disease. *Kidney Int. Suppl.* **2018**, *8*, 18–25. [CrossRef]
140. Bloomgarden, Z. The kidney and cardiovascular outcome trials. *J. Diabetes* **2018**, *10*, 88–89. [CrossRef]
141. Yaribeygi, H.; Atkin, S.L.; Katsiki, N.; Sahebkar, A. Narrative review of the effects of antidiabetic drugs on albuminuria. *J. Cell Physiol.* **2019**, *234*, 5786–5797. [CrossRef]
142. León Jiménez, D.; Cherney, D.Z.I.; Bjornstad, P.; Guerra, L.C.; Miramontes González, J.P. Antihyperglycemic agents as novel natriuretic therapies in diabetic kidney disease. *Am. J. Physiol. Renal Physiol.* **2018**, *315*, F1406–F1415. [CrossRef] [PubMed]
143. Cosentino, F.; Grant, P.J.; Aboyans, V.; Bailey, C.J.; Ceriello, A.; Delgado, V.; Federici, M.; Filippatos, G.; Grobbee, D.E.; Hansen, T.B.; et al. 2019 ESC Guidelines on diabetes, pre-diabetes, and cardiovascular diseases developed in collaboration with the EASD. *Eur. Heart J.* **2019**. [CrossRef] [PubMed]

14

The Anti-Inflammatory, Anti-Oxidative and Anti-Apoptotic Benefits of Stem Cells in Acute Ischemic Kidney Injury

Kuo-Hua Lee [1,2,3], Wei-Cheng Tseng [1,2,3], Chih-Yu Yang [1,2,3] and Der-Cherng Tarng [1,2,3,4,*]

1 Division of Nephrology, Department of Medicine, Taipei Veterans General Hospital, Taipei 11217, Taiwan
2 Institute of Clinical Medicine, National Yang-Ming University, Taipei 11217, Taiwan
3 Center for Intelligent Drug Systems and Smart Bio-devices (IDS2B), Hsinchu 30010, Taiwan
4 Department and Institute of Physiology, National Yang-Ming University, Taipei 11217, Taiwan
* Correspondence: dctarng@vghtpe.gov.tw

Abstract: Ischemia-reperfusion injury (IRI) plays a significant role in the pathogenesis of acute kidney injury (AKI). The complicated interaction between injured tubular cells, activated endothelial cells, and the immune system leads to oxidative stress and systemic inflammation, thereby exacerbating the apoptosis of renal tubular cells and impeding the process of tissue repair. Stem cell therapy is an innovative approach to ameliorate IRI due to its antioxidative, immunomodulatory, and anti-apoptotic properties. Therefore, it is crucial to understand the biological effects and mechanisms of action of stem cell therapy in the context of acute ischemic AKI to improve its therapeutic benefits. The recent finding that treatment with conditioned medium (CM) derived from stem cells is likely an effective alternative to conventional stem cell transplantation increases the potential for future therapeutic uses of stem cell therapy. In this review, we discuss the recent findings regarding stem cell-mediated cytoprotection, with a focus on the anti-inflammatory effects via suppression of oxidative stress and uncompromised immune responses following AKI. Stem cell-derived CM represents a favorable approach to stem cell-based therapy and may serve as a potential therapeutic strategy against acute ischemic AKI.

Keywords: ischemia-reperfusion; acute kidney injury; stem cell; conditioned medium; inflammation

---

1. Introduction

Acute kidney injury (AKI) involves a complex interaction between the kidney parenchyma and immune system that leads to inflammation at the site of the injured tissue and impaired renal function [1]. Renal ischemia is a significant cause of AKI and is characterized by reduced tissue perfusion, which leads to acute tubular injury. Re-establishing the blood supply after prolonged ischemia activates vascular endothelial cells and enhances the generation of reactive oxygen species (ROS). This triggers a myriad of inflammatory consequences and induces apoptosis of tubular epithelial cells (TECs) [2]. This phenomenon is referred to as ischemia-reperfusion induced AKI (IR-AKI) and is characterized by elevated oxidative stress and activation of the immune system in response to ischemic tissue injury [3,4].

In the early stages of renal ischemia, the circulating neutrophils and monocytes rapidly infiltrate the ischemic kidney and release lysosomal enzymes, leading to tubular epithelial cell injury [2]. Subsequent crosstalk between the injured TECs, activated endothelial cells, and tissue macrophages induces oxidative stress and complement activation, aggravating cell damaging processes, such as mitochondrial dysfunction and lipid peroxidation [5].

Furthermore, the extensive release of pro-inflammatory cytokines, such as tumor necrosis factor (TNF)-α, interleukin (IL)-6, and monocyte chemoattractant protein 1 (MCP-1), attract an immune response involving monocytes, dendritic cells (DC), natural killer (NK) cells, and lymphocytes [6]. Subsequent ROS-mediated mitogen-activated protein kinase (MAPK) and nuclear factor (NF)-κB cascades amplify the inflammatory response. The signaling transduction pathways induce extensive TEC apoptosis and upregulate several important inflammatory mediators, such as IL-6, TNF-α, IL-1β, interferon (IFN)-γ, and IL-17 [2,4,7]. These immune reactions establish a continuous positive feedback loop, or a vicious circle, resulting in constant stimulation. As a consequence, IR-AKI is not merely a localized kidney insult, but also a trigger for a cascade of systemic inflammation (Figure 1).

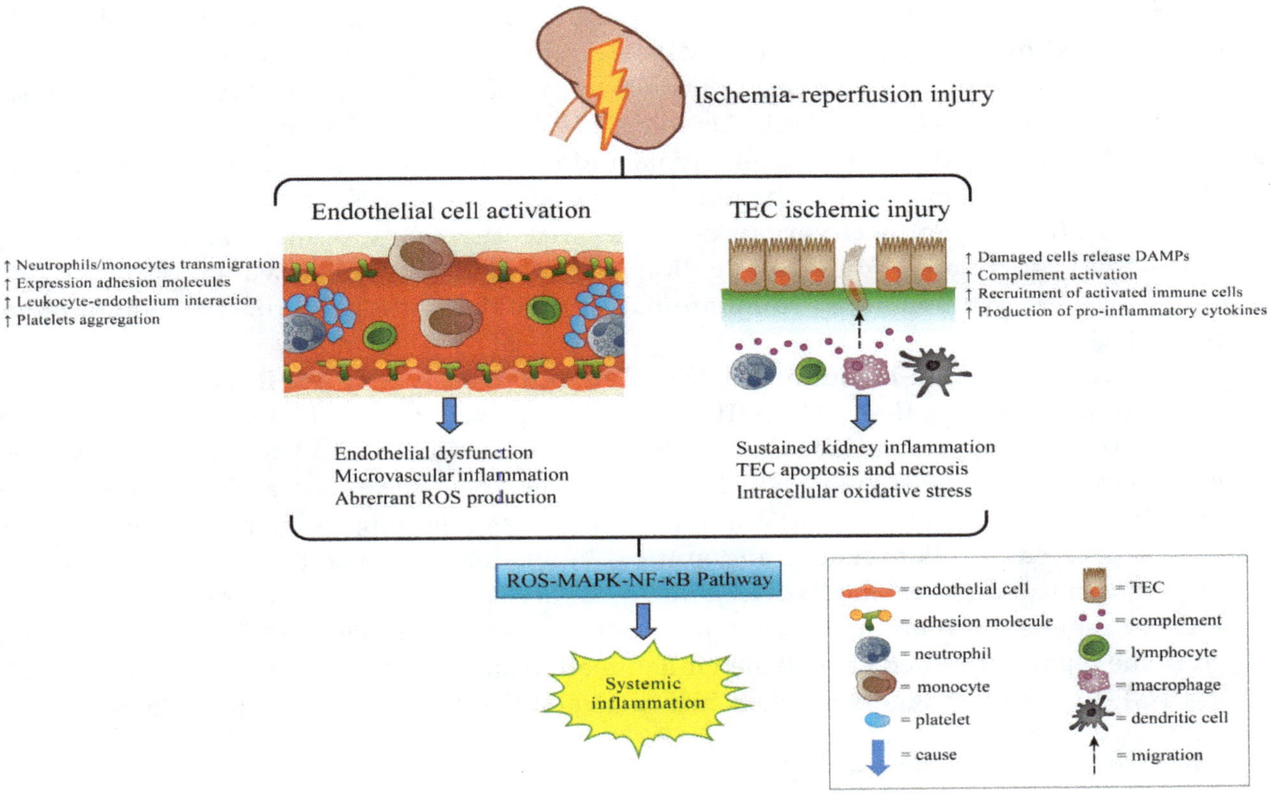

Figure 1. Pathogenesis of ischemia-reperfusion induced acute kidney injury. Ischemia-reperfusion-induced acute kidney injury involves endothelial cell activation (1). The increased leukocyte adhesion molecules on the activated endothelial cells induce leukocyte transmigration and platelet aggregation, which both cause microvascular inflammation. In tubular epithelial cell injury (2), the injured tubular cells release danger signals, which activate immune cells involved in local and systemic inflammation. The substantial amount of reactive oxygen species generated by this process activates the MAPK-NF-κB pathway and induces systemic inflammation. Abbreviations: DAMPs, damage-associated molecular patterns; TECs, tubular epithelial cells; ROS, reactive oxygen species; MAPK, mitogen-activated protein kinase; NF-κB, nuclear factor-κB.

In contrast to previous therapeutic approaches for AKI, which were mainly supportive, innovative treatments targeting AKI-induced inflammation, including stem cell therapy, have elicited a great deal of interest. In experimental models, administration of stem cells has proven effective in the treatment of AKI. One of the critical mechanisms of stem cell therapy is the anti-inflammatory effect caused by interaction with immune cells in the inflamed microenvironment [8–10]. Furthermore, stem cells may minimize the magnitude of tissue damage by secreting soluble cytoprotective factors in a paracrine manner [11,12].

Given that oxidative stress and inflammation have been implicated in the pathogenesis of IR-AKI, it is imperative to discuss these anti-inflammatory and immunoregulatory properties of stem cells. In this review, we focus on the therapeutic potential of stem cells in IR-AKI and illustrate the underlying antioxidant and anti-inflammatory mechanisms of this therapy. Because stem cells release soluble factors and microvesicles in a paracrine manner [13], we also discuss the effectiveness of stem cell-derived conditioned medium (CM) as an alternative to stem cell transplantation in the treatment of IR-AKI.

2. Immune Responses and Inflammation in IR-AKI

In IR-AKI, damaged cells are thought to be the critical trigger of inflammation. During the reperfusion phase, TECs are vulnerable to oxidative stress, and apoptotic and necrotic TECs release damage-associated molecular patterns (DAMPs) into the extracellular space. Endogenous DAMP molecules include DNA, RNA, and several intracellular proteins such as S100, heat-shock proteins, and high-mobility group box 1 (HMGB1) [14]. The so-called "danger signals" stimulate pattern recognition receptors (PRRs) expressed on renal parenchyma and immune cells, like epithelial and endothelial cells, DCs, lymphocytes, and macrophages. This recognition process initiates the host's defense mechanisms and further produces various cytokines that attract neutrophils and macrophages [15]. Signaling pathways activated by DAMP ligation of PRRs also result in activation of NF-κB, which further promotes the expression of pro-inflammatory cytokines and perpetuates the inflammatory response in IR-AKI.

The balance between pro-inflammatory (e.g., TNF-α, IFN-γ, IL-6, IL-1β, IL-17, C3, C5a, and C5b) and anti-inflammatory (e.g., IL-4, TGF-β, IL-10, and heme oxygenase-1 (HO-1)) mediators secreted by the participating cell populations determines the status of injury and repair [16]. HO-1 is an endogenous stress-inducible enzyme, which modulates leukocyte adhesion and migration, immune cell maturation, and production of inflammatory cytokines following ischemia. Up-regulation of HO-1 represents an anti-inflammatory and anti-oxidative defense capacity against IRI [17]. Under ideal conditions, a regulated balance between inflammatory and anti-inflammatory mediators ensures healthy tissue regeneration and reversal of homeostatic conditions. However, AKI often results in impeded tissue repair attributed to sustained inflammation and secretion of profibrotic cytokines (e.g., IL-13 and TGF-β1), which triggers myofibroblast activation and progressive kidney fibrosis [18].

Immunomodulatory Effects of Stem Cells

Considered an innovative anti-inflammatory treatment, the immunomodulatory effects of mesenchymal stem cells (MSCs) have been extensively investigated among other types of stem cells [19–21]. Firstly, MSCs are hypoimmunogenic as a result of reduced major histocompatibility complex (MHC) class I expression and a complete lack of expression of MHC class II and costimulatory molecules CD80 and CD86 [22]. This indicates that they can likely evade innate immunity processes, such as NK cell-mediated cytotoxicity, and lack the antigen presentation pathway essential for activation of the adaptive immune system [23]. To elicit an immunological balance, MSCs act as an immunomodulator by reducing the functional capacities and proliferation of all types of immune cells. MSCs have been proven to suppress lymphocyte activation and regulate their survival in a quiescent state [24]. Inhibition of T cell proliferation occurs through expression of inducible nitric oxide synthase (iNOS) and indoleamine 2,3-dioxygenase (IDO) in rodent and human MSCs, respectively [25]. More specifically, MSCs suppress $CD4^+$ T helper (Th) cells from differentiating into their Th1 and Th17 subsets, which are the causal agents in the pathogenesis of autoimmunity [26]. On the other hand, MSCs enhance the proliferation of regulatory T cells (Tregs) and strengthen their immune modulating capacities [27,28]. MSCs also inhibit the differentiation, maturation, and activation of DCs by downregulating the surface expression of CD80, CD86, and MHC class II molecules, retaining the DCs in a tolerogenic phenotype. In this state, they express various factors, such as IDO and prostaglandin E2 (PGE2), which lower DC immunogenicity, reduce T cell proliferation, and induce Treg differentiation [29,30]. Simultaneously,

MSCs induce macrophages to secrete immunosuppressive cytokines, like IL-4, IL-10 and transforming growth factor-β (TGF-β). It has also been shown that MSCs suppress NK cell proliferation and protect against perforin/granzyme-mediated cytotoxicity [31]. Furthermore, MSCs have inhibitory effects on B-cell proliferation, differentiation, and antibody production [32]. Given that HO-1 has significant anti-inflammatory therapeutic potential, recent research has pointed out HO-1-modified MSCs have an enhanced ability to attenuate inflammatory responses in ischemic heart disease [33], acute ischemic liver failure [34], lipopolysaccharide (LPS)-induced microvascular injury [35], and cisplatin-induced AKI [36]. Taken together, the administration of MSCs prevents immune cell activation and modulates kidney inflammation progression by managing cytokine secretion to promote anti-inflammatory processes.

It is noteworthy that the environment surrounding the MSCs is of critical importance to regulate the immunomodulatory effects. Liu et al. reported that MSCs derived from inflamed periodontal ligaments exhibit an impaired immunosuppressive capacity, with less inhibition of T cell proliferation, less induction of regulatory T cell, and less IL-10 production. The inflamed microenvironment also diminishes the immunomodulatory benefits of MSCs by reducing Th17 differentiation and IL-17 production [37]. Furthermore, Waterman et al. disclosed that MSCs could undergo functional polarization by differential Toll-like receptor (TLR) downstream signaling. Activation through TLR4 induced the pro-inflammatory MSC1, mostly producing pro-inflammatory mediators (IL-6, IL-8, and IFN-γ), can induce T cell activation. On the other hand, the TLR3-primed MSC2 mainly express anti-inflammatory factors such as IDO, PGE2, and HO-1, leading to T cell inhibition [38,39]. Moreover, to explain the diverse response of MSCs to TLR activation, Levin et al. suggested the level of co-cultured LPS-binding protein as a predictive factor in determining the secretomes of MSCs in response to TLR activation [40].

Similar to MSCs, Schnabel et al. found that induced pluripotent stem cells (iPSCs) possess immunomodulatory capacities evidenced by reducing responder T-cell proliferation in modified mixed leukocyte reactions in vitro [41]. Their findings echo our previous study [42], in which iPSCs without c-Myc were introduced into IR-AKI rat kidneys. This approach was not only safe, but also resulted in a substantial decrease in the levels of ROS and inflammatory cytokines. Furthermore, iPSCs have been shown to have strong immunomodulation effects through suppression of lymphocyte proliferation, NK cell-directed cytotoxicity, and DC differentiation and function [43–45]. This information is critical in considering the use of iPSCs in place of MSCs for both regenerative medicine and transplant medicine.

3. Oxidative Stress in IR-AKI

After the occurrence of acute ischemia, restoration of renal perfusion rapidly activates vascular endothelial cells, which trigger the production of pro-inflammatory cytokines and ROS, including superoxide (•$O2^-$), hydrogen peroxide (HOOH), and hydroxyl radical (•OH) [46]. Following IR-AKI, defective antioxidant processes cause depletion of endogenous antioxidants and reduced activity of redox-regulated enzymes, exacerbating the accumulation of intracellular ROS. This increased ROS production associated with reduced antioxidant capacity leads to a state of oxidative stress, which ultimately results in mitochondrial damage, depletion of ATP, increased lipid peroxidation, and activation of cell death pathways. Another harmful effect of ROS is oxidative modification of cell membrane proteins; this impairs ion and nutrient transport, energy metabolism, and organelle function essential for cellular homeostasis [47]. Furthermore, ROS-mediated activation of NF-κB continues to exacerbate systemic inflammation, triggering TEC apoptosis and kidney fibrosis, which have a detrimental impact on renal function [48].

Antioxidant Effects of Stem Cells

As a promising regenerative approach, stem cell therapy has been demonstrated to ameliorate various inflammatory diseases via its antioxidative activity [49–52]. MSCs can be isolated from bone marrow, umbilical cord blood, adipose tissue, placenta, periosteum, trabecular bone, synovium, skeletal muscle, and deciduous teeth [53], and their administration has been widely reported to upregulate the expression of the antioxidative enzyme HO-1 [35,54–57]. Increased HO-1 enzymatic activity is not only essential for MSC maturation, but is also cytoprotective against oxidative stress [58,59]. The antioxidant effects of HO-1 arise from its ability to increase reduced glutathione levels and degrade heme, as well as its ability to increase biliverdin and bilirubin, which have potent antioxidant properties [60,61]. In IR-AKI models, the increased production of HO-1 after MSC administration correlated with decreased levels of 8-hydroxy-2-deoxyguanosine (8-OHdG) and ROS [62]. The pro-angiogenic effects of MSCs lacking HO-1 expression are impaired; this triggers post-ischemic neovascularization and tissue repair, demonstrated by decreased secretion of several crucial pro-angiogenic growth factors, such as stromal cell-derived factor-1, vascular endothelial growth factor-A (VEGF-A), and hepatocyte growth factor (HGF) [36]. Similarly, CM derived from HO-1 knockout MSCs lacked therapeutic effects and failed to restore the functional and morphological changes in AKI [63]. A recent study also showed that modification with HO-1 significantly attenuated cell-cycle arrest, activated the PI3K/Akt and MEK/ERK pathways, and enhanced the survival of MSCs, all of which improved the therapeutic effects of MSCs against IR- AKI [64].

In addition to its impact on HO-1, IR-AKI also reduces the activity of antioxidant enzymes that scavenge ROS, including superoxide dismutase (SOD), catalase (CAT), glutathione-S-transferase (GST), and glutathione peroxidase (GPX), in post-ischemic kidney tissue [65]. MSC therapy increases the antioxidant capacity of post-ischemic kidney tissue by enhancing the activity of these ROS-scavenging enzymes, thereby reducing the levels of tissue malondialdehyde (MDA) [66–68]. Zhang et al. applied MSC-derived extracellular vesicles (MSC-EV) into an IR-AKI model and found that MSC-EV treatment reduced oxidative stress, and subsequently attenuated IR-AKI. This antioxidant effect is likely a result of activation of the NF-E2-related factor 2 (Nrf2)/antioxidant responsive element (ARE) pathway [69], but may also be due to decreased expression of NADPH oxidase 2 (NOX2) and ROS in injured kidney tissues [57,70].

In addition to MSCs, induced pluripotent stem cells (iPSC) are also equipped with antioxidative properties. In rats with IR- AKI, our previous study showed that the administration of iPSCs into kidneys via an intrarenal arterial route not only ameliorated the severity of tubular damage and kidney failure by reducing the expression of oxidative markers, pro-inflammatory cytokines, and apoptotic factors, but also improved the survival of IR-AKI rats [42]. We further showed that treatment of iPSC-CM in rats with IR-AKI significantly diminished oxidative stress and protected tubular cells against apoptosis [71], supporting the innovation occurring in this field of research.

4. Apoptosis of TEC in IR-AKI

Apoptosis is known to be a relevant mechanism of tubular cell death in IR-AKI. Kidney biopsies from IR-AKI animal models and humans have consistently shown apoptotic changes in TECs. There are several mechanisms of the pathogenesis of apoptosis of TECs. During ischemia, the pro-apoptotic protein Bax is upregulated in TECs, which results in a reduction of the anti-apoptotic protein Bcl-2, thus, promoting the initiation of apoptosis [72]. Another important stress kinase activated in the setting of ischemia is glycogen synthase kinase 3-β (GSK3β), which has been linked to mitochondrial dysfunction after exposure to oxidative stress [73]. During ischemia and ATP depletion, GSK3β upregulates Bax to activate caspase cascades, thus, promoting TEC apoptosis. Active GSK3β also positively regulates NF-κB leading to the inhibition of TNF-mediated apoptosis [74].

Other mechanisms of the activation of apoptotic pathways during IR-AKI have been proposed. The extrinsic apoptotic pathway is triggered by the binding of TNF-α and Fas ligands to death receptors, including Fas, tumor necrosis factor receptor 1 (TNFR1), and TNF-related apoptosis-inducing ligand receptors (TRAIL-Rs), expressed on TECs. Binding to these ligands results in receptor aggregation and recruitment of adaptor proteins, which, in turn, initiates a proteolytic cascade by activating initiator caspase-8 and caspase-10 [75]. The intrinsic apoptotic pathway is characterized by permeabilization of the mitochondrial outer membrane, resulting in the release of cytochrome c into the cytoplasm [76]. Cytochrome c then forms a multiprotein complex known as the "apoptosome" and initiates activation of the caspase cascade through caspase-9 [77]. Due to the significant consequences of TEC apoptosis and the complexity of its pathogenesis, reduction of tubular apoptosis is an essential requirement for the successful treatment of IR-AKI by stem cell therapy.

Anti-Apoptotic Effects of Stem Cells

To date, the anti-apoptotic property of stem cells seems to be the most widely recognized beneficial effect of MSCs [49,78–80]. In experimental models of AKI, administration of MSCs displayed a renoprotective effect by preventing tissue apoptosis, which accelerated the repair of injured tissue. MSC-treated AKI mice showed increased expression of the anti-apoptotic gene BCL2 and downregulation of the pro-apoptotic gene BAX [81]. Regarding the mechanisms of these treatment processes, MSCs modulate tubular apoptosis and regeneration through production of soluble paracrine factors and trophic growth factors, including VEGF, HGF, insulin-like growth factor 1 (IGF-1), stanniocalcin-1, TGF-β, and fibroblast growth factor 2 [82,83]. Cumulating evidence indicates that MSCs release extracellular vesicles (EVs) that deliver genes, microRNAs, exosomes, and proteins to recipient cells, thus, acting as mediators of MSC paracrine action and conferring resistance to apoptosis [84,85]. These EVs are also thought to communicate intercellularly and influence the function of progenitor cells to stimulate angiogenesis and other reparative processes and, consequently, accelerate tissue repair [11,86].

iPSCs present a promising new therapeutic approach for AKI [87], and several studies have illustrated their anti-apoptotic effects against IR-AKI. Subcapsular transplantation of human-iPSCs in rodent kidneys attenuated TEC apoptosis and ameliorated histological alterations resulting in renal function improvements following IR-AKI [88]. Li et al. also demonstrated the therapeutic effect of iPSC-derived renal progenitor cells (RPC) in IR-AKI; they observed the reduction of tubular apoptosis and renal function recovery in a rat model of IR-AKI. Simultaneously, increased expression of anti-inflammatory mediators and growth factors involved in kidney repair were observed after transplantation of iPSC-derived RPCs and MSCs in injured kidneys [88–90]. Shen et al. also showed that iPSC-derived endothelial progenitor cells ameliorated apoptosis of TECs and cardiomyocytes while treating IR-AKI in mice [91]. Regarding the mechanisms of the anti-apoptotic properties of stem cells, our previous study suggested that iPSC-derived CM provided a protective effect against IR-AKI by reducing ROS generation, suppressing p38-MAPK activation, and inhibiting TNF-induced cell death and its downstream effect of NF-κB-induced systemic inflammation [71]. Therefore, we have demonstrated that iPSCs exerted renoprotective effects via the secretion of paracrine factors and suggest that iPSC-CM is a potential resource for stem cell-based therapy against IR-AKI.

The therapeutic potential of spermatogonial stem cells (SSC) in AKI has been explored in the preclinical setting. Unlike the production of soluble cytokines and growth factors by MSCs and iPSCs, the mechanism governing SSCs to accelerate tissue regeneration is through direct differentiation into renal parenchymal cells. To prove this phenomenon, Wu et al. injected mouse SSCs into adult female mice kidneys. Three months after SSC administration, the histological analysis revealed the transplanted SSCs migrated to the basement membrane and trans-differentiated into mature renal TECs. The most convincing evidence for self-renewal and multipotency of SSCs came from the presence of the Y chromosome in the nucleolus of TECs and glomerular podocytes isolated from the SSC-transplanted kidneys in female mice [92].

Under specific conditions, SSCs can spontaneously transform into germline cell-derived pluripotent stem cells (GPSCs), which can be readily frozen and thawed without loss of cell viability. Using a novel renal epithelial differentiation protocol, Chiara et al. generated GPSC-derived tubular-like cells (GTCs) resembling renal TEC phenotypes and biological functions. After administration of GTCs intravenously in IR-AKI mice, these cells were able to home in on sites of inflammation and showed long-term engraftment in the injured kidney. Histological analysis disclosed less extent of cortical damage, inflammatory infiltrate, and interstitial fibrosis in the GTC-treated kidney. The GTCs also elicit cytoprotective functions in reducing renal oxidative stress, tubular apoptosis, and upregulation tubular expression of HO-1. Accordingly, GPSCs could be considered as a potential stem cell therapy against IR-AKI and subsequent chronic kidney damage [93].

5. Stem Cells in the Context of Clinical Use

Clinical applications of stem cell therapy are widely under investigation, as they possess anti-inflammatory, anti-fibrotic, and anti-apoptotic properties. However, clinical trials evaluating the therapeutic potentials of stem cells in AKI are still in the evolving stage, and their promise in preclinical models is yet to be translated. Dating back to 2008, the first phase 1 clinical trial (NTC00733876) evaluated the safety and efficacy of MSCs in AKI initiated with open-heart surgery. This study enrolled 16 open-heart surgical patients, and bone marrow-derived MSCs were administered into the suprarenal aorta through a femoral catheter after completion of surgery. The inclusion criteria were patients at high risk for postoperative AKI, such as old age, underlying diabetes mellitus, congestive heart failure, chronic obstructive lung disease, and pre-existing CKD stage 1-4. The exclusion criteria were active infection, evolving myocardial infarction, cardiogenic shock, history of malignancy, or advanced CKD stage 5/5D. The primary outcome was the absence of MSC-specific adverse events. During the six-month follow-up period, there were no specific or serious adverse effects observed, and this study concluded that infusions of MSCs might provide a novel and safe approach for inducing renal protection [94]. Based on this positive result, a subsequent multicenter randomized controlled trial in 2017 (NCT01602328) was conducted to determine the efficacy of allogeneic human MSCs in accelerating kidney recovery from established AKI. This phase 2 study enrolled patients who developed AKI within 48 h after cardiac surgery, and they randomized a total 156 participants to receive allogeneic MSCs (AC607, in a single dose of 2×10^6 cells/kg) or placebo administration through an intra-aortic route. The primary outcome was the time to recovery of kidney function. At the end of follow-up, although treatment with MSCs was found to be safe and tolerated well, this study concluded that administration of MSCs did not decrease the time to renal function recovery or provision for dialysis. Besides, the 30-day all-cause mortality was comparable between MSCs group and placebo group, and the rates of other major adverse kidney events were similar [95]. From these two early-phase clinical trials, the role of administering allogeneic MSCs for postcardiac surgery AKI is initially recognized. Although MSCs may be of no value as a therapy to recover renal function in established AKI, the preliminary analysis showed that MSC administration is safe at all tested doses. Unfortunately, there are no other ongoing registered clinical trials for the treatment of postcardiac surgery AKI, thus leaving unexplored the possibility of a potential beneficial effect of MSC therapy at doses higher than those reported so far.

Other clinical trials regarding AKI situation include administration of MSC to kidney transplant recipients. In a single-site, prospective, open-label, randomized study in China (NCT00658073), a total of 159 adult subjects underwent kidney transplants with allografts from living donors were divided into three groups: The standard dose ($n = 53$) and lower dose (80% of standard, $n = 52$) calcineurin inhibitors (CNI), in combination with a double intravenous infusion of autologous bone marrow-derived MSCs ($1–2 \times 10^6$/kg) at kidney reperfusion and 2 weeks later. Patients ($n = 51$) in the control group were given the anti-IL-2 receptor antibody basiliximab induction therapy, plus standard dose CNI. The main outcome included the one-year incidence of acute rejection, adverse events, patient and graft survival. Compared to the basiliximab group, this study demonstrated that the use of autologous MSC resulted in a lower incidence of acute rejection, lower risk of opportunistic infection, and better graft function at one year [96]. Another trial also suggested MSCs enable 50% reduction of CNI maintenance immunosuppression in living donor kidney transplant recipients [97]. Therefore, MSC-based therapy has proven to reduce induction and maintenance of immunosuppressive drugs without compromising patient safety and graft outcome. This may be due to the immunomodulatory activity of MSCs, but these studies, unfortunately, did not address the underlying mechanism.

A clinical trial using stem cells in treating AKI receiving continuous renal replacement therapy (CRRT) is ongoing (NCT03015623) [98]. AKI participants were treated with extracorporeal therapy with hemofiltration device containing millions of allogeneic MSCs (SBI-101) up to 24 h, designed to regulate inflammation and promote repair of injured tissue. Instead of intravenous infusion of allogeneic MSCs that are diluted rapidly throughout the body, SBI-101 allows delivery of a stable dose of cells by exposing the blood ultrafiltrate to MSCs that are immobilized on the extraluminal side of membranes within the hollow fiber dialyzer. This provides AKI patients with both standard-of-care hemofiltration as well as MSC-mediated blood conditioning in a single session. The conditioned ultrafiltrate is then delivered back to the subject, which allows for continuous exposure of the MSCs to patient blood during the CRRT treatment. In this trial, the recruitment is currently active, and subjects will be randomized into three different doses: Low dose SBI-101 containing 250 million MSCs, high dose SBI-101 containing 750 million MSCs, or sham control to characterize the pharmacokinetics and pharmacodynamics of SBI-101. In this first-in-human clinical trial, the primary outcome is its safety and tolerability. Measures of SBI-101 efficacy could be reduced patient time on dialysis or reduced patient time in the ICU.

There are still some barriers in the utilization of stem cells in clinical settings for AKI. Although MSC therapy has multiple benefits with no detrimental side effects, so far it still lacks both long-term follow-up data and the consensus in therapeutic protocols. Furthermore, the collection of MSCs from bone marrow is relatively invasive and the source is not available in a large volume. Similarly, SSC-based therapies in AKI have some limitations. Although SSCs are recognized to differentiate into renal lineages, their promise in preclinical AKI models is not yet translated in humans. Furthermore, even though SSCs can be administered in both genders, they can only be harvested from the testis and require a somewhat invasive procedure on male donors. In regard to iPSCs, c-Myc, one of the reprogramming factors to induce pluripotency, is a well-known oncogene leading to tumorigenesis. Therefore, the adverse effect of teratoma or tumor formation derived from iPSC treatment warrants significant concern. Our previous study demonstrated that rats treated with iPSCs without c-Myc effectively blocked the teratoma formation [42]. Alternatively, therapy utilizing iPSC-CM showed the promising anti-inflammatory benefits for IR-AKI and eliminated the concern of tumorigenesis as well [71]. Until now, there are few clinical trials of iPSC or stem cell-derived CM containing soluble factors and EVs in the treatment of AKI, and the future outcomes are highly expected [99].

6. Conclusions

In summary, animal experiments have provided compelling evidence to support a renoprotective role for stem cells in rescuing IR-AKI. Multiple mechanisms have been proposed to explain the beneficial effects of stem cells and their derived CM, including antioxidant, immunomodulatory, and anti-apoptotic effects (Figure 2). Another essential component of the beneficial effects of stem cells is their production of soluble paracrine factors and trophic growth factors. Moreover, recent investigations have found that stem cell-derived EVs may carry pro-regenerative micro-RNA molecules that stabilize vascular and tubular function, which has therapeutic potential for rescuing IR-AKI. Although the majority of studies in the field of IR-AKI show remarkable benefits of stem cell therapy, they are mostly confined to experimental animal models. More translational studies are needed to provide a more comprehensive understanding of stem cell-based therapies and to ensure their safety for future clinical applications.

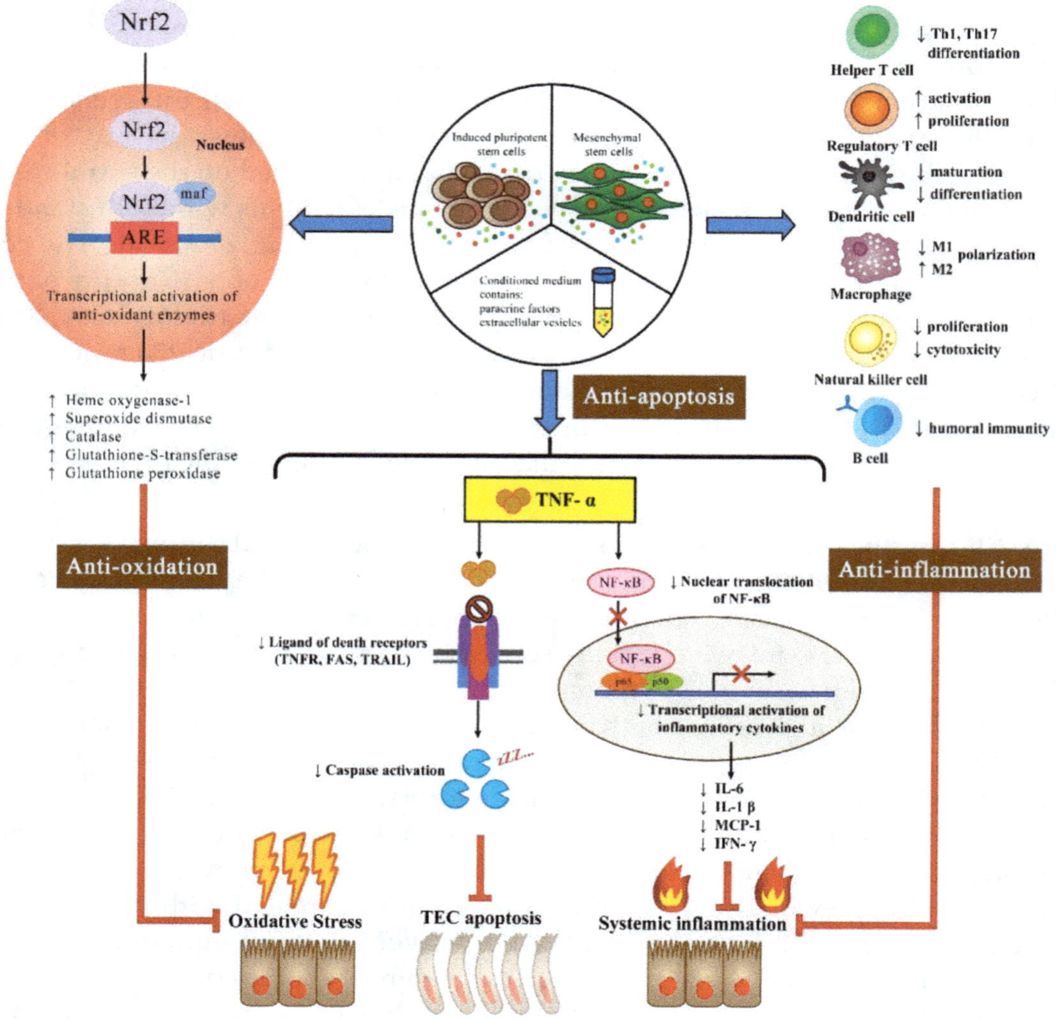

Figure 2. Illustration of proposed mechanisms of stem cell therapy in rescuing ischemia-reperfusion induced acute kidney injury. The therapeutic effects of mesenchymal stem cells, induced pluripotent stem cells, and their conditioned medium containing soluble factors and extracellular vesicles include: (1) Anti-oxidation, which may act through activation of the Nrf2/ARE pathway and, subsequently, upregulation of antioxidative enzymes against oxidative stress; (2) anti-inflammation, via immunosuppressive effects on immune cells and inhibition of NF-κB transcriptional activity; and (3) anti-apoptosis, possibly through decreased tumor necrosis factor-induced intrinsic apoptosis signaling. Abbreviations: Nrf2, NF-E2-related factor 2; ARE, antioxidant responsive element; TNF-α, tumor necrosis factor-α; TNFR, tumor necrosis factor receptor; TRAIL, TNF-related apoptosis-inducing ligand; TEC, tubular epithelial cell; NF-κB, nuclear factor-κB; MCP-1, monocyte chemoattractant protein 1; IFN-γ, Interferon-γ.

Author Contributions: K.-H.L. and D.-C.T. were involved in the planning and data collection for this review. K.-H.L., W.-C.T., C.-Y.Y., and D.-C.T. all participated in the drafting/editing of the manuscript. All of the abovementioned authors have approved the final draft of the manuscript.

References

1. Rabb, H.; Griffin, M.D.; McKay, D.B.; Swaminathan, S.; Pickkers, P.; Rosner, M.H.; Kellum, J.A.; Ronco, C.; Acute Dialysis Quality Initiative Consensus, X.W.G. Inflammation in AKI: Current Understanding, Key Questions, and Knowledge Gaps. *J. Am. Soc. Nephrol.* **2016**, *27*, 371–379. [CrossRef] [PubMed]
2. Malek, M.; Nematbakhsh, M. Renal ischemia/reperfusion injury; from pathophysiology to treatment. *J. Ren. Inj. Prev.* **2015**, *4*, 20–27. [CrossRef] [PubMed]

3. Bonventre, J.V.; Yang, L. Cellular pathophysiology of ischemic acute kidney injury. *J. Clin. Investig.* **2011**, *121*, 4210–4221. [CrossRef] [PubMed]
4. Mulay, S.R.; Holderied, A.; Kumar, S.V.; Anders, H.J. Targeting Inflammation in So-Called Acute Kidney Injury. *Semin. Nephrol.* **2016**, *36*, 17–30. [CrossRef] [PubMed]
5. Huen, S.C.; Cantley, L.G. Macrophages in Renal Injury and Repair. *Annu. Rev. Physiol.* **2017**, *79*, 449–469. [CrossRef] [PubMed]
6. Bonavia, A.; Singbartl, K. A review of the role of immune cells in acute kidney injury. *Pediatr. Nephrol.* **2018**, *33*, 1629–1639. [CrossRef]
7. Chen, L.; Deng, H.; Cui, H.; Fang, J.; Zuo, Z.; Deng, J.; Li, Y.; Wang, X.; Zhao, L. Inflammatory responses and inflammation-associated diseases in organs. *Oncotarget* **2018**, *9*, 7204–7218. [CrossRef]
8. Pino, C.J.; Humes, H.D. Stem cell technology for the treatment of acute and chronic renal failure. *Transl. Res.* **2010**, *156*, 161–168. [CrossRef]
9. Pavyde, E.; Usas, A.; Maciulaitis, R. Regenerative pharmacology for the treatment of acute kidney injury: Skeletal muscle stem/progenitor cells for renal regeneration? *Pharmacol. Res.* **2016**, *113*, 802–807. [CrossRef]
10. Zhao, H.; Alam, A.; Soo, A.P.; George, A.J.T.; Ma, D. Ischemia-Reperfusion Injury Reduces Long Term Renal Graft Survival: Mechanism and Beyond. *EBioMedicine* **2018**, *28*, 31–42. [CrossRef]
11. Aghajani Nargesi, A.; Lerman, L.O.; Eirin, A. Mesenchymal stem cell-derived extracellular vesicles for kidney repair: Current status and looming challenges. *Stem Cell Res. Ther.* **2017**, *8*, 273. [CrossRef] [PubMed]
12. Hu, H.; Zou, C. Mesenchymal Stem Cells in Renal Ischemia-Reperfusion Injury: Biological and Therapeutic Perspectives. *Curr. Stem Cell Res. Ther.* **2017**, *12*, 183–187. [CrossRef] [PubMed]
13. Yang, Y.; Song, M.; Liu, Y.; Liu, H.; Sun, L.; Peng, Y.; Liu, F.; Venkatachalam, M.A.; Dong, Z. Renoprotective approaches and strategies in acute kidney injury. *Pharmacol. Ther.* **2016**, *163*, 58–73. [CrossRef] [PubMed]
14. Agarwal, A.; Dong, Z.; Harris, R.; Murray, P.; Parikh, S.M.; Rosner, M.H.; Kellum, J.A.; Ronco, C.; Acute Dialysis Quality Initiative XIII Working Group. Cellular and Molecular Mechanisms of AKI. *J. Am. Soc. Nephrol.* **2016**, *27*, 1288–1299. [CrossRef] [PubMed]
15. Lu, L.; Zhou, H.; Ni, M.; Wang, X.; Busuttil, R.; Kupiec-Weglinski, J.; Zhai, Y. Innate Immune Regulations and Liver Ischemia-Reperfusion Injury. *Transplantation* **2016**, *100*, 2601–2610. [CrossRef] [PubMed]
16. Mulay, S.R.; Kumar, S.V.; Lech, M.; Desai, J.; Anders, H.J. How Kidney Cell Death Induces Renal Necroinflammation. *Semin. Nephrol.* **2016**, *36*, 162–173. [CrossRef] [PubMed]
17. Bolisetty, S.; Zarjou, A.; Agarwal, A. Heme Oxygenase 1 as a Therapeutic Target in Acute Kidney Injury. *Am. J. Kidney Dis.* **2017**, *69*, 531–545. [CrossRef]
18. Chung, S.; Overstreet, J.M.; Li, Y.; Wang, Y.; Niu, A.; Wang, S.; Fan, X.; Sasaki, K.; Jin, G.N.; Khodo, S.N.; et al. TGF-beta promotes fibrosis after severe acute kidney injury by enhancing renal macrophage infiltration. *JCI Insight* **2018**, *3*. [CrossRef]
19. Yi, T.; Song, S.U. Immunomodulatory properties of mesenchymal stem cells and their therapeutic applications. *Arch. Pharm. Res.* **2012**, *35*, 213–221. [CrossRef]
20. Casiraghi, F.; Perico, N.; Cortinovis, M.; Remuzzi, G. Mesenchymal stromal cells in renal transplantation: Opportunities and challenges. *Nat. Rev. Nephrol.* **2016**, *12*, 241–253. [CrossRef]
21. Gao, F.; Chiu, S.M.; Motan, D.A.; Zhang, Z.; Chen, L.; Ji, H.L.; Tse, H.F.; Fu, Q.L.; Lian, Q. Mesenchymal stem cells and immunomodulation: Current status and future prospects. *Cell Death Dis.* **2016**, *7*, e2062. [CrossRef] [PubMed]
22. Ankrum, J.A.; Ong, J.F.; Karp, J.M. Mesenchymal stem cells: Immune evasive, not immune privileged. *Nat. Biotechnol.* **2014**, *32*, 252–260. [CrossRef] [PubMed]
23. McTaggart, S.J.; Atkinson, K. Mesenchymal stem cells: Immunobiology and therapeutic potential in kidney disease. *Nephrology* **2007**, *12*, 44–52. [CrossRef] [PubMed]
24. Benvenuto, F.; Ferrari, S.; Gerdoni, E.; Gualandi, F.; Frassoni, F.; Pistoia, V.; Mancardi, G.; Uccelli, A. Human mesenchymal stem cells promote survival of T cells in a quiescent state. *Stem Cells* **2007**, *25*, 1753–1760. [CrossRef] [PubMed]
25. Su, J.; Chen, X.; Huang, Y.; Li, W.; Li, J.; Cao, K.; Cao, G.; Zhang, L.; Li, F.; Roberts, A.I.; et al. Phylogenetic distinction of iNOS and IDO function in mesenchymal stem cell-mediated immunosuppression in mammalian species. *Cell Death Differ.* **2014**, *21*, 388–396. [CrossRef] [PubMed]
26. Castro-Manrreza, M.E.; Montesinos, J.J. Immunoregulation by mesenchymal stem cells: Biological aspects and clinical applications. *J. Immunol. Res.* **2015**, *2015*, 394917. [CrossRef] [PubMed]

27. Duffy, M.M.; Ritter, T.; Ceredig, R.; Griffin, M.D. Mesenchymal stem cell effects on T-cell effector pathways. *Stem Cell Res. Ther.* **2011**, *2*, 34. [CrossRef] [PubMed]
28. Fitzsimmons, R.E.B.; Mazurek, M.S.; Soos, A.; Simmons, C.A. Mesenchymal Stromal/Stem Cells in Regenerative Medicine and Tissue Engineering. *Stem Cells Int.* **2018**, *2018*, 8031718. [CrossRef] [PubMed]
29. Cahill, E.F.; Tobin, L.M.; Carty, F.; Mahon, B.P.; English, K. Jagged-1 is required for the expansion of $CD4^+$ $CD25^+$ $FoxP3^+$ regulatory T cells and tolerogenic dendritic cells by murine mesenchymal stromal cells. *Stem Cell Res. Ther.* **2015**, *6*, 19. [CrossRef]
30. Ethokic, J.M.; Tomic, S.Z.; Colic, M.J. Cross-Talk Between Mesenchymal Stem/Stromal Cells and Dendritic Cells. *Curr. Stem Cell Res. Ther.* **2016**, *11*, 51–65.
31. Reinders, M.E.; Hoogduijn, M.J. NK Cells and MSCs: Possible Implications for MSC Therapy in Renal Transplantation. *J. Stem Cell Res. Ther.* **2014**, *4*, 1000166. [CrossRef] [PubMed]
32. Rosado, M.M.; Bernardo, M.E.; Scarsella, M.; Conforti, A.; Giorda, E.; Biagini, S.; Cascioli, S.; Rossi, F.; Guzzo, I.; Vivarelli, M.; et al. Inhibition of B-cell proliferation and antibody production by mesenchymal stromal cells is mediated by T cells. *Stem Cells Dev.* **2015**, *24*, 93–103. [CrossRef] [PubMed]
33. Jiang, Y.B.; Zhang, X.L.; Tang, Y.L.; Ma, G.S.; Shen, C.X.; Wei, Q.; Zhu, Q.; Yao, Y.Y.; Liu, N.F. Effects of heme oxygenase-1 gene modulated mesenchymal stem cells on vasculogenesis in ischemic swine hearts. *Chin. Med. J.* **2011**, *124*, 401–407. [PubMed]
34. Wang, X.; Wang, S.; Zhou, Y.; Obulkasim, H.; Zhang, Z.H.; Dai, B.; Zhu, W.; Shi, X.L. BMMSCs protect against liver ischemia/reperfusion injury via HO1 mediated autophagy. *Mol. Med. Rep.* **2018**, *18*, 2253–2262. [CrossRef] [PubMed]
35. Chen, X.; Zhang, Y.; Wang, W.; Liu, Z.; Meng, J.; Han, Z. Mesenchymal Stem Cells Modified with Heme Oxygenase-1 Have Enhanced Paracrine Function and Attenuate Lipopolysaccharide-Induced Inflammatory and Oxidative Damage in Pulmonary Microvascular Endothelial Cells. *Cell. Physiol. Biochem.* **2018**, *49*, 101–122. [CrossRef]
36. Zarjou, A.; Kim, J.; Traylor, A.M.; Sanders, P.W.; Balla, J.; Agarwal, A.; Curtis, L.M. Paracrine effects of mesenchymal stem cells in cisplatin-induced renal injury require heme oxygenase-1. *Am. J. Physiol. Ren. Physiol.* **2011**, *300*, F254–F262. [CrossRef]
37. Liu, D.; Xu, J.; Liu, O.; Fan, Z.; Liu, Y.; Wang, F.; Ding, G.; Wei, F.; Zhang, C.; Wang, S. Mesenchymal stem cells derived from inflamed periodontal ligaments exhibit impaired immunomodulation. *J. Clin. Periodontol.* **2012**, *39*, 1174–1182. [CrossRef]
38. Najar, M.; Krayem, M.; Meuleman, N.; Bron, D.; Lagneaux, L. Mesenchymal Stromal Cells and Toll-Like Receptor Priming: A Critical Review. *Immune Netw.* **2017**, *17*, 89–102. [CrossRef]
39. Waterman, R.S.; Tomchuck, S.L.; Henkle, S.L.; Betancourt, A.M. A new mesenchymal stem cell (MSC) paradigm: Polarization into a pro-inflammatory MSC1 or an Immunosuppressive MSC2 phenotype. *PLoS ONE* **2010**, *5*, e10088. [CrossRef]
40. Levin, S.; Pevsner-Fischer, M.; Kagan, S.; Lifshitz, H.; Weinstock, A.; Gataulin, D.; Friedlander, G.; Zipori, D. Divergent levels of LBP and TGFbeta1 in murine MSCs lead to heterogenic response to TLR and proinflammatory cytokine activation. *Stem Cell Rev.* **2014**, *10*, 376–388. [CrossRef]
41. Schnabel, L.V.; Abratte, C.M.; Schimenti, J.C.; Felippe, M.J.; Cassano, J.M.; Southard, T.L.; Cross, J.A.; Fortier, L.A. Induced pluripotent stem cells have similar immunogenic and more potent immunomodulatory properties compared with bone marrow-derived stromal cells in vitro. *Regen. Med.* **2014**, *9*, 621–635. [CrossRef]
42. Lee, P.Y.; Chien, Y.; Chiou, G.Y.; Lin, C.H.; Chiou, C.H.; Tarng, D.C. Induced pluripotent stem cells without c-Myc attenuate acute kidney injury via downregulating the signaling of oxidative stress and inflammation in ischemia-reperfusion rats. *Cell Transplant.* **2012**, *21*, 2569–2585. [CrossRef]
43. Yen, B.L.; Chang, C.J.; Liu, K.J.; Chen, Y.C.; Hu, H.I.; Bai, C.H.; Yen, M.L. Brief report—Human embryonic stem cell-derived mesenchymal progenitors possess strong immunosuppressive effects toward natural killer cells as well as T lymphocytes. *Stem Cells* **2009**, *27*, 451–456. [CrossRef]
44. Gao, W.X.; Sun, Y.Q.; Shi, J.; Li, C.L.; Fang, S.B.; Wang, D.; Deng, X.Q.; Wen, W.; Fu, Q.L. Effects of mesenchymal stem cells from human induced pluripotent stem cells on differentiation, maturation, and function of dendritic cells. *Stem Cell Res. Ther.* **2017**, *8*, 48. [CrossRef]
45. Tan, Z.; Su, Z.Y.; Wu, R.R.; Gu, B.; Liu, Y.K.; Zhao, X.L.; Zhang, M. Immunomodulative effects of mesenchymal stem cells derived from human embryonic stem cells in vivo and in vitro. *J. Zhejiang Univ. Sci. B* **2011**, *12*, 18–27. [CrossRef]

46. Korthuis, R.J. Mechanisms of I/R-Induced Endothelium-Dependent Vasodilator Dysfunction. *Adv. Pharmacol.* **2018**, *81*, 331–364. [CrossRef]
47. Gonzalez-Vicente, A.; Garvin, J.L. Effects of Reactive Oxygen Species on Tubular Transport along the Nephron. *Antioxidants* **2017**, *6*, 23. [CrossRef]
48. Marko, L.; Vigolo, E.; Hinze, C.; Park, J.K.; Roel, G.; Balogh, A.; Choi, M.; Wubken, A.; Cording, J.; Blasig, I.E.; et al. Tubular Epithelial NF-kappaB Activity Regulates Ischemic AKI. *J. Am. Soc. Nephrol.* **2016**, *27*, 2658–2669. [CrossRef]
49. Shih, Y.C.; Lee, P.Y.; Cheng, H.; Tsai, C.H.; Ma, H.; Tarng, D.C. Adipose-derived stem cells exhibit antioxidative and antiapoptotic properties to rescue ischemic acute kidney injury in rats. *Plast. Reconstr. Surg.* **2013**, *132*, 940e–951e. [CrossRef]
50. Zhang, J.B.; Wang, X.Q.; Lu, G.L.; Huang, H.S.; Xu, S.Y. Adipose-derived mesenchymal stem cells therapy for acute kidney injury induced by ischemia-reperfusion in a rat model. *Clin. Exp. Pharmacol. Physiol.* **2017**, *44*, 1232–1240. [CrossRef]
51. Havakhah, S.; Sankian, M.; Kazemzadeh, G.H.; Sadri, K.; Bidkhori, H.R.; Naderi-Meshkin, H.; Ebrahimzadeh Bideskan, A.; Niazmand, S.; Bahrami, A.R.; Khajavi Rad, A. In vivo effects of allogeneic mesenchymal stem cells in a rat model of acute ischemic kidney injury. *Iran. J. Basic Med. Sci.* **2018**, *21*, 824–831. [CrossRef]
52. Lee, K.W.; Kim, T.M.; Kim, K.S.; Lee, S.; Cho, J.; Park, J.B.; Kwon, G.Y.; Kim, S.J. Renal Ischemia-Reperfusion Injury in a Diabetic Monkey Model and Therapeutic Testing of Human Bone Marrow-Derived Mesenchymal Stem Cells. *J. Diabetes Res.* **2018**, *2018*, 5182606. [CrossRef]
53. Orbay, H.; Tobita, M.; Mizuno, H. Mesenchymal stem cells isolated from adipose and other tissues: Basic biological properties and clinical applications. *Stem Cells Int.* **2012**, *2012*, 461718. [CrossRef]
54. Zhang, Z.H.; Zhu, W.; Ren, H.Z.; Zhao, X.; Wang, S.; Ma, H.C.; Shi, X.L. Mesenchymal stem cells increase expression of heme oxygenase-1 leading to anti-inflammatory activity in treatment of acute liver failure. *Stem Cell Res. Ther.* **2017**, *8*, 70. [CrossRef]
55. Sung, P.H.; Chang, C.L.; Tsai, T.H.; Chang, L.T.; Leu, S.; Chen, Y.L.; Yang, C.C.; Chua, S.; Yeh, K.H.; Chai, H.T.; et al. Apoptotic adipose-derived mesenchymal stem cell therapy protects against lung and kidney injury in sepsis syndrome caused by cecal ligation puncture in rats. *Stem Cell Res. Ther.* **2013**, *4*, 155. [CrossRef]
56. Du, T.; Cheng, J.; Zhong, L.; Zhao, X.F.; Zhu, J.; Zhu, Y.J.; Liu, G.H. The alleviation of acute and chronic kidney injury by human Wharton's jelly-derived mesenchymal stromal cells triggered by ischemia-reperfusion injury via an endocrine mechanism. *Cytotherapy* **2012**, *14*, 1215–1227. [CrossRef]
57. Zhang, D.; Fu, L.; Wang, L.; Lin, L.; Yu, L.; Zhang, L.; Shang, T. Therapeutic benefit of mesenchymal stem cells in pregnant rats with angiotensin receptor agonistic autoantibody-induced hypertension: Implications for immunomodulation and cytoprotection. *Hypertens. Pregnancy* **2017**, *36*, 247–258. [CrossRef]
58. Camara, N.O.; Soares, M.P. Heme oxygenase-1 (HO-1), a protective gene that prevents chronic graft dysfunction. *Free Radic. Biol. Med.* **2005**, *38*, 426–435. [CrossRef]
59. Liu, N.; Wang, H.; Han, G.; Tian, J.; Hu, W.; Zhang, J. Alleviation of apoptosis of bone marrow-derived mesenchymal stem cells in the acute injured kidney by heme oxygenase-1 gene modification. *Int. J. Biochem. Cell Biol.* **2015**, *69*, 85–94. [CrossRef]
60. Turkseven, S.; Kruger, A.; Mingone, C.J.; Kaminski, P.; Inaba, M.; Rodella, L.F.; Ikehara, S.; Wolin, M.S.; Abraham, N.G. Antioxidant mechanism of heme oxygenase-1 involves an increase in superoxide dismutase and catalase in experimental diabetes. *Am. J. Physiol. Heart Circ. Physiol.* **2005**, *289*, H701–H707. [CrossRef]
61. Tsai, M.T.; Tarng, D.C. Beyond a Measure of Liver Function-Bilirubin Acts as a Potential Cardiovascular Protector in Chronic Kidney Disease Patients. *Int. J. Mol. Sci.* **2018**, *20*, 117. [CrossRef]
62. Liu, H.; McTaggart, S.J.; Johnson, D.W.; Gobe, G.C. Anti-oxidant pathways are stimulated by mesenchymal stromal cells in renal repair after ischemic injury. *Cytotherapy* **2012**, *14*, 162–172. [CrossRef]
63. Agarwal, A.; Bolisetty, S. Adaptive responses to tissue injury: Role of heme oxygenase-1. *Trans. Am. Clin. Climatol. Assoc.* **2013**, *124*, 111–122.
64. Liu, N.; Wang, H.; Han, G.; Cheng, J.; Hu, W.; Zhang, J. Enhanced proliferation and differentiation of HO-1 gene-modified bone marrow-derived mesenchymal stem cells in the acute injured kidney. *Int. J. Mol. Med.* **2018**, *42*, 946–956. [CrossRef]
65. Mates, J.M. Effects of antioxidant enzymes in the molecular control of reactive oxygen species toxicology. *Toxicology* **2000**, *153*, 83–104. [CrossRef]
66. Zhuo, W.; Liao, L.; Xu, T.; Wu, W.; Yang, S.; Tan, J. Mesenchymal stem cells ameliorate ischemia-reperfusion-induced renal dysfunction by improving the antioxidant/oxidant balance in the

ischemic kidney. *Urol. Int.* **2011**, *86*, 191–196. [CrossRef]
67. Fahmy, S.R.; Soliman, A.M.; El Ansary, M.; Elhamid, S.A.; Mohsen, H. Therapeutic efficacy of human umbilical cord mesenchymal stem cells transplantation against renal ischemia/reperfusion injury in rats. *Tissue Cell* **2017**, *49*, 369–375. [CrossRef]
68. Inan, M.; Bakar, E.; Cerkezkayabekir, A.; Sanal, F.; Ulucam, E.; Subasi, C.; Karaoz, E. Mesenchymal stem cells increase antioxidant capacity in intestinal ischemia/reperfusion damage. *J. Pediatr. Surg.* **2017**, *52*, 1196–1206. [CrossRef]
69. Zhang, G.; Zou, X.; Huang, Y.; Wang, F.; Miao, S.; Liu, G.; Chen, M.; Zhu, Y. Mesenchymal Stromal Cell-Derived Extracellular Vesicles Protect Against Acute Kidney Injury Through Anti-Oxidation by Enhancing Nrf2/ARE Activation in Rats. *Kidney Blood Press. Res.* **2016**, *41*, 119–128. [CrossRef]
70. Zhang, G.; Zou, X.; Miao, S.; Chen, J.; Du, T.; Zhong, L.; Ju, G.; Liu, G.; Zhu, Y. The anti-oxidative role of micro-vesicles derived from human Wharton-Jelly mesenchymal stromal cells through NOX2/gp91(phox) suppression in alleviating renal ischemia-reperfusion injury in rats. *PLoS ONE* **2014**, *9*, e92129. [CrossRef]
71. Tarng, D.C.; Tseng, W.C.; Lee, P.Y.; Chiou, S.H.; Hsieh, S.L. Induced Pluripotent Stem Cell-Derived Conditioned Medium Attenuates Acute Kidney Injury by Downregulating the Oxidative Stress-Related Pathway in Ischemia-Reperfusion Rats. *Cell Transplant.* **2016**, *25*, 517–530. [CrossRef]
72. Borkan, S.C. The Role of BCL-2 Family Members in Acute Kidney Injury. *Semin. Nephrol.* **2016**, *36*, 237–250. [CrossRef]
73. Plotnikov, E.Y.; Kazachenko, A.V.; Vyssokikh, M.Y.; Vasileva, A.K.; Tcvirkun, D.V.; Isaev, N.K.; Kirpatovsky, V.I.; Zorov, D.B. The role of mitochondria in oxidative and nitrosative stress during ischemia/reperfusion in the rat kidney. *Kidney Int.* **2007**, *72*, 1493–1502. [CrossRef]
74. Jacobs, K.M.; Bhave, S.R.; Ferraro, D.J.; Jaboin, J.J.; Hallahan, D.E.; Thotala, D. GSK-3beta: A Bifunctional Role in Cell Death Pathways. *Int. J. Cell Biol.* **2012**, *2012*, 930710. [CrossRef]
75. Devarapu, S.K.; Grill, J.F.; Xie, J.; Weidenbusch, M.; Honarpisheh, M.; Vielhauer, V.; Anders, H.J.; Mulay, S.R. Tumor necrosis factor superfamily ligand mRNA expression profiles differ between humans and mice during homeostasis and between various murine kidney injuries. *J. Biomed. Sci.* **2017**, *24*, 77. [CrossRef]
76. Wu, C.C.; Bratton, S.B. Regulation of the intrinsic apoptosis pathway by reactive oxygen species. *Antioxid. Redox Signal.* **2013**, *19*, 546–558. [CrossRef]
77. Dorstyn, L.; Akey, C.W.; Kumar, S. New insights into apoptosome structure and function. *Cell Death Differ.* **2018**, *25*, 1194–1208. [CrossRef]
78. Humphreys, B.D.; Cantaluppi, V.; Portilla, D.; Singbartl, K.; Yang, L.; Rosner, M.H.; Kellum, J.A.; Ronco, C.; Acute Dialysis Quality Initiative XIII Working Group. Targeting Endogenous Repair Pathways after AKI. *J. Am. Soc. Nephrol.* **2016**, *27*, 990–998. [CrossRef]
79. Rowart, P.; Erpicum, P.; Detry, O.; Weekers, L.; Gregoire, C.; Lechanteur, C.; Briquet, A.; Beguin, Y.; Krzesinski, J.M.; Jouret, F. Mesenchymal Stromal Cell Therapy in Ischemia/Reperfusion Injury. *J. Immunol. Res.* **2015**, *2015*, 602597. [CrossRef]
80. Fleig, S.V.; Humphreys, B.D. Rationale of mesenchymal stem cell therapy in kidney injury. *Nephron Clin. Pract.* **2014**, *127*, 75–80. [CrossRef]
81. Bianchi, F.; Sala, E.; Donadei, C.; Capelli, I.; La Manna, G. Potential advantages of acute kidney injury management by mesenchymal stem cells. *World J. Stem Cells* **2014**, *6*, 644–650. [CrossRef]
82. Naji, A.; Favier, B.; Deschaseaux, F.; Rouas-Freiss, N.; Eitoku, M.; Suganuma, N. Mesenchymal stem/stromal cell function in modulating cell death. *Stem Cell Res. Ther.* **2019**, *10*, 56. [CrossRef]
83. Gnecchi, M.; Danieli, P.; Malpasso, G.; Ciuffreda, M.C. Paracrine Mechanisms of Mesenchymal Stem Cells in Tissue Repair. *Methods Mol. Biol.* **2016**, *1416*, 123–146. [CrossRef]
84. Borger, V.; Bremer, M.; Ferrer-Tur, R.; Gockeln, L.; Stambouli, O.; Becic, A.; Giebel, B. Mesenchymal Stem/Stromal Cell-Derived Extracellular Vesicles and Their Potential as Novel Immunomodulatory Therapeutic Agents. *Int. J. Mol. Sci.* **2017**, *18*, 1450. [CrossRef]
85. Li, N.; Long, B.; Han, W.; Yuan, S.; Wang, K. microRNAs: Important regulators of stem cells. *Stem Cell Res. Ther.* **2017**, *8*, 110. [CrossRef]
86. Nargesi, A.A.; Lerman, L.O.; Eirin, A. Mesenchymal Stem Cell-derived Extracellular Vesicles for Renal Repair. *Curr. Gene Ther.* **2017**, *17*, 29–42. [CrossRef]
87. Osafune, K. Cell therapy for kidney injury: Different options and mechanisms–kidney progenitor cells. *Nephron Exp. Nephrol.* **2014**, *126*, 64. [CrossRef]
88. Toyohara, T.; Mae, S.; Sueta, S.; Inoue, T.; Yamagishi, Y.; Kawamoto, T.; Kasahara, T.; Hoshina, A.; Toyoda, T.;

Tanaka, H.; et al. Cell Therapy Using Human Induced Pluripotent Stem Cell-Derived Renal Progenitors Ameliorates Acute Kidney Injury in Mice. *Stem Cells Transl. Med.* **2015**, *4*, 980–992. [CrossRef]

89. Li, Q.; Tian, S.F.; Guo, Y.; Niu, X.; Hu, B.; Guo, S.C.; Wang, N.S.; Wang, Y. Transplantation of induced pluripotent stem cell-derived renal stem cells improved acute kidney injury. *Cell Biosci.* **2015**, *5*, 45. [CrossRef]
90. Ko, S.F.; Chen, Y.T.; Wallace, C.G.; Chen, K.H.; Sung, P.H.; Cheng, B.C.; Huang, T.H.; Chen, Y.L.; Li, Y.C.; Chang, H.W.; et al. Inducible pluripotent stem cell-derived mesenchymal stem cell therapy effectively protected kidney from acute ischemia-reperfusion injury. *Am. J. Transl. Res.* **2018**, *10*, 3053–3067.
91. Shen, W.C.; Chou, Y.H.; Huang, H.P.; Sheen, J.F.; Hung, S.C.; Chen, H.F. Induced pluripotent stem cell-derived endothelial progenitor cells attenuate ischemic acute kidney injury and cardiac dysfunction. *Stem Cell Res. Ther.* **2018**, *9*, 344. [CrossRef]
92. Wu, D.P.; He, D.L.; Li, X.; Liu, Z.H. Differentiations of transplanted mouse spermatogonial stem cells in the adult mouse renal parenchyma in vivo. *Acta Pharmacol. Sin.* **2008**, *29*, 1029–1034. [CrossRef]
93. De Chiara, L.; Fagoonee, S.; Ranghino, A.; Bruno, S.; Camussi, G.; Tolosano, E.; Silengo, L.; Altruda, F. Renal cells from spermatogonial germline stem cells protect against kidney injury. *J. Am. Soc. Nephrol.* **2014**, *25*, 316–328. [CrossRef]
94. Togel, F.E.; Westenfelder, C. Kidney protection and regeneration following acute injury: Progress through stem cell therapy. *Am. J. Kidney Dis.* **2012**, *60*, 1012–1022. [CrossRef]
95. Swaminathan, M.; Stafford-Smith, M.; Chertow, G.M.; Warnock, D.G.; Paragamian, V.; Brenner, R.M.; Lellouche, F.; Fox-Robichaud, A.; Atta, M.G.; Melby, S.; et al. Allogeneic Mesenchymal Stem Cells for Treatment of AKI after Cardiac Surgery. *J. Am. Soc. Nephrol.* **2018**, *29*, 260–267. [CrossRef]
96. Tan, J.; Wu, W.; Xu, X.; Liao, L.; Zheng, F.; Messinger, S.; Sun, X.; Chen, J.; Yang, S.; Cai, J.; et al. Induction therapy with autologous mesenchymal stem cells in living-related kidney transplants: A randomized controlled trial. *JAMA* **2012**, *307*, 1169–1177. [CrossRef]
97. Pan, G.H.; Chen, Z.; Xu, L.; Zhu, J.H.; Xiang, P.; Ma, J.J.; Peng, Y.W.; Li, G.H.; Chen, X.Y.; Fang, J.L.; et al. Low-dose tacrolimus combined with donor-derived mesenchymal stem cells after renal transplantation: A prospective, non-randomized study. *Oncotarget* **2016**, *7*, 12089–12101. [CrossRef]
98. Miller, B.L.K.; Garg, P.; Bronstein, B.; LaPointe, E.; Lin, H.; Charytan, D.M.; Tilles, A.W.; Parekkadan, B. Extracorporeal Stromal Cell Therapy for Subjects With Dialysis-Dependent Acute Kidney Injury. *Kidney Int. Rep.* **2018**, *3*, 1119–1127. [CrossRef]
99. Rota, C.; Morigi, M.; Imberti, B. Stem Cell Therapies in Kidney Diseases: Progress and Challenges. *Int. J. Mol. Sci.* **2019**, *20*, 2790. [CrossRef]

Permissions

All chapters in this book were first published by MDPI; hereby published with permission under the Creative Commons Attribution License or equivalent. Every chapter published in this book has been scrutinized by our experts. Their significance has been extensively debated. The topics covered herein carry significant findings which will fuel the growth of the discipline. They may even be implemented as practical applications or may be referred to as a beginning point for another development.

The contributors of this book come from diverse backgrounds, making this book a truly international effort. This book will bring forth new frontiers with its revolutionizing research information and detailed analysis of the nascent developments around the world.

We would like to thank all the contributing authors for lending their expertise to make the book truly unique. They have played a crucial role in the development of this book. Without their invaluable contributions this book wouldn't have been possible. They have made vital efforts to compile up to date information on the varied aspects of this subject to make this book a valuable addition to the collection of many professionals and students.

This book was conceptualized with the vision of imparting up-to-date information and advanced data in this field. To ensure the same, a matchless editorial board was set up. Every individual on the board went through rigorous rounds of assessment to prove their worth. After which they invested a large part of their time researching and compiling the most relevant data for our readers.

The editorial board has been involved in producing this book since its inception. They have spent rigorous hours researching and exploring the diverse topics which have resulted in the successful publishing of this book. They have passed on their knowledge of decades through this book. To expedite this challenging task, the publisher supported the team at every step. A small team of assistant editors was also appointed to further simplify the editing procedure and attain best results for the readers.

Apart from the editorial board, the designing team has also invested a significant amount of their time in understanding the subject and creating the most relevant covers. They scrutinized every image to scout for the most suitable representation of the subject and create an appropriate cover for the book.

The publishing team has been an ardent support to the editorial, designing and production team. Their endless efforts to recruit the best for this project, has resulted in the accomplishment of this book. They are a veteran in the field of academics and their pool of knowledge is as vast as their experience in printing. Their expertise and guidance has proved useful at every step. Their uncompromising quality standards have made this book an exceptional effort. Their encouragement from time to time has been an inspiration for everyone.

The publisher and the editorial board hope that this book will prove to be a valuable piece of knowledge for researchers, students, practitioners and scholars across the globe.

List of Contributors

Kurt T. K. Giuliani, Helen Healy and Pedro H. F. Gois
Kidney Health Service, Royal Brisbane and Women's Hospital, Brisbane, QLD 4029, Australia
Conjoint Kidney Research Laboratory, Chemical Pathology – Pathology Queensland, Brisbane, QLD 4029, Australia
Faculty of Medicine, University of Queensland, Brisbane, QLD 4006, Australia

Andrew J. Kassianos
Kidney Health Service, Royal Brisbane and Women's Hospital, Brisbane, QLD 4029, Australia
Conjoint Kidney Research Laboratory, Chemical Pathology – Pathology Queensland, Brisbane, QLD 4029, Australia
Faculty of Medicine, University of Queensland, Brisbane, QLD 4006, Australia
Institute of Health and Biomedical Innovation/School of Biomedical Sciences, Queensland University of Technology, Brisbane, QLD 4059, Australia

Paola Romagnani and Francesco Guzzi
Excellence Centre for Research, Transfer and High Education for the development of DE NOVO Therapies (DENOTHE), University of Florence, 50139 Florence, Italy Department of Experimental and Clinical Biomedical Sciences "Mario Serio", University of Florence, 50134 Florence, Italy
Nephrology and Dialysis Unit, Meyer Children's University Hospital, 50139 Florence, Italy

Luigi Cirillo and Rosa Maria Roperto
Nephrology and Dialysis Unit, Meyer Children's University Hospital, 50139 Florence, Italy

Elena Lazzeri
Excellence Centre for Research, Transfer and High Education for the development of DE NOVO Therapies (DENOTHE), University of Florence, 50139 Florence, Italy Department of Experimental and Clinical Biomedical Sciences "Mario Serio", University of Florence, 50134 Florence, Italy

Tianqi Wang
Traditional Chinese Medicine History and Literature, Institute for Literature and Culture of Chinese Medicine, Shandong University of Traditional Chinese Medicine, Jinan 250355, China
Institute for Literature and Culture of Chinese Medicine, Shandong University of Traditional Chinese Medicine, Jinan 250355, China

Xianjun Fu
Institute for Literature and Culture of Chinese Medicine, Shandong University of Traditional Chinese Medicine, Jinan 250355, China
Key Laboratory of Traditional Chinese Medicine for Classical Theory, Ministry of Education, Shandong University of Traditional Chinese Medicine, Jinan 250355, China

Zhenguo Wang
Institute for Literature and Culture of Chinese Medicine, Shandong University of Traditional Chinese Medicine, Jinan 250355, China

Zhibo Gai
Key Laboratory of Traditional Chinese Medicine for Classical Theory, Ministry of Education, Shandong University of Traditional Chinese Medicine, Jinan 250355, China

Qingfa Chen
The Institute for Tissue Engineering and Regenerative Medicine, The Liaocheng University, Liaocheng 252000, China

Jayanta Kumar Patra
Research Institute of Biotechnology & Medical Converged Science, Dongguk University-Seoul, Goyangsi 10326, Korea

Dongdong Wang
Institute of Clinical Chemistry, University Hospital Zurich, University of Zurich, Wagistrasse 14, 8952 Schlieren, Switzerland
Guizhou University of Traditional Chinese Medicine, Fei Shan Jie 32, Guiyang 550003, China

Jia-Feng Chang
Division of Nephrology, Department of Internal Medicine, En Chu Kong Hospital, New Taipei City 237, Taiwan
Renal Care Joint Foundation, New Taipei City 220, Taiwan
Department of Nursing, Yuanpei University of Medical Technology, Hsinchu 300, Taiwan
Graduate Institution of Biomedical and Pharmaceutical Science, College of Medicine, Fu Jen Catholic University, New Taipei City 242, Taiwan
Division of Nephrology, Department of Internal Medicine, Shuang Ho Hospital, Taipei Medical University, New Taipei City 235, Taiwan

Jih-Chen Yeh
Renal Care Joint Foundation, New Taipei City 220, Taiwan
Department of Dentistry, Far Eastern Memorial Hospital, New Taipei City 220, Taiwan

Chun-Ta Ho
Renal Care Joint Foundation, New Taipei City 220, Taiwan

Chih-Yu Hsieh
Division of Nephrology, Department of Internal Medicine, En Chu Kong Hospital, New Taipei City 237, Taiwan
Renal Care Joint Foundation, New Taipei City 220, Taiwan

Jen-Yu Wang and Wei-Ning Lin
Graduate Institution of Biomedical and Pharmaceutical Science, College of Medicine, Fu Jen Catholic University, New Taipei City 242, Taiwan

Shih-Hao Liu
Division of Pathology, En-Chu-Kong Hospital, New Taipei City 237, Taiwan

Ting-Ming Wang
Department of Orthopaedic Surgery, School of Medicine, National Taiwan University, Taipei 106, Taiwan Department of Orthopaedic Surgery, National Taiwan University Hospital, Taipei 106, Taiwan

Shu-Wei Chang
Department of Civil Engineering, National Taiwan University, Taipei 106, Taiwan

I-Ta Lee
School of Dentistry, College of Oral Medicine, Taipei Medical University, Taipei 110, Taiwan

Kuo-Yang Huang
Graduate Institute of Pathology and Parasitology, National Defense Medical Center, Taipei 114, Taiwan

Marta Tapparo, Stefania Bruno, Gabriele Togliatto and Giovanni Camussi
Department of Medical Sciences and Molecular Biotechnology Center, University of Torino, 10126 Torino, Italy

Federica Collino
Department of Biomedical Sciences and Paediatric Research Institute "Citta della Speranza", University of Padova, 35129 Padova, Italy

Maria Chiara Deregibus
2i3T Società per la gestione dell'incubatore di imprese e per il trasferimento tecnologico Scarl, University of Torino, 10126 Torino, Italy

Paolo Provero
Department of Molecular Biotechnology and Health Sciences and Molecular Biotechnology Center, University of Torino, 10126 Torino, Italy

Sicheng Wen and Peter J. Quesenberry
Division of Hematology/Oncology, Brown University, Rhode Island Hospital, Providence, Rhode Island, RI 02912, USA

Kai-Uwe Eckardt
Department of Nephrology and Medical Intensive Care, Charité-Universitätsmedizin Berlin, 13353 Berlin, Germany

Laura Katharina Sievers
Department of Nephrology and Medical Intensive Care, Charité-Universitätsmedizin Berlin, 13353 Berlin, Germany
Max-Delbrück Center for Molecular Medicine in the Helmholtz Association, 13125 Berlin, Germany
Experimental and Clinical Research Center, a joint cooperation of Max-Delbrück Center for Molecular Medicine and Charité-Universitätsmedizin Berlin, 13125 Berlin, Germany
Berlin Institute of Health (BIH), 10178 Berlin, Germany

Benjamin Bochon
Psychiatric Services of Thurgovia, Academic Teaching Hospital of the Medical University of Salzburg, 8596 Münsterlingen, Switzerland

Magdalena Kozubska
General Practice, 43-426 Dębowiec, Poland

Grzegorz Surygała
Regional Blood Donation and Blood Treatment Centre, 40-074 Katowice, Poland

Agnieszka Witkowska
DaVita Dialysis, 42-700 Lubliniec, Poland

Roman Kuźniewicz, Władysław Grzeszczak and Grzegorz Wystrychowski
Department of Internal Medicine, Diabetology and Nephrology, School of Medicine with the Division of Dentistry in Zabrze, Medical University of Silesia in Katowice, 41-800 Zabrze, Poland

Chul Won Yun
Medical Science Research Institute, Soonchunhyang University Seoul Hospital, Seoul 04401, Korea

Sang Hun Lee
Medical Science Research Institute, Soonchunhyang University Seoul Hospital, Seoul 04401, Korea
Department of Biochemistry, Soonchunhyang University College of Medicine, Cheonan 34538, Korea

Giuseppe Castellano, Alessandra Stasi, Rossana Franzin, Chiara Divella, Alessandra Spinelli, Simona Simone, Giovanni Battista Pertosa and Loreto Gesualdo
Nephrology, Dialysis and Transplantation Unit, Department of Emergency and Organ Transplantation, University of Bari, 70124 Bari, Italy

Fabio Sallustio
Nephrology, Dialysis and Transplantation Unit, Department of Emergency and Organ Transplantation, University of Bari, 70124 Bari, Italy
Department of Basic Medical Sciences, Neuroscience and Sense Organs, University of Bari, 70124 Bari, Italy

Giuseppe Stefano Netti and Giuseppe Grandaliano
Nephrology, Dialysis and Transplantation Unit, Department of Medical and Surgical Sciences, University of Foggia, 71122 Foggia, Italy

Enrico Fiaccadori
Nephrology Unit, Department of Medicine and Surgery, University of Parma, 43121 Parma, Italy

Vincenzo Cantaluppi
Department of Translational Medicine, University of Piemonte Orientale, 28100 Novara, Italy

Antonio Crovace, Francesco Staffieri and Luca Lacitignola
Veterinary Surgery Unit, Department of Emergency and Organ Transplantation, University of Bari, 70010 Bari, Italy

Jenny Frese and Oliver Gross
Clinic of Nephrology and Rheumatology, University Medical Center Goettingen, 37075 Goettingen, Germany

Matthias Kettwig and Hildegard Zappel
Clinic of Pediatrics and Adolescent Medicine, University Medical Center Goettingen, 37075 Goettingen, Germany

Johannes Hofer
Department of Pediatrics, Pediatrics I, Innsbruck Medical University, 6020 Innsbruck, Austria

Hermann-Josef Gröne
Department of Cellular and Molecular Pathology, German Cancer Research Center, 69120 Heidelberg, Germany

Mato Nagel
Center for Nephrology and Metabolic Disorders, Molecular Diagnostics, 02943 Weißwasser, Germany

Gere Sunder-Plassmann
Division of Nephrology and Dialysis, Department of Medicine III, Medical University of Vienna, 1090 Vienna, Austria

Renate Kain
Department of Pathology, Medical University of Vienna, 1090 Vienna, Austria

Jörg Neuweiler
Institute of Pathology, Kantonsspital, 9007 St. Gallen, Switzerland

Juan Antonio Moreno and Melania Guerrero-Hue
Renal, Vascular and Diabetes Research Laboratory. Fundacion Jimenez Diaz University Hospital-Health Research Institute (FIIS-FJD), Autonoma University of Madrid (UAM), 28040 Madrid, Spain
Department of Cell Biology, Physiology, and Immunology, Maimonides Biomedical Research Institute of Cordoba (IMIBIC), University of Cordoba, 14014 Cordoba, Spain

Cristina Vázquez-Carballo, Carmen Herencia and Cristina García-Caballero
Renal, Vascular and Diabetes Research Laboratory. Fundacion Jimenez Diaz University Hospital-Health Research Institute (FIIS-FJD), Autonoma University of Madrid (UAM), 28040 Madrid, Spain

Ángel Sevillano, Eduardo Gutiérrez, Manuel Praga and Claudia Yuste
Department of Nephrology, Hospital 12 de Octubre, 28040 Madrid, Spain

Jesús Egido
Renal, Vascular and Diabetes Research Laboratory. Fundacion Jimenez Diaz University Hospital-Health Research Institute (FIIS-FJD), Autonoma University of Madrid (UAM), 28040 Madrid, Spain
Spanish Biomedical Research Centre in Diabetes and Associated Metabolic Disorders (CIBERDEM), 28040 Madrid, Spain

Mary Taub
Biochemistry Dept, Jacobs School of Medicine and Biomedical Sciences, University at Buffalo, 955 Main Street Suite 4102, Buffalo, NY 14203, USA

Vjera Ninčević, Martina Smolić and Tea Omanović Kolarić
Department of Pharmacology, Faculty of Medicine, Josip Juraj Strossmayer University of Osijek, J. Huttlera 4, 31000 Osijek, Croatia
Department of Pharmacology and Biochemistry, Faculty of Dental Medicine and Health, Josip Juraj Strossmayer University of Osijek, Crkvena 21, 31000 Osijek, Croatia

Hrvoje Roguljić
Department of Pharmacology, Faculty of Medicine, Josip Juraj Strossmayer University of Osijek, J. Huttlera 4, 31000 Osijek, Croatia
Department for Cardiovascular Disease, University Hospital Osijek, 4, 31000 Osijek, Croatia

Tomislav Kizivat
Clinical Institute of Nuclear Medicine and Radiation Protection, University Hospital Osijek, 31000 Osijek, Croatia
Department for Nuclear Medicine and Oncology, Faculty of Medicine, Josip Juraj Strossmayer University of Osijek; J. Huttlera 4, 31000 Osijek, Croatia

Ines Bilić Ćurčić
Department of Pharmacology, Faculty of Medicine, Josip Juraj Strossmayer University of Osijek, J. Huttlera 4, 31000 Osijek, Croatia
Department of Diabetes, Endocrinology and Metabolism Disorders, University Hospital Osijek, 31000 Osijek, Croatia

Kuo-Hua Lee, Wei-Cheng Tseng and Chih-Yu Yang
Division of Nephrology, Department of Medicine, Taipei Veterans General Hospital, Taipei 11217, Taiwan Institute of Clinical Medicine, National Yang-Ming University, Taipei 11217, Taiwan
Center for Intelligent Drug Systems and Smart Bio-devices (IDS2B), Hsinchu 30010, Taiwan

Der-Cherng Tarng
Division of Nephrology, Department of Medicine, Taipei Veterans General Hospital, Taipei 11217, Taiwan Institute of Clinical Medicine, National Yang-Ming University, Taipei 11217, Taiwan
Center for Intelligent Drug Systems and Smart Bio-devices (IDS2B), Hsinchu 30010, Taiwan
Department and Institute of Physiology, National Yang-Ming University, Taipei 11217, Taiwan

Index

Printed in the USA
CPSIA information can be obtained
at www.ICGtesting.com
LVHW080053211023
761596LV00010BA/2043